Fundamental Orthopedic
Management for the
Physical Therapist Assistant

Fundamental Orthopedic Management for the Physical Therapist Assistant

Gary A. Shankman, PTA

NovaCare
Atlanta, Georgia

with 443 illustrations

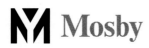 Mosby

St. Louis Baltimore Boston Carlsbad Chicago Naples New York Philadelphia Portland
London Madrid Mexico City Singapore Sydney Tokyo Toronto Wiesbaden

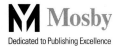

Dedicated to Publishing Excellence

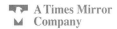

Publisher: Don Ladig
Executive Editor: Martha Sasser
Developmental Editor: Kellie F. White
Editorial Assistant: Laura A. MacAdam
Project Manager: Mark Spann
Production Editor: Julie Eddy
Designer: Jeanne Wolfgeher
Manufacturing Supervisor: Tony McAllister

Printed in the United States of America
Composition by Carlisle Communications, Ltd.
Printing/binding by R. R. Donnelley & Sons Company

Mosby-Year Book, Inc.
11830 Westline Industrial Drive
St. Louis, Missouri 63146

Library of Congress Cataloging in Publication Data

Shankman, Gary A.
    Fundamental orthopedic management for the physical therapist
assistant / Gary A. Shankman.
     p. cm.
    Includes bibliographical references and index.
    ISBN 0–8151–7541–8 (alk. paper)
    1. Orthopedics.   2. Physical therapy.   3. Physical therapy
assistants.   I. Title.
    [DNLM: 1. Orthopedics. 2. Allied Health Personnel. 3. Physical
Therapy.   WE 168 S527f 1997]
    RD731.S5513   1997
    617.3—dc20
    DNLM/DLC
    for Library of Congress   96–16046
                                                  CIP

97 98 99 00 01 / 9 8 7 6 5 4 3 2 1

Dedication

To my mother, Yvonne, who taught me the meaning of perseverance and personal achievement. To my brothers, Harry and Ryan, who continue to inspire me with their love and devotion. To my wife, Judy, and my sons, Kyle, Tyler, and Jordan, who all stood by me and encouraged me during the many long months, late hours, and lost weekends in the preparation of this book. And to the memory of my late father, Arthur; All my love and respect.

Foreword

In the past, the duties and activities that surrounded the orthopedic management of a patient have existed solely within the purview of the physical therapist. The physical therapist assistant had little or no contribution to the process of evaluating a patient's functional status and usually was expected to follow the directions of the attending physical therapist with little room for modification. Tradition dictated that the physical therapist assume responsibility for the majority of a patient's treatment, with the delegation of only minor tasks to the physical therapist assistant. In the past, the physical therapist assistant did not really need to be concerned with the processes for the appropriate orthopedic management of a patient as such matters were handled exclusively by the physical therapist. The present, however, requires a different mode of operation and a different set of expectations for the physical therapist assistant.

The contemporary scheme of orthopedic management has evolved from the traditional system to a newer system of managed care. The physical therapist is still directly responsible for the disposition of a patient's treatment, but delegates as many clinical management duties as are possible to the physical therapist assistant. The current real world expectation for orthopedic management is this "evaluate and delegate" model for physical therapist and physical therapist assistant practice. Although this new model certainly expands the scope of practice for the physical therapist assistant, it also requires much more clinical responsibility in the management of patients who have orthopedic disorders. Such new responsibility requires knowledge, which is the purpose of this book.

Fundamental Orthopedic Management for the Physical Therapist Assistant is the first text that consolidates the orthopedic knowledge expected of the physical therapist assistant under the new "evaluate and delegate" model of clinical physical therapy care. The author, Gary A. Shankman, PTA, is very well experienced and qualified as an expert in the arena of orthopedic management and does an excellent job of presenting the important information contained in this book in a clear and comprehensive manner. Mastery of the knowledge presented in this text will help to ensure that physical therapist assistants meet, if not exceed, the expectations for their clinical role in the modern system of orthopedic health care.

Kent E. Timm, PhD, PT, SCS,
OCS, ATC, FACSM
St. Luke's Healthcare Association
Saginaw, Michigan

Preface

Within the discipline of physical therapy, "orthopaedics has emerged as the largest specialty group,"[1] requiring that the physical therapist assistant play a key role in the care of patients suffering from injury or disease of the musculoskeletal system. An introduction to basic concepts and applied principles of orthopedics is necessary for the physical therapist assistant (PTA), who needs a source for learning the key elements consistent with responsible, appropriate rehabilitation team management of patient care. Yet there have been very few texts written specifically for the PTA student and the practicing PTA clinician. This text responds to the absence of appropriate textbooks, intending to fill this long-neglected void in PTA education, and will serve as a primary resource, supplemental guide, and valuable reference.

Current popular orthopedic texts used in both physical therapy and physical therapist assistant education focus on comprehensive, objective evaluation procedures, differential diagnosis, and the development of treatment plans related to anatomy, biomechanics, and pathophysiology of injury. Care has been taken throughout this text to focus instead on fundamental, basic scientific principles, as well as on clinical applications of physical therapy interventions related to the scope and use of the physical therapist assistant. It is the intent and design of this text that the reader immediately recognize this focus on the application of fundamental orthopedic physical therapy principles.[1,2,4,5]

Additionally, this text seeks to show the student and the clinician that individual differences exist between patients experiencing the same general pathology. A consistent effort is made to clearly identify the interrelationship between soft tissue and bone healing time constraints, severity of injury, methods of immobilization or bone fixation, as well as the ongoing evaluation and reassessment procedures used to design a precise, individualized treatment plan. This element necessitates the introduction of individual criteria-based rehabilitation programs applying tissue healing mechanisms and the patient's individual tolerance (or intolerance) to advances in physical therapy interventions.[6] Yet a specific presentation of a clearly defined treatment protocol does not expose the PTA to the many complex variables the physical therapist takes into account when designing an appropriate plan of care for each patient. For this reason specific protocols have been omitted throughout this text. In the presence of so many conflicting opinions about how to manage the same injury or disease, it becomes necessary to define the intent of specific protocols rather than the protocols themselves.

Those familiar with physical therapy departments or outpatient clinics recognize that many different protocols exist for the same pathology, each influenced by the training and practical experiences of the physicians and physical therapists involved. In order to minimize conflicts of opinion on this subject, I decided to focus on aiding the physical therapist assistant in understanding the fact that many complex factors dictate patient care following injury, surgery, or disease of the musculoskeletal system. Most important for the PTA is the ability to first recognize the patient's individual response to treatment and then, after consultation with the physical therapist, to modify, add, or delete the treatment procedures of the physical therapy plan of care.

To achieve this result, the text strives to actively involve the reader in the concept of *teamwork* in the care of all patients. An often overused term and under-applied concept, *teamwork,* is necessary to successful patient care. In each chapter the need for immediate, open, accurate, and purposeful communication between the physical therapist assistant, physical therapist, physician, patient, and others is made clear to highlight the interdependence of all team members in patient care. In all, the PTA must realize that the elements of effective and responsible patient supervision, understanding the mechanisms affecting musculoskeletal tissue healing, and communicating with other rehab team members all play a critical role in developing individual treatment plans. This text gives the instructor, student, and clinician greater freedom to investigate and critically analyze rationale for treatment progression.

The body of the text is organized into eighteen chapters, each evolving to include more complex and practical applications. Chapter one, "Patient Supervision and Observation During Treatment," introduces a concept vital to the assistant's scope of practice: patient care is a *shared responsibility,* and the physical therapist assistant must assume a proactive role in that responsibility. Chapters two through five move on to develop rudimentary concepts of flexibility, strength, endurance, balance, and coordination, with specific references to applying these basic scientific principles to orthopedic physical therapy.

Because it is clinically relevant for the assistant to appreciate the magnitude of the events and factors that influence healing and, ultimately, the course of physical therapy treatment, chapters six through nine introduce appropriate concepts of injury and repair of musculoskeletal tissue. The relationships of injury, disease, surgery, and immobilization to restoration of motion, strength, and function are consistently emphasized. Chapter eleven outlines and describes fundamentals of peripheral joint mobilization. The appropriate use of specific joint mobilization techniques are quite useful for pain reduction and for enhancing joint motion, and in clinical practice the physical therapist may elect to have the assistant perform patient set-up and provide select techniques to peripheral joints. Clinical instructors, students, and practicing clinicians may effectively use the fundamental principles found in this chapter to enhance specific goals of treatment.

The foundation of this text appears in chapters twelve through eighteen. In these chapters the foot and ankle, knee, hip, spine and pelvis, shoulder, elbow, and the wrist and hand are reviewed in sequence. The chapters introduce the reader to the common soft tissue injuries, fractures, and diseases of each area. Although examples of surgery for specific injuries are included, the emphasis is on rehabilitation treatment options used to reduce pain and swelling, increase motion and strength, enhance balance and proprioception, and, ultimately, to restore purposeful function.

As important as it is to discuss what this text is, it is equally important to identify what it is not. Although this text provides essential, practical information related to afflictions of the musculoskeletal system appropriate to the scope of the physical therapist assistant, it does not substantially cover anatomy, physiology, kinesiology, or include a comprehensive review of all musculoskeletal injuries. It is imperative, therefore, that the student or practicing clinician thoroughly study and review these essential subjects prior to and throughout the study of this text.[1–5] Those who have already acquired, or are in the process of acquiring, familiarity with these fundamental areas will find this text's focus on the application of fundamental orthopedic physical therapy principles a great compliment to the pursuit of increased information, awareness, and knowledge. This textbook was written solely for the physical therapist assistant using the experience, education, and clinical perspective of a practicing physical therapist assistant, and I hope this book will be judged by instructors and readers to be the solution to the problem of finding appropriate textbooks for PTA curricula.

Gary A. Shankman

Suggested Reading

1. Donatelli R, Wooden MJ: *Orthopaedic physical therapy,* New York, 1989, Churchill-Livingstone.

2. Kisner C, Colby LA: *Therapeutic exercise: foundations and techniques,* ed 2, Philadelphia, 1990, FA Davis.

3. Lippert L: *Clinical kinesiology for physical therapist assistants,* ed 2, Philadelphia, 1994, FA Davis.

4. Norkin C, Levangie P: *Joint structure and function, a comprehensive analysis,* ed 2, Philadelphia, 1992, FA Davis.

5. Richardson JK, Iglarsh ZA: *Clinical orthopaedic physical therapy,* Philadelphia, 1994, WB Saunders.

6. Timm KE: Knee. In Richardson JK, Iglarsh ZA, editors: *Clinical orthopaedic physical therapy,* Philadelphia, 1994, WB Saunders.

Acknowledgments

The process of completing this text was truly a team effort. I am grateful to Lil Daley, who typed the manuscript and who demonstrated great reserve and determination during the many months of typing and revisions. A great deal of thanks goes to Dan Nichols, CMI, for the many outstanding drawings and for offering very insightful and creative artistic suggestions. Thank you to my brother, Ryan Beckett, for taking the photographs in this text and for his enduring patience and attention to detail. A special thanks to Tara Adkins for appearing as the model-subject in many of the photographs.

A heart-felt thank you goes to my colleagues, Cindy Knupp, PT, Leah O'Brien, MS, PT, Gail Pickle, OTR, Tammy Davis, COTA, Jopi Duke, MS, CCC-SLP, and Jill Decorso, MS, CCC-SLP, who collectively literally had to endure my journey.

I also wish to give thanks to Al Jones, PT, who nineteen years ago became my friend and mentor, and whom I will forever honor, dignify, and respect. I am also grateful to Kent Timm, PhD, PT, OCS, SCS, FACSM, for writing the foreword to this text.

This book could not be possible without the combined talents, wisdom, experience, and direction from the many people at Mosby. I acknowledge and give sincere thanks to Martha Sasser, Executive Editor, who had faith in this project and who demonstrated a great deal of enthusiasm from the very beginning. To my "right hand," Kellie White, Developmental Editor, and her Editorial Assistant, Laura A. MacAdam; I give thanks and gratitude for their endless patience, encouragement, and skills to see this project through. To Julie Eddy and Jenny Doll, Production Editors, thank you for your attention to the smallest detail and for keeping me on schedule and on time.

And finally to Rick Hammesfahr, MD, who many years ago wrote a short note encouraging me to pursue writing as a way to communicate and express my ideas. From the bottom of my heart, thank you. Thank you to everyone who helped make this book possible.

Gary A. Shankman

Contents

Basic Concepts of Orthopedic Management

The foundations for the appropriate application of skills and therapeutic techniques related to orthopedic physical therapy are based on the interdependence of basic science principles and the relationships between patient and therapist. The physical therapist assistant, while responsible for proper patient supervision and clinical observation during treatment, is frequently guided and directed to modify or adjust therapeutic interventions in consultation with the physical therapist based on specific physiologic responses from the patient. Keen observation skills and properly directed patient supervision techniques, and a thorough understanding of physiologic and therapeutic adaptations to exercise techniques will serve the physical therapist assistant to effectively and skillfully apply rudimentary as well as advanced rehabilitation techniques.

Therefore this section will introduce basic orthopedic physical therapy components of patient supervision; flexibility and soft tissue contracture management; muscular strength, power, plyometrics and closed kinetic chain exercise; cardiovascular and muscular endurance, peripheral neuromuscular fatigue; as well as balance, coordination, and the enhancement of the afferent neural input system related to orthopedic physical therapy management. The focus and specific intent of this section is to provide a sound, practical, and purposeful introduction to the principles of basic orthopedic management as well as the therapeutic application of these critical components related to specific tissue healing constraints, immobilization, and post-surgical recovery following orthopedic injury.

Patient Supervision and Observation During Treatment

LEARNING OBJECTIVES

1. Identify and discuss the rationale for clear and concise communication among all members of the rehabilitation team.
2. Discuss the skills required to provide patient supervision.
3. Define objective scales of measurements used to communicate changes in a patient's status to the physical therapist.
4. Apply proactive listening skills and objective scales of measurement to provide appropriate, accountable, and responsible observation and supervision of the patient during treatment.
5. Define open-end and closed-end questioning.
6. Define the quadrants of the basic dimensional model.
7. Discuss the four categories of behavior of the physical therapist assistant: dominance, submission, hostility, and warmth.
8. Describe the differences between "prompting" and "cueing."

KEY TERMS

Responsibility
Communication
Listening
Accountability
Proactive
Probing questions
Open-end questions
Closed-end questions
Dominance
Submission
Hostility
Warmth
Basic dimensional model
Recognition

CHAPTER OUTLINE

SUPERVISING THE PATIENT DURING TREATMENT

Among the many challenges for the physical therapist assistant are supervision of the patient during treatment and the making of appropriate decisions. The assistant must recognize that interpersonal communication skills, patient supervision methods, and responsive clinical decision making must be learned, practiced, and demonstrated to function efficiently and effectively.

Initial contact with a patient establishes a framework of rapport and sets the stage for all future interactions with that individual. The assistant has the opportunity to convey confidence, capability, and sensitivity during the initial introductions by the physical therapist. This leads the patient to trust the assistant and minimizes fear and anxiety in the patient.

The physical therapist assistant is responsible for carrying out prescribed treatments in patient supervision and appropriate clinical decision making. For proper care to be given, the physical therapist assistant must monitor the patient's response to therapeutic interventions and accurately and swiftly report changes to the supervising therapist. This involves constant patient interaction, observation, palpation, reassessment of initial data, and responsive action to clarify and enhance the effectiveness of prescribed treatments. Changes in the patient's status, both positive and negative, can occur throughout the treatment program, whether during a single visit or over the span of multiple treatments. Some of these changes are subtle and require keen awareness of the initial objective data and acute sensitivity to the patient's subjective reports. Other changes are profound and sudden. In either situation, the physical therapist assistant observes a patient's range of motion, strength, pain, balance, coordination, swelling, endurance, or gait deviations. When reported to the supervising therapist, these changes will dictate and significantly affect the course of treatment.

Components of Patient Supervision

Clinical patient supervision can be viewed as a process whose purposes are as follows:[3]
- To gather relevant information
- To establish and enhance rapport, trust, and confidence
- To facilitate understanding of the physical therapist assistant's concept of the patient's problem as outlined, described, and initially determined by the physical therapist
- To assist in the management of the patient
- To provide a conduit or therapeutic outlet for the patient to voice concerns about his or her problem

Clearly, gathering information from the patient and interpreting those data during the initial evaluation are functions primarily done by the physical therapist. However, the physical therapist assistant must help the patient understand the problem throughout the course of rehabilitation. The assistant must recognize how difficult it is for patients to grasp all the components of the situation well enough to fully appreciate the rationale for the prescribed treatment. Therefore the physical therapist assistant's role is to help the patient understand the disorder being treated and reassure him or her concerning the appropriateness of care.[3] In so doing, the assistant must be keenly aware of and sensitive to subtle or overt signs of patient apprehension, fear, and anxiety.

Although direct patient supervision is frequently the task of one individual, **responsibility** for the patient's care is shared by the entire rehabilitation team. In addition, the patient must be actively involved in the treatment and accept shared responsibility for his or her own care.

During treatment the assistant makes observations of the patient and develops an objective assessment using appropriate scales of measurement (Box 1-1). Using applicable questioning techniques ensures that the patient is actively involved. This interactive approach to supervision, as well as the skills of the physical therapist assistant to seek, understand, and accurately relay information related to the patient's status, distinguishes the assistant from a physical therapist aide.[4]

Patient Supervision by the Rehabilitation Team

The assistant must be aware of the key members of the rehabilitation team. The physical therapist and the rehabilitation aide are involved with direct patient care on a daily basis. The occupational therapist and occupational therapy assistant, along with the speech language pathologist, audiologist, rehabilitation counselors, nurses, respiratory therapists, psychologists, and dietitians, play significant roles in daily patient care. This network of rehabilitation specialists seeks to maximize recovery for each patient and must always be regarded as resources to meet specific patient needs as those needs are identified by any member of the team. Thus the assistant charged with direct patient care and supervision is only one vital member of the team, and he or she can take comfort in knowing that every member of the team is prepared to provide appropriate skills so that the patient can achieve the highest functional gains in recovery. Developing a team mindset helps the physical therapist assistant to be responsible and accountable to the other members of the team for his or her own contribution and to reach out to others when their expertise is required.[5]

BOX 1-1   General Scales of Measurements

Strength: Manual muscle testing

$5/5$ *Normal*: Full resistance against gravity
$4/5$ *Good*: Some resistance against gravity
$3/5$ *Fair*: No resistance against gravity
$2/5$ *Poor*: No movement against gravity
$1/5$ *Trace*: Slight contraction, no movement
$0/5$ *Zero*: No contraction

Pain: Analog scale

Graded from zero to ten (10 severe, 0 absent)

Swelling: Generally measured by:

Circumferential measurement
Water displacement
Blood pressure: $120/80$ normal, use sphygmomanometer and stethoscope
Pulse: Average 72 BPM. Pulse can be lower (i.e., 55) for trained athletes
Respirations: Average 12–16 per minute.

Coordination:

Tapping foot or hand
Finger to nose
Heel on shin
Coordination activities are tested first with eyes open, then with eyes closed. All events are described as degrees of rhythmic, symmetrical, even, and consistent.

Stretch reflex (DTR):

0 = Areflexia
+ = Hyperreflexia
1 to 3 = Average
3 + to 4+ = Hyperreflexia

Range of motion: Standard goniometry

Shoulder:

Flexion 0 - 180°
Extention 0 - 60°
Abduction 0 - 180°
Int Rot 0 - 70°
Ext Rot 0 - 90°

Hip:

Flexion 0 - 120°
Extension 0 - 30°
Abduction 0 - 45°
Abduction 0 - 30°
Ext Rot 0 - 45°
Int Rot 0 - 45°

Ankle:

Dorsiflexion 0 - 20°
Plantarflexion 0 - 50°
Inversion 0 - 35°
Eversion 0 - 15°

Knee:

Flexion 0 - 135°

Elbow:

Flexion 0 - 150°

Effective **communication** is the hallmark of a great team and should be maximized. To effectively supervise and provide the greatest care for the patient, the assistant must learn to communicate openly and freely, with honesty and respect, and in a professional manner with every member of the team.[5] It is important to differentiate between the language used for communicating among peers and that used to define and explain injury, disease, and physical therapy procedures to a patient. The assistant must employ appropriate and professional medical language to outline and describe an orthopedic problem to a physical therapist and must be able to use familiar terms to describe the same pathologic condition to a patient or family member. If the assistant uses medical jargon inappropriately, the patient or family member could perceive the therapist as insensitive, aloof, and impersonal. Generally, use of language appropriate to the patient's comprehension conveys understanding, sensitivity, warmth, and reassurance and removes uncomfortable and unnecessary barriers to communication.[3]

The physical therapist assistant must also be aware that **listening** is an effective communication tool. Listening demonstrates interest and provides the opportunity for a better understanding of the patient's concept of the problem. By active listening, the assistant is better able to integrate verbal and nonverbal messages that the patient may have received.[3] In addition, patients may be more comfortable and trusting with a good listener, be more at ease, and be more willing to provide information.

Supervision of patients by the physical therapist assistant must be done systematically and reliably with an emphasis on **accountability.** Appropriate and responsible investigative questioning of the patient during treatment will help the assistant focus on which areas to probe, which findings to quantify, and which objective changes to assess. The assistant is responsible for reporting all findings to the physical therapist so that modifications can be made in accordance with changes in patient status.*

Basic Patient Supervision Skills

Communication skills. The physical therapist assistant can be most effective if he or she develops an understanding of human behavior and adopts a **proactive** role in supervising patients. With a proactive role, the assistant does not wait to be placed in a reactive position. Use of appropriate **probing questions** is a proactive method to use during patient supervision. Questioning patients during treatment can be insightful, rewarding, and helpful for both the physical therapist and the assistant. The format of asking probing questions is critical and strongly influences the responses received (Fig. 1-1). Using **open-end questions** invites the patient to share feelings, thoughts, and opinions. Examples are as follows:

"Tell me about your pain."
"How does that feel?"
"What do you think about this exercise?"

These types of questions are generally not answered by "yes" or "no." They open discussions and prompt the patient to express a wide range of views and opinions.

Open-end questions for patients have been described as "a good medium for facilitating rapport and, as such, are particularly useful. . . ."[3] Using open-end questions will promote personal interactions between the client and patient, may allow the patient to give a more in-depth explanation of the problem, and may lead to discussions of what the patient identifies as important. Although this type of questioning does not enable the patient to give precise, clear answers, it is appropriate in situations that require compassion and empathy from the assistant and shared feelings between the assistant and patient.

Closed-end questions are directed toward finding facts, obtaining specific responses, and filling in details. By asking the patient questions such as, "Where is your pain?", "When does your knee feel unstable?", or "Does your back hurt when you bend forward?", the assistant proactively directs the discussion and the se-

quence of questions instead of sifting out pertinent information from among all the data gathered in open-end questioning.

Summary-type statements check understanding, help the patient clarify thinking, and provide direction for the therapist. Examples include the following: "So your back hurts only at night?" and "Then your knee doesn't hurt with this exercise." Using precise closed-end questions with summary statements will elicit information that can lead to an objective assessment of the patient. The approach the assistant takes will influence the balance of questioning between open-end and closed-end questions.

Behavior. The behavior of the physical therapist assistant during supervision can either reassure the patient and demonstrate appropriate responsive professional care or create a sense of indifference. Four broad categories of behavior are: **dominance, submission, hostility,** and **warmth.**[1] Buzzotta and Lefton[1] define these four categories as follows:

Dominance: Exercising control or influence. People showing dominant behavior are forceful, dynamic, and assertive. They push their ideas forward or try to sway the way other people think or behave. They take charge, guide, lead, and move other people to action.

Submission: Being passive. People showing submissive behavior are willing to take a back seat. They are ready to comply, quick to give in, and reluctant to try exerting influence.

Hostility: Unresponsiveness or insensitivity to others and their needs. People showing hostile behavior tend to care only about themselves, and they lack regard for other people's feelings and ideas. Although anger is a form of hostility, people can be hostile while showing no open anger at all.

Warmth: Responsiveness and sensitivity to others and their needs. People showing warm behavior are open and caring and have a high regard for other people's ideas and feelings. This does not mean they automatically gush with affection. A person can be warm without being openly affectionate.

These four categories of behavior are used to describe the extremes of the **basic dimensional model** (Fig. 1-2). Quadrants (Q) are formed (Fig. 1-3) and certain patterns of behavior exist when two dimensions are combined, as follows:

Q1 Dominant hostile
Q2 Submissive hostile
Q3 Submissive warm
Q4 Dominant warm

---

*From Guide for Conduct of the Affiliate Member: American Physical Therapy Association.

Probe	Definition	Objectives	Characteristics	Examples
Opened-end questions	A question or statement that invites a wide-ranging response, often asks for ideas, opinions, or views.	• Open up discussion • Invite broad response • Give other freedom to talk • Gets involvement	• Can't be answered "yes" or "no" • Gets at feelings, opinions, thoughts	• "What do you think about. . . ?" • "Tell me about. . . " • "Why do you feel. . .?" • "What's your opinion?"
Pause	An intentional, purposeful period of silence.	• Give other a chance to think and respond • Slow down pace • Draw out other	• Usually follows open-end • Deliberate	• "Why do you say that?" (silence) • "Tell me more." (silence)
Reflective	A statement that describes and reflects a feeling or emotion (without implying agreement or disagreement).	• Identify emotions • Show you understand • Vent interfering emotions	• Names a feeling or emotion • Usually uses the word "you" or "you're" • May state cause of the emotion	• "You're pretty mad about it." • "You seem reluctant to talk about it." • "Sounds like you're excited."
Neutral phrase or question	A question or statement that encourages other to elaborate.	• Get other to tell more about a subject	• Few words • About subject under discussion	• "Tell me more." • "Please elaborate." • "Explain that." • "Amplify on that."
Brief assertion	A short statement, sound, or gesture, which shows involvement.	• Encourage other to continue • Increase receptivity	• Elicits additional information • Occurs automatically	• "Oh, okay." • "Yes, sure." • "I see." • Nodding your head.
Summary statements	A brief statement, in your own words, of the content of what was said.	• Check understanding • Prove you're listening • Give structure and direction • Help other clarify thinking • Invite other to comment or expand	• Summarizes content, not feelings • Restatement of essential ideas • In own words	• "So you disagree about. . . ." • "The way you see it is. . . ." • "You prefer working overtime. . . ." • "Let me summarize how I. . . ."
Closed-end questions	A question that limits the answer by requesting specific facts, or a "yes" or "no" answer.	• Find out details, specifics • Check understanding • Direct the discussion • Get other to take a stand	• Often starts with "Who", "Which", "When", "Where", "How many", etc. • Can sometimes be answered with a simple "yes" or "no"	• "Who is. . . ?" • "Which order. . . ?" • "When will you. . . ?" • "Do you think. . . ?"
Leading questions	A question that implies only one answer, or a rhetorical question—no answer is needed.	• Pin down positions or agreements • Can verify assumptions • Can be threatening	• The question gives the answer • No answer is required	• "Shouldn't we discuss. . . ?" • "This is the best way to go, isn't it?"

FIG. 1-1 Probes and probing questions: The use of questions, statements, and pauses to elicit information, thoughts, and opinions. The type of questions used will elicit a characteristic response. (From Buzzotta VR, Lefton RE: *Dimensional management training,* St. Louis, 1989, Psychological Associates, Inc).

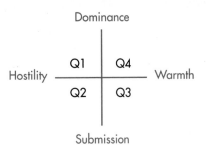

Dominance—Active behavior: leading, controlling, making things happen

Submission—Passive behavior: following, letting things happen, reacting

Hostility—A lack of concern or regard, and unresponsiveness for other people and their position/ideas

Warmth—Concern, regard, and responsiveness for other people and their position/ideas

FIG. 1-2 The dimensional model: A tool to size up behavior. The model applies to subordinates, peers, and superiors. General behavior characteristics are dominance, submission, hostility, and warmth. (From Buzzotta VR, Lefton RE: *Dimensional management training,* St. Louis, 1989, Psychological Associates, Inc).

Dominance

Quadrant 1 (Q1)	**Quadrant 4 (Q4)**
Dominance plus hostility	Dominance plus warmth

Hostility ——————— Warmth

Quadrant 2 (Q2)	**Quadrant 3 (Q3)**
Submission plus hostility	Submission plus warmth

Submission

FIG. 1-3 Quadrants are formed between dominance, submission, hostility and warmth, which create certain patterns of behavior. (From Buzzotta VR, Lefton RE: *Dimensional management training,* St. Louis, 1989, Psychological Associates, Inc).

From this comes four patterns, or types of human behavior (Fig. 1-4).

Applying this model when asking open-end and closed-end questions shows such questions to be equally

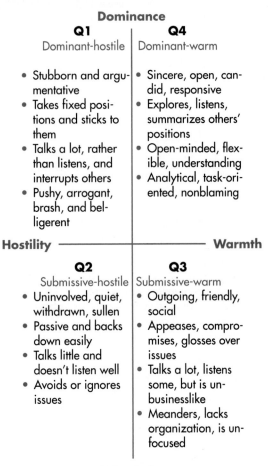

FIG. 1-4 Four distinct patterns and characteristics are formed between the four quadrants: Q1, dominant-hostile; Q2, submissive-hostile; Q3, submissive-warm; and Q4, dominant-warm. (From Buzzotta VR, Lefton RE: *Dimensional management training,* St. Louis, 1989, Psychological Associates, Inc).

balanced within Quadrant 4 (Q4). The goal of the physical therapist assistant during supervision of the patient is to consistently demonstrate those qualities found in Q4. For example, being appropriately friendly, attentive, responsive, involved, exploring, analytical, and task oriented.

While supervising patients according to the Q4 model, the assistant must understand the differences between prompting and cueing a patient to perform a specific task. Prompting a patient to perform a task can be viewed as the presentation of a question. For example, when instructing a patient to ambulate with a standard walker, the assistant should prompt the patient by asking, "After you move the walker, what foot do you move next?" Prompting allows patients to decipher information, solve problems, and provide solutions to activities they must overcome during recovery. Cueing can be viewed as a direction. An example would be, "After you move the walker, move your injured leg." Although the solution is provided for the patient, he or she must still demonstrate appropriate follow-through and proper understanding of the command.

MODIFICATIONS DURING TREATMENT

Using attentive Q4 behavior with balanced open-end and closed-end questioning of the patient helps the physical therapist assistant identify and quantify changes in the patient's condition. After consulting the physical therapist and receiving direction, the assistant can effectively modify a specific treatment procedure in accordance with changes in patient status.*

The following example will help clarify the scope of treatment modifications during postoperative rehabilitation after anterior cruciate ligament (ACL) reconstruction.

Swelling (joint effusion) after knee surgery is common, and occurs in about 12% of cases after ACL reconstruction.[6] Usually the effusion is a hemarthrosis (blood within the joint). As little as 60 ml of fluid within a joint can cause a 30% to 50% inhibition of voluntary muscle contraction. In such a case, the physical therapist would provide baseline evaluation data about the degree of swelling present by making comparative circumferential measurements at mid-patella, 2 inches superior to the mid-patella, and 2 inches inferior to the midpatella. The physical therapist assistant maintains daily records of the three comparative circumferential measurements. Because reeducation and strengthening of muscle is influenced negatively by postoperative swelling, any increase or decrease in swelling will necessitate a modification in the initial program outlined by the physical therapist. Thus the degree of swelling documented will influence the adjustment made in the exercise prescription.

As the physical therapist assistant identifies objective changes in the patient's status each day, the concept of visual, nonresponsive, and noninteractive supervision is altered to one of appropriate, responsive, and accountable supervision.

Isometric exercises are generally used early in the rehabilitation of acute postoperative knee injuries. As rehabilitation proceeds, concentric and eccentric exercises are introduced. Concentric and eccentric exercises are defined as dynamic, producing work, and creating changes in joint angles and muscle length.[2] The progression from isometric to dynamic exercise produces an increase in force generated, increases muscle soreness, and causes greater articular stresses.[7] If swelling and pain increase as the patient progresses from isometric to concentric and eccentric contractions, the physical therapist assistant, with direction and input from the physical therapist, can adjust or modify the program back to isometrics, reduce the amount of resistance, reduce the joint angle of exercise, reduce the volume of exercise, or reduce the velocity of movement. The specific sequence or combination of these modifications will depend on the patient's specific needs, the surgical procedure, and the patient's tolerance to exercise. It is usually prudent to begin with the least drastic change in exercise prescription and then progress (Box 1-2).

The clinical decision-making process used by the physical therapist assistant involves recognizing that a problem exists, then taking orderly and specific steps to notify the therapist and adjust the program accordingly. Thus the assistant takes an active, participatory role while supervising patients, using his or her training and skills to the fullest extent.

BOX 1-2   Knee Extension—Isotonic Exercise Modifications

If pain and swelling develops during full range of motion isotonic knee extension:

- Adjust the resistance. Reduce the amount of weight being used.
- Adjust the range of motion to limit full knee flexion. Example: Begin knee extension exercises from 45° of flexion or less instead of 90° or greater. *Note:* some acute, chronic, and post- surgical conditions prohibit terminal knee extension (0°). In this case limit full extension to −10° or greater.
- Adjust the speed or velocity of the performance of the exercise. Closely observe the speed of the exercise. Perform slow, controlled, nonballistic exercise.
- Adjust the volume of exercise
  a. Reduce the number of repetitions being performed.
  b. Reduce the number of sets being performed.
  c. Reduce the number of days per week performing the exercise.
- Change the performance of exercise
  a. Perform only isometric holds followed by eccentric loads. No concentric lifting.

---

*Guide for Conduct of the Affiliate Member: American Physical Therapy Association.

Note that the **recognition** of changes in patient status does not imply interpretation of objective, measurable data by the assistant. The assistant's task is to provide information to the Physical Therapist on a daily basis, to keep the therapist informed concerning patient status, and to provide insightful and meaningful suggestions for modifications.

The objective data supplied to the therapist by the assistant include goniometric measurements, circumferential measurements, manual muscle testing, endurance grading, heart rate, blood pressure, respirations, dynamic balance, and coordination measurements, according to the scope of the assistant's training.

UNDERSTANDING DIFFERENT PHILOSOPHIES OF THERAPISTS

Fundamental differences exist between therapists concerning the methods, protocols, and directives they use to treat patients. In addition, just as the physical therapist assistant is directed by the therapist, the physical therapist is often directed by the physician. Within a hospital physical therapy department, the assistant may have contact with many therapists and physicians, each with different backgrounds, experiences, and education. The assistant will see the same pathologic condition managed differently using various protocols between therapists and physicians. It is not the task of the assistant to change or modify treatment plans or protocols without the therapist's direction. Opinions and controversies exist concerning how best to manage various orthopedic pathologic conditions. Changes in surgery and physical therapy occur because of advanced technology and rigorous research in rehabilitation medicine and orthopedic surgery. New procedures in arthroscopic ACL surgery allow a more rapid return to function, motion, and strength than ever before. Although ideally we presume all surgical procedures and rehabilitation techniques to be universally accepted, in fact the specialties of orthopedics and physical therapy are both art and science. Therefore diversity is accepted.

The physical therapist assistant can be placed in frustrating and confusing situations when dealing with therapists with different backgrounds and opinions concerning the management of patients. To minimize the confusing array of treatment protocols, the assistant must communicate with the supervising therapist to clarify differences in patient care, always remembering that the responsibility for patient care is a shared one. The assistant does not divest interest in the care of any patient because of a disagreement in strategy with the therapist. The assistant's task requires a broader perspective and understanding that there are many ways to effectively manage the same pathology.

Having strong opinions on how to care for orthopedic patients is appropriate and shows passion, interest, and confidence in a certain method or protocol that has demonstrated good results. However, particular experience with the successful management of patients by one therapist may in fact conflict with the course of treatment prescribed by another therapist. On the surface, this situation may seem particularly frustrating and stressful. To better understand this difference, the assistant must identify the key elements of disagreement and seek an appropriate explanation from the therapist. This gives each therapist the opportunity to teach and explain the rationale for the particular treatment and exposes the assistant to new information. The assistant can then observe and learn new methods that may actually prove equally or more successful than the previous plan of care.

Fully understanding the rationale and purpose of each treatment allows for improved delivery of service to the patient. During direct patient supervision, the assistant can reinforce any procedure the therapist directs him or her to perform as long as the safety and welfare of the patient are not compromised.

The well-adapted assistant views any apparent roadblocks as learning opportunities. The assistant is advised to take advantage of the broad knowledge and experience of many therapists, to constantly inquire about the rationale and scientific basis for a particular program, and to establish himself or herself as an eager learning participant who is open to innovative ways of managing various pathologic conditions.

REFERENCES

1. Buzzotta VR, Lefton RE: *Dimensional management training,* St. Louis, 1989, Psychological Associates, Inc.
2. Jokl PJ: Muscle. In Albright JA, Brand RA, editors: *The scientific bases of orthopaedics,* ed 2, Norwalk, Conn., 1987, Appleton & Lange.
3. Lombardo P, Stolberg S: Interviewing and communication skills. In Ballweg R, Stolberg S, Sullivan EM, editors: *Physician assistant a guide to clinical practice,* Philadelphia, 1994, WB Saunders Co.
4. Lupi-Williams FA: The PTA, role and function. An analysis in three parts. I. Education, *Clinical Management* 3(3).
5. Mallory C: *Team Building.* Leadership Series, 1991, National Press Publications.
6. Sacks RA et al: Complications of knee ligament surgery. In Daniel D, Akeson W, O'Connor J, editors: *Knee ligaments structure, function surgery and repair,* New York, 1990, Raven Press.
7. Sapaga AA: Muscle performance evaluation in orthopaedic practice, *J Bone & Joint Surg* 72A: 1562–1574 1990.

Flexibility

LEARNING OBJECTIVES

1. Define and discuss range of motion and flexibility.
2. Identify the properties of connective tissue.
3. Explain the differences between stress and strain.
4. Describe plastic deformation and elastic deformation.
5. Discuss how temperature affects connective tissue.
6. Identify and describe various stretching techniques.
7. Define Golgi tendon organs (GTO) and muscle spindles.
8. Describe the clinical applications for stretching soft tissue contractures.
9. Describe and contrast the differences and similarities between scar tissue and adhesions.
10. Outline various methods used to measure flexibility.

KEY TERMS

Flexibility
Range of motion (ROM)
Collagen
Stress
Strain
Elastic deformation
Plastic deformation
Static stretching
Ballistic stretching
Proprioceptive
    neuromuscular
    facilitation (PNF)
Specificity
Golgi tendon organs
    (GTO)
Muscle spindles
Scar tissue
Contracture
Adhesions
Low-load, prolonged
    stretch

CHAPTER OUTLINE

Flexibility
Properties of Connective Tissue
Practical Applications
    Static stretching
    Ballistic stretching
    Proprioceptive neuromuscular facilitation

Stretching of Soft Tissue Contractures
Measuring Flexibility

FLEXIBILITY

Flexibility can be defined as the ability of a muscle to relax and yield to a stretch force.[13] Kisner and Colby[13] assert that "flexibility exercises are stretching exercises designed to increase range of motion." Therefore flexibility can refer to various measurable components of joint motion. Muscles, tendons, ligaments, skin, joint capsule, and bone geometry all influence the degree of movement in joints. For example, a muscle can stretch or elongate, creating a measurable effect on the joint or joints upon which it acts. If a muscle becomes damaged by trauma or disease, or becomes shortened because of immobilization, its ability to stretch and allow freedom of joint motion is affected.

The amount of movement available to a joint moving within its anatomic range is called its **range of motion (ROM).** The stretching or elongating of muscle and joint ROM are two components of flexibility. An understanding of the properties and components of various connective tissues is fundamental in delivering various stretching and flexibility regimens.

PROPERTIES OF CONNECTIVE TISSUE

Just as amino acids are the building blocks of protein, tropocollagen is the building block of **collagen** (Fig. 2-1). Collagen is found in all connective tissues: bone, tendon, muscle, skin, hyaline cartilage, and joint capsule.[4,23] Collagen is a protein building block of connective tissue, and it provides the strength needed to withstand high levels of tension and force during movement and exercise. Five separate types of collagen have been identified: I, II, III, IV, and V. These are found in varying amounts within the different connective tissues. Types I and III collagen are the most common types found within joint capsule and muscle tissue.

Elastin is a structural protein present in tendons in amounts of less than 1%.[4,9] Tissues with greater amounts of elastin usually demonstrate greater degrees of flexibility. Elastin assists collagen in the "recovery" of tissues after stress.[4]

Stress is defined as the amount of tension or load placed on tissues.[4,23,24] **Strain** is the proportional degree of elongation that occurs during stress.[4,24] The ability of tissues to recover after stress is extremely important in relation to flexibility. Woo et al[28] have shown that increasing the levels of stress produces an increase in collagen within ligaments and tendons, whereas reducing the levels of stress causes weakening in connective tissues.

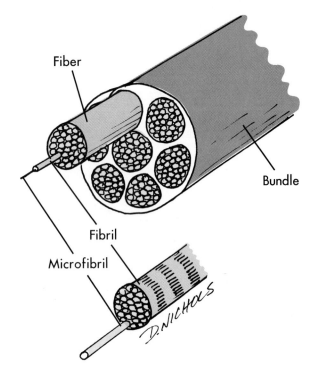

FIG. 2-1 Collagen bundle.

Recovery is the ability of tissues to return to their previous resting state. It does not imply that permanent elongation or microscopic damage has not occurred. Lehman et al[15] and Warren et al[27] have demonstrated that recovery of the tissue's resting length had occurred after microscopic failure had begun.

The rate at which tissues are stretched has a profound effect on the degree or percent of strain. Slower rates of stress produce greater amounts of strain or elongation, whereas faster rates of stretch produce much more smaller amounts of elongation.[4,23,24]

When tissues are subjected to constant stress, or when there is repeated stress to tissues over a long duration, they gradually lengthen. This slow response to stress is called *creep*.[25]

Two viscoelastic properties of connective tissue are elastic and plastic deformation. **Elastic deformation** is similar to the changes that occur in a rubber band under high rates of strain. The rubber band rapidly conforms to a new length and is able to return to its original resting length when the stress is removed. However, if the degree of stress exceeds the strain capabilities, the rubber band breaks (Fig. 2-2). **Plastic deformation** is force dependent under slow rates of stress. For example,

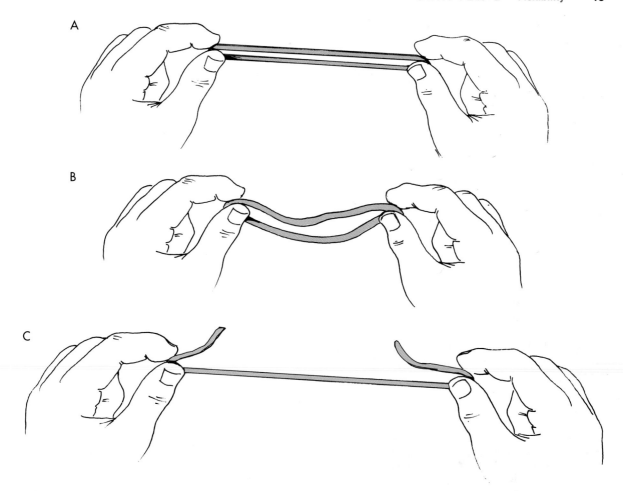

FIG. 2-2 Elastic deformation. **A,** Stress applied to a rubber band. **B,** When stress is removed the rubber band returns to its original length. **C,** If the stress exceeds the strain capabilities of the band, it can break.

when a low degree of stress is applied to a plastic spoon, the spoon slowly deforms to a new shape. If the stress is applied too fast, the spoon breaks (Fig. 2-3).

Along with stress and the rate of stress applied to tissues, temperature also affects connective tissue extensibility. Temperatures in the range of 37°C (98.6°F) to 40°C (104°F) affect the viscoelastic properties of connective tissue.[24] The higher the temperature (approximately 45°C [113°F] is the therapeutic upper limit), the greater the degree of elongation with stress before tissue failure.[29] Because connective tissue's viscoelastic and plastic changes occur at higher temperatures, there is less microscopic damage under stress at these temperatures. Studies by Warren et al[26] have demonstrated that a temperature of 45°C is needed to reduce tissue damage during strains of 2.6% or less.

Muscle or contractile tissue responds to stretch by elastic and plastic deformation properties in ways similar to connective tissue. Obviously, the contractile properties of muscle allow for the greatest degree of freedom of movement around a joint. The arrangements and relationships of the microscopic elements of the sarcomere, actin, myosin, A-band, Z-band, I-band, and H-zone will be addressed in Chapter 3 (Strength).

Although connective tissue is considered a passive resistant to joint motion, muscle tissue, by virtue of its elastic and contractile elements, is considered an active restraint to joint motion.

Active exercise (muscular contractions) affects intramuscular temperature. Increases to approximately 39°C are observed in exercised muscle.[3] Commonly used passive thermal agents that increase tissue temperature

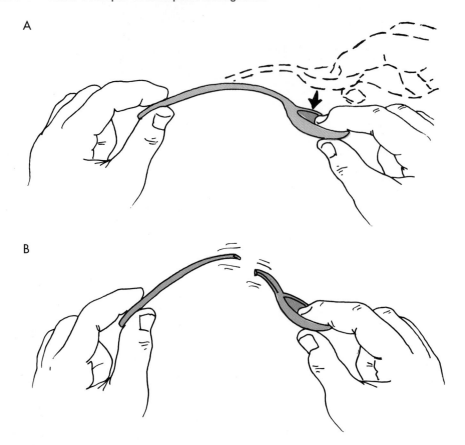

FIG. 2-3 Plastic deformation. **A,** A low degree of stress is applied to a plastic spoon. The spoon will deform slowly and accommodate to a new shape. **B,** If stress is applied suddenly and with great force, the spoon will break.

are moist heat and ultrasound. The judicious use of active exercise and passive thermal agents before and during stretching programs enhances the effectiveness of the prescribed program.

PRACTICAL APPLICATIONS

When discussing flexibility and associated stretching programs, the stretching of nonpathologic muscle must be separated from stretching noncontractile connective tissue. Improving muscle extensibility in nonpathologic conditions and in adaptive muscle shortening after injury or immobilization requires a complement of active exercise techniques and thermal agents.

Types of active stretching exercises are **static stretching, ballistic stretching,** and **proprioceptive neuromuscular facilitation (PNF)** techniques (contract-relax, hold-relax, and slow-reversal-hold).

Static stretching. Static stretching involves placing a muscle in a fully elongated position and holding that position for a period of time (Figs. 2-4 & 2-5). Athletes use static stretching before sports activities as part of a warm-up prior to a workout and as part of a cool-down after a workout. Because intramuscular temperature rises to approximately 39°C during exercise,[3] active general body movements can improve muscle temperature before stretching is done.

Studies on rat tail tendons[14] demonstrate that ruptures occur with 31% of normal loads when temperatures are at 25°C, whereas increasing temperatures to 45°C delays tendon rupture until 102% of normal load. This demonstrates that stretching at normal body temperatures damages tissue,[27] but elevating tissue temperature before and during prolonged stretch is less damaging.[26,27]

Static stretching has distinct advantages such as reduced chance of exceeding strain limits of tissues, reduced energy requirements compared with other forms of stretching, and reduced potential for muscle soreness.[9,24,29] The ease and practicality of teaching patients

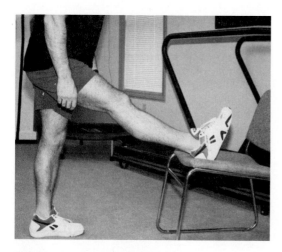

FIG. 2-4 Static stretching. Initial starting position for standing hamstring stretch.

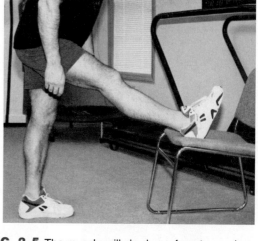

FIG. 2-5 The muscle will slowly conform to an elongated position by maintaining stress on the tissue for a period time.

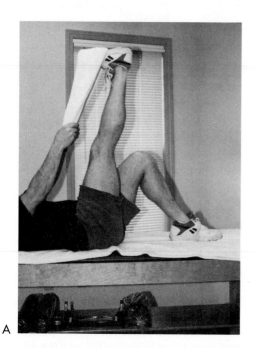

A

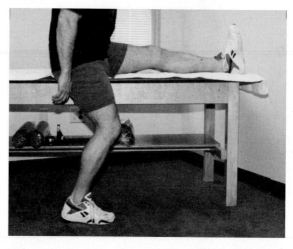

B

FIG. 2-6 A, Supine static hamstring stretch using a towel. **B,** Sitting hamstring stretch.

to perform static stretching is another advantage. For example, hamstring stretches can be taught with the patient in various positions (Fig. 2-6). When teaching the proper execution of static stretching programs, it is important to outline and describe general and specific goals and expected outcomes for the patient. The general goals of static stretching are to prevent or minimize the risk of soft tissue injury from participation in sports or

physical activities, to improve movement and increase flexibility, and to prevent contracture.[1,13]

Generally, static stretches are "held" in a fully elongated position for 10 to 60 seconds.[1,12] After a short rest (5 to 10 seconds), an attempt is made to extend the stretched position farther within tolerable limits (Fig. 2-7). Multiple repetitions are performed (5 to 15), with one "set" of stretches generally equal to 10 repetitions.

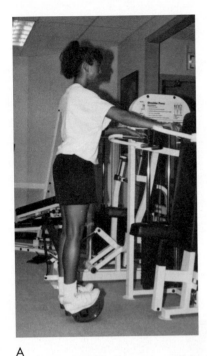
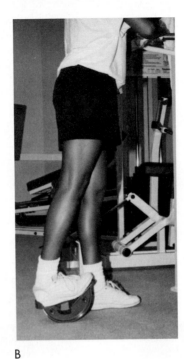
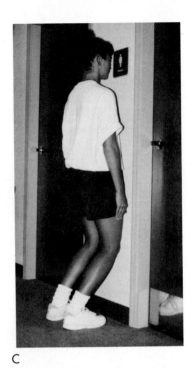

A   B   C

FIG. 2-7 Examples of static stretching positions and techniques for the Grastroc-soleus complex. **A,** Standing bilateral calf stretch. **B,** Single limb static calf stretch. **C,** Grastroc-soleus stretch.

The limits of motion achieved during a stretching program depend on the patient's tolerance, age, pathologic condition, if any, and level of motivation and commitment. The muscle's ability to adapt is a prolonged process. Patients must be cautioned not to exceed their pain limits and must receive counseling regarding the fact that many sessions of stretching are needed to produce change and lasting improvement. Approximately 6 weeks of stretching are required to demonstrate significant increases in muscular flexibility.[30] To improve flexibility, an individual must stretch at least three times per week. To maintain the flexibility gained during the program, the patient must stretch at least 1 day per week.[29]

Ballistic stretching. Athletes use dynamic, high velocity, and even violent motions during sporting events and require extraordinary flexibility to prevent or reduce the risk of potential musculoskeletal injury. A concept applicable to conditioning athletes to better defend against injury is specificity. **Specificity** is described as training an organism in a way that most closely duplicates the desired application or functional goal. In other words, if you want to improve an athlete's ability to move dynamically with rapid changes in direction and velocity, you must train and condition the athlete in that manner.

Dynamic or ballistic stretching involves a "bounce" at the end of the ROM (Fig. 2-8). Relatively high velocity, or quick bouncing may not be appropriate for many patients. The potential for tissue damage exists in all forms of exercise, but ballistic stretching may increase the risk of connective tissue and contractile tissue trauma, although a narrow segment of patients may benefit. Ballistic stretching is used as a part of a progression of stretching and never as a single treatment. In training, a general body warm up is needed first. The beneficial effects of a warm up before strenuous activities include the following:

- Blood flow to working muscles is increased
- Temperature in working muscles is increased
- Cardiovascular response to sudden, dynamic exercise is improved
- Breakdown of oxyhemoglobin for the delivery of oxygen to the working muscles is increased
- The risk of connective tissue and contractile tissue damage is reduced

After a warm up of 5 or 10 minutes, a progressive static stretching program is begun. After a few repetitions of

spindle. The GTOs are inhibitory sensory receptors located within the myotendinous junction (Fig. 2-9). GTOs are activated by excessive or prolonged stretches and by muscular contractions. When a muscle is stretched, the GTOs send messages to the spinal cord to inhibit contraction. This causes a reflex relaxation, which protects against damage to the muscle fibers.

Muscle spindles are excitatory specialized fibers within the muscle (Fig. 2-10) that are sensitive to rapid changes in muscle length. When a muscle is stretched quickly, the spindles send messages to the spinal cord, which in turn signals the muscle to contract. The classic

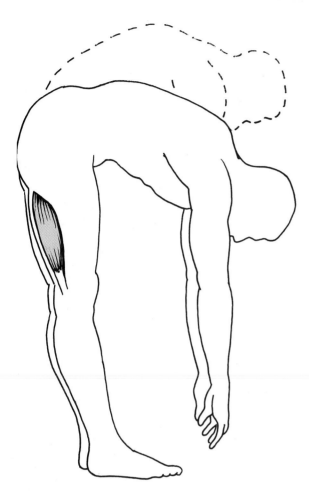

FIG. 2-8 Dynamic or ballistic stretching requires a relatively high velocity "bounce" at the end-range of motion. Typically, ballistic stretching techniques are reserved for an athletic population in preparation for high velocity, ballistic, and sometimes violent physical activity.

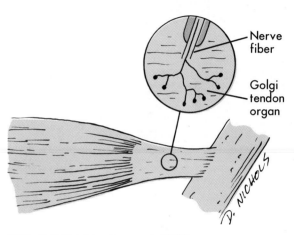

FIG. 2-9 Golgi tendon organ (GTO).

static stretches, a gradually increasing period of ballistic stretching is started.

Ballistic stretching does not imply aggressive, violent, high-velocity stretches throughout the ROM; instead it involves a slight but progressively greater bounce at the end of the range achieved through static stretching.

Proprioceptive neuromuscular facilitation. PNF stretching techniques have been found to be superior to other forms of active stretching.[5,18-21] They are based on the stretch reflex.[1,21] Two neurophysiological sensory receptors involved with the stretch reflex are the **Golgi tendon organs (GTOs)** and the muscle

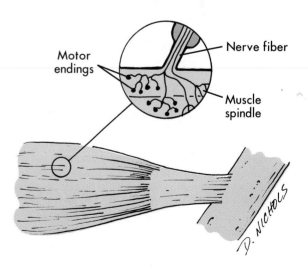

FIG. 2-10 Muscle spindle.

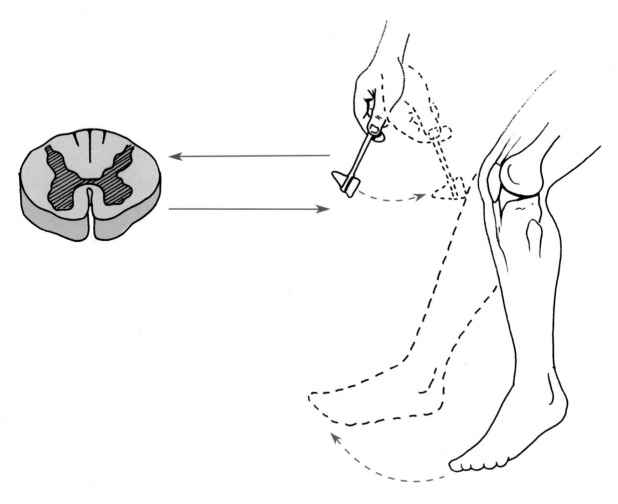

FIG. 2-11 Muscle spindle activation by quick stretch-reflex between the spinal cord and quadriceps.

clinical demonstration of the stretch reflex is produced by tapping the relaxed patellar tendon, which causes the reflexive contraction of the quadriceps. The muscle spindles within the quadriceps are activated by the quick stretch of the patellar tendon, causing the quadriceps to contract reflexively (Fig. 2-11).

A few drawbacks to PNF stretching are that it is more time consuming than other methods, it requires skillful application by trained professionals to be effective, and it may lead to complaints of discomfort by the patient.[29]

Three effective PNF stretching techniques are contract-relax, hold-relax, and slow-reversal-hold. The *contract-relax technique* involves instructing the patient to relax the affected muscle while the therapist passively moves the limb to the limit of motion. The patient is instructed to actively contract the antagonist against the

isotonic, manually applied resistance of the therapist for 10 seconds. The patient is then instructed to relax while the therapist passively moves the limb to the new limits of motion (Fig. 2-12). Relaxation of the antagonist muscle during contraction is called autogenic inhibition.[1,21]

The *hold-relax technique* is similar to contract-relax. However, instead of an active, isotonic contraction of the antagonist, the patient isometrically contracts against the force applied by the therapist at the end of the ROM. After a 10 second isometric contraction, the patient is instructed to relax. The therapist then passively stretches the limb to the new limits of motion (Fig. 2-13).

The *slow-reversal-hold technique* requires the patient to actively move the affected limb to the limits of motion. The patient then applies an isometric 30 second

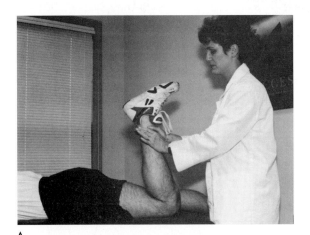

A

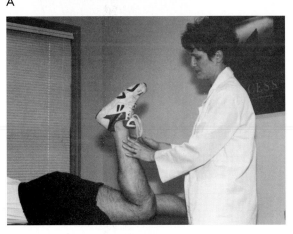

B

FIG. 2-12 Proprioceptive neuromuscular facilitation (PNF), contract-relax technique. **A,** The patient actively contracts against manually applied resistance for 10 seconds. **B,** The patient then relaxes while the therapist passively moves the limb to the new limits of motion.

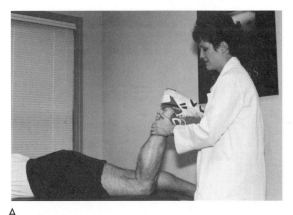

A

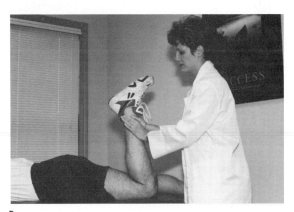

B

FIG. 2-13 PNF hold-relax technique. **A,** The patient isometrically contracts against the force applied by the therapist for 10 seconds. **B,** The patient relaxes, and the therapist passively moves the limb to new limits of motion.

contraction of the antagonist against the force applied by the therapist. The patient is instructed to relax the antagonist, then actively contract the antagonist to bring the limb to the new limits of motion (Fig. 2-14). The reflexive relaxation of the antagonist during contraction of the agonist is termed *reciprocal inhibition.*[1,21]

STRETCHING OF SOFT TISSUE CONTRACTURES

The stretching of soft tissue contractures involves muscle, capsule, tendon, ligament, bursa, and skin. The stretching of joint contractures differs significantly from static, ballistic, or PNF stretching. Many options exist

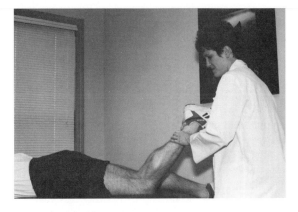

FIG. 2-14 PNF slow-reversal-hold technique (see text for description of technique).

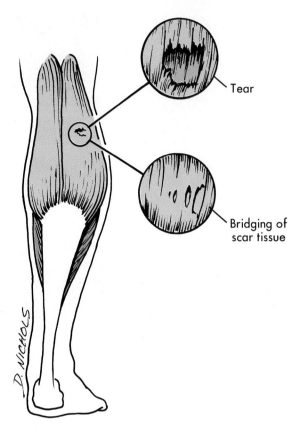

FIG. 2-15 Scar tissue formation.

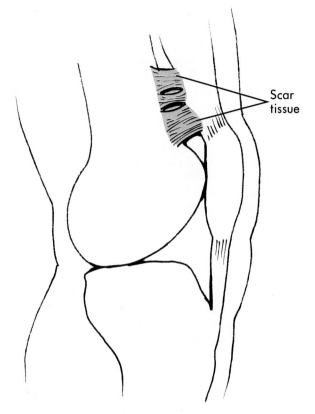

FIG. 2-16 Adhesions formed between quad tendon and underlying bone results in a limitation of function.

for the therapist when prescribing stretching exercises for patients after immobilization or injury. Long-duration, low-load static stretching has been an effective technique that produces long-lasting connective tissue changes[8,14,26,27] The physical therapist assistant must recognize adaptive changes that occur in various soft tissues after injury or immobility. First, **scar tissue** is formed and a **contracture** develops. For our purposes, a contracture will be defined as a permanent or transient limitation of movement or shortening of muscle or other soft tissues.[6] Scar tissue is the same as an adhesion and results from healing or union of two injured or torn parts (Fig. 2-15). An adhesion involves a limitation of function resulting from scar tissue that forms between structures.[6] For example, when scar tissue forms after knee surgery, it can "bind down" and form **adhesions** between the patella, suprapatellar pouch, and quadriceps tendon (Fig. 2-16).

Generally, immature scar is defined as adaptable for up to 8 weeks and becomes progressively less change-able for up to 14 weeks.[7] Scar becomes quite inexten-sible at 14 weeks and is termed *unadaptable,* or mature, scar.[2] According to Cummings,[7] adaptable scar is highly

vascular, with many cells, including myofibrocytes, which give the scar the ability to contract. Immature scar tissue also has a high rate of remodeling,[2,7] which is the process of tissue restructuring in response to stress or immobilization.[8]

Adaptable or immature scar tissue becomes increas-ingly organized and oriented, with specific directional lines of stress.[7] As new scar tissue is formed, the collagen fibers become highly unorganized and arranged randomly, creating an immobile structure.[17]

The critical components for the physical therapist assistant to appreciate with regard to stretching are as follows:

- The time dependent and stress reactive nature of scar tissue
- The fragility of immature adaptable scar:
  At 5 days, new scar is only 10% of its maximum potential strength
  At 40 days, new scar is 40% of its maximum strength
  At 60 days, new scar is 70% of its maximum strength
  At 12 months, new scar is approximately 100% of its maximum strength

- New scar tissue will organize and align itself along lines of stress, so appropriately applied stress helps to remodel unorganized scar

Low-load, long-duration stretching of joint contractures in combination with thermal agents to preheat extensible connective tissue has proved effective in the treatment of soft tissue contracture.[10,15,16] Long-duration stretching means stretching over a period of 20 to 60 minutes.[7]

Clinically, the following areas are involved in a **low-load, prolonged stretch** technique:

1. Preheating the involved structures with moist heat and/or ultrasound.[8]
2. Placing the involved structures in a position of comfort, not maximum stretch. This is an extremely important point. To elicit relaxation, the involved structures must be placed in a supported and comfortable gravity-assisted position.
3. Maintaining moist heat application during the entire course of treatment (between 20 and 60 minutes).
4. Applying stress or load gradually and minimally. With new immature scar, gravity alone may be enough to clinically effect change. With mature scar, only slightly greater loads should be used. This is a critical point. Lentell et al[15] found that the magnitude of force used in their study (0.5% of body weight) to create a significant long-lasting change in motion fostered such relaxation that many subjects "did not even feel a sensation of stretch during the procedure." In efforts to gain knee extension after surgery, for example, it is wise to use this technique to avoid reflexive splinting or muscle guarding (Fig. 2-17).
5. Allowing the patient to rest or recover for a few minutes during the course of treatment if the sensation of stretch becomes too uncomfortable.
6. Maintaining heat application for 5 to 10 minutes after removal of the loads. Some researchers[22] have advocated the use of ice packs after stretch in this protocol. Lentell et al[15] did not find cooling to be effective in their study. However, cooling the involved structures after stress may be effective in selected cases where pain and an inflammatory response are present.
7. Initiating isometric contractions after the application of heat and passive stretching to enhance strength gains at the new end of ROM.

Lentell et al[15] demonstrated the effectiveness of applying heat before and during low-load, prolonged stretching and external rotation of nonpathologically involved shoulders. Heat application before and during such stretching was clinically superior to bouts of stretching alone, stretching plus ice, and a heat-stretch-ice protocol. Clinically, few contraindications exist when attempting to gain motion after specific surgical procedures.

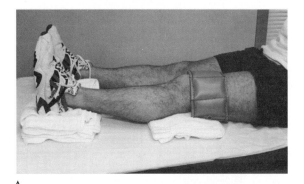

A

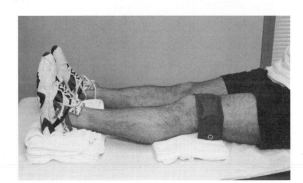

B

FIG. 2-17 External force is applied to enhance passive low-load prolonged stretch. **A,** Excessive weight causes reflexive muscle splinting and guarding. **B,** Only very light resistance is required to elicit appropriate relaxation.

In selected cases, adhesions are desirable and are, in fact, a surgical goal. In some knee surgeries and in surgical correction of some shoulder instabilities, desirable, permanent shortening of connective tissue is needed to prevent a functional loss of movement. If an attempt is made to fully regain external shoulder rotation after surgery to correct recurrent dislocation, the intent to "scar down" and protect the joint from further dislocation may be derailed. In this case it is wise to gain functional motion very slowly to allow enough time for mature scar to form (14 weeks).

The clinical application of low-load, prolonged stretch can be modified to varying degrees depending on the surgical procedure, time constraints of healing, and goals of the rehabilitation program. For example, supine wall slides are a modified technique that uses some of the points of low-load, prolonged stretch (Fig. 2-18). When attempting to gain knee flexion range, it is wise to preheat the quadriceps muscles and suprapatellar pouch before stretching. Next, the patient is placed in a supine position and the foot of the involved limb put on a towel

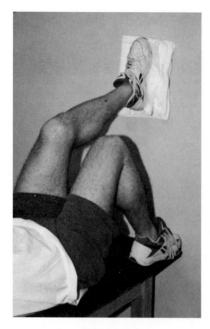

FIG. 2-18 Supine wall slides to gain knee flexion motion.

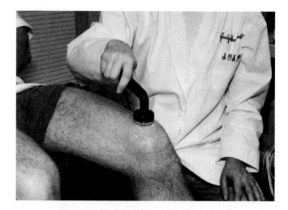

FIG. 2-19 Thermal agents of moist heat and ultrasound applied prior to passive stretching techniques help elevate tissue temperature and aid in soft-tissue extensibility and patient relaxation.

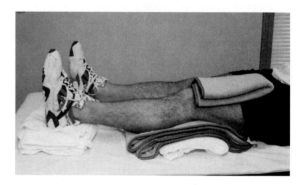

FIG. 2-20 Gaining knee extension using thermal agents (moist heat) and low-load prolonged stretch.

against a wall. To reduce friction against the wall, the contact surface of the towel is lightly coated with baby powder so it will slide more easily against the wall. As the patient relaxes, gravity assists in knee flexion and the foot slides down the wall.

This concept can be modified further. In keeping with the example of gaining knee flexion range, the use of isotonic exercise equipment can be helpful. With the patient in a seated position on a knee extension machine, moist heat and/or ultrasound can be used before and during the stretch (Fig. 2-19). Many knee extension machines are manufactured with an adjustable range-limiting device that allows the patient to adjust the starting and stopping angle of the exercise. To begin the stretch the patient's hips are secured with straps to keep them from rising during the treatment. An angle is selected that is comfortable to the patient. As the tissues are continually heated, a very gradual increase in the flexion angle is initiated. The angle does not have to be excessive to be effective. Thus the protocol remains essentially the same, but the equipment and the position of the patient are changed.

The knee serves as an excellent example to further describe and clarify methods to improve ROM by prolonged static stretching. To gain knee extension range, the patient can be supine with moist heat applied behind the knee (popliteal fossa) and on the hamstring and quadriceps. The heel of the involved limb is placed on a small folded towel (Fig. 2-20). If the knee is contracted to −20°; for example, towels are added under the hot packs under the knee to ensure a very comfortable starting position. During the course of treatment, very small layers of towel can be gradually removed to allow for improved range of knee extension. As a progression to this technique, a very small vertical force can be applied on the knee. Care should be taken to ensure that this force is very small (1 to 2 pounds or lighter) and that it is applied superior to the patella to avoid compressive forces between the patella and the femur (Fig. 2-21).

To enhance this stretch further, the patient is brought to a sitting position. A towel is used to dorsiflex the involved foot, and the patient is instructed to slowly lean forward to stretch the hamstrings (Fig. 2-22). Simultaneous isometric quadriceps sets are also used to improve strength at the new limits of knee extension.

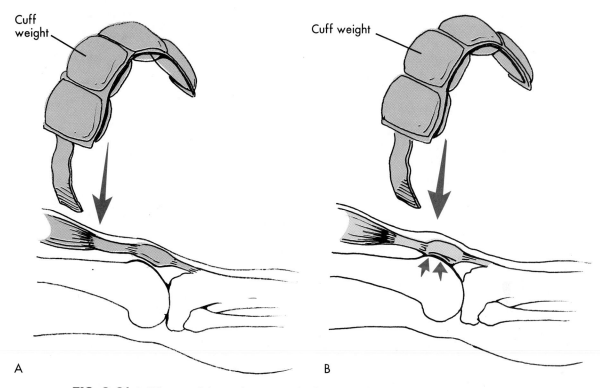

FIG. 2-21 **A,** When applying resistance on the knee to gain extension, it is essential that the resistance be placed superior to the patella. **B,** If resistance is placed directly on the patella, there is a sharp concentration of force, which increases patellofemoral compression.

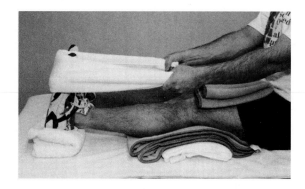

FIG. 2-22 Seated passive towel stretch.

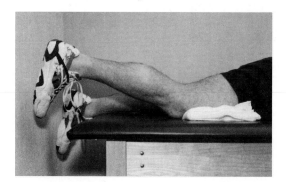

FIG. 2-23 Passive prone knee extension stretch. Note the use of towels placed under the quadriceps to elevate the patella off the table to reduce patellofemoral compression.

Gaining knee extension can be achieved in a prone position as well (Fig. 2-23). However, care must be taken to elevate the patella off of the table and thereby prevent excessive patellofemoral compression. This is done by placing a small folded towel superior to the patella. This position works well when only slight degrees of motion are needed (5 to 10 degrees of knee extension). This procedure can also be done on an isotonic exercise apparatus fol-

lowing the same process as described with gaining knee flexion on an isotonic exercise machine.

Knee extension range can also be improved in a sitting position with or without the aid of isotonic exercise equipment (Fig. 2-24).

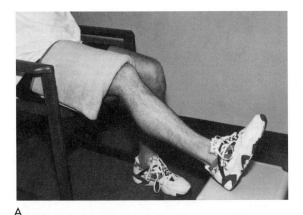

A

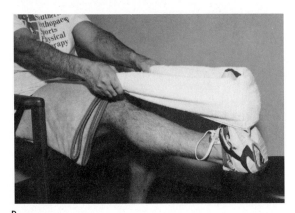

B

FIG. 2-24 A, Seated knee extension stretch with moist heat application to the quadriceps. **B,** The stretch is enhanced by using a towel to dorsiflex the foot of the involved limbs and to instruct the patient to flex the trunk forward.

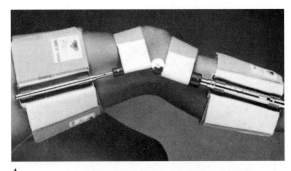

A

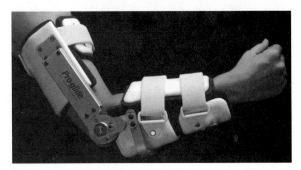

B

FIG. 2-25 A, Dynasplint® commercial appliance for low-load prolonged stretch. (Courtesy of Dynasplint Systems® Inc., Severna Park, Md.). **B,** Proglide appliance. (Courtesy of LMB Hand Rehab Products, Inc., San Luis Obispo, Calif.).

There are many commercially available tools that use the concept of low-load, prolonged stretch. Dynasplint® (Dynasplint Systems®, Inc) and Proglide (manufactured by LMB) are two examples of dynamic splints used to progressively "load" selected joints to gain motion (Fig. 2-25). An arrangement of pivot points and incrementally adjustable degrees of tension provides the levels of stress needed to effect change in joint motion.

The selection of patients for use of one of these splints must be made carefully. In the elderly population, skin integrity is an issue that must be addressed. Metal hinges and spring-loaded tension flanges may not be appropriate for this population because of the weight of the devices and the patient's potential for skin breakdown.

Simple tools for dynamic stretching can be used at home. A wand, cane, or shortened broomstick can be used for general shoulder flexibility (Fig. 2-26A). In-creased mobility can be gained by using the unaffected arm to assist the affected extremity (Fig. 2-26B).

Codman's pendulum exercises are effective for gaining relaxation and small degrees of motion in the shoulder. Relaxation is paramount to the effectiveness of this exercise. In one exercise technique, the patient is placed prone on a treatment table and a very light weight is held in the hand of the affected extremity. This light distraction force is used in conjunction with gradual, light oscillations in various directions (Fig. 2-27). Relaxation is enhanced by applying moist heat followed by ultrasound to the affected joint before pendulum exercise.

When teaching the oscillation component of this exercise, it must be made clear that muscular contractions must not be used to initiate and maintain the prescribed motions. The oscillation movements can be initiated by gently swinging the upper body or torso.

MEASURING FLEXIBILITY

Measuring joint ROM is accomplished by using standard goniometric instruments. Joint stability differs from joint

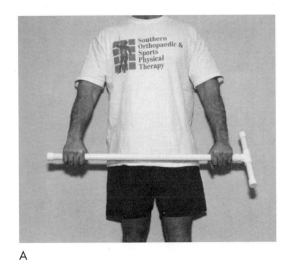

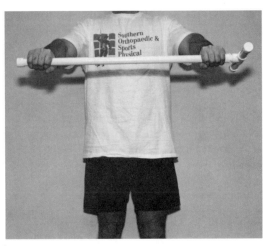

FIG. 2-26 A wand or cane can be used to enhance motion of the shoulder (**A** & **B**).

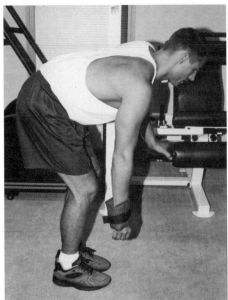

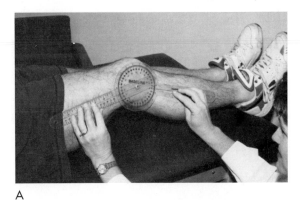

A

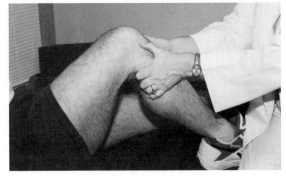

B

FIG. 2-27 Codman's pendulum exercise. For the exercise to be effective, the patient must relax completely and allow the affected arm to hang and gently oscillate in various directions.

ROM in that the ligaments and surface geometry of joint articulations dictate static joint integrity (stability). A patient may demonstrate limited ROM in knee flexion and extension (by goniometry); however, anterior and posterior joint motion may be excessive and unstable (Fig. 2-28). On the other hand, a patient may demonstrate

FIG. 2-28 A, Measuring joint motion with a goniometer. **B,** Joint stability is measured by manually applied clinical tests. Anterior drawer test of the knee is shown.

"normal" joint ROM, yet when tested statically the joint may be very stable, "tight," and unyielding to pressure.

Generally less specific flexibility tests are the sit and reach test (Fig. 2-29), the standing toe touch for back and hamstring flexibility (Fig. 2-30), the seated hip external rotation test (Fig. 2-31), and the standing knee recurvatum test. These and other tests are used to provide very general assessment of multijoint flexibility. Such tests can also be used as stretching techniques to improve limitations in movement. However, objective clinical documentation of joint ROM is made by joint goniometry.

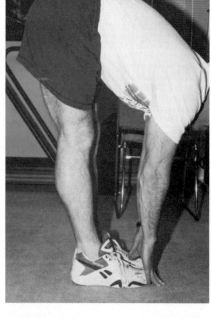

FIG. 2-30 General, nonspecific standing toe-touch flexibility test for the hamstring and low back.

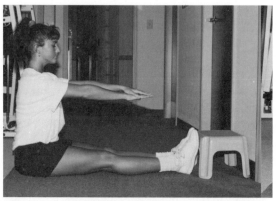

A

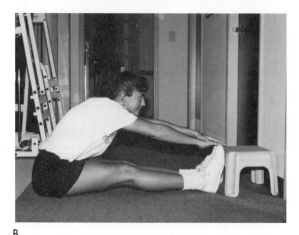

B

FIG. 2-29 General, nonspecific flexibility test. **A,** Sit and reach test for hamstrings and low-back flexibility, starting position. **B,** End position of sit and reach test.

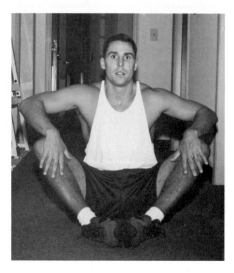

FIG. 2-31 Seated hip external rotation "butterfly" stretch.

REFERENCES

1. Allerheiligen WB: Stretching and warm-up, In Baechle TR editor: *Essentials of strength training and conditioning,* Champaign, Ill., 1994, Human Kinetics.

2. Aram AJ, Madden JW: Effects of stress on healing wounds: intermittent noncyclical tension, *J of Surg Res 20: 93–102, 1976.*

3. Asmussen E, Boje E: Body temperature and capacity for work, *Acta Physiological Scand* 10:12, 1945.

4. Best TM, Garrett WE: Basic science of soft tissue. In DeLee & Drez, editors: *Muscle and tendon, in orthopaedic sports medicine: principles and practice,* vol I, Philadelphia, 1994, WB Saunders.

5. Cornelius W, Jackson A: The effects of cryotherapy and PNF on hip extensor flexibility, *Athletic Training* 19:183, 1984.

6. Cummings GS, Crutchfield CA, Barnes MR: *Orthopedic physical therapy series,* vol I, Soft tissue changes in contractures, Atlanta, 1983, Stokesville Publishing.

7. Cummings GS, Crutchfield CA, Barnes MR: *Orthopedic physical therapy series,* vol 2, Soft tissue changes in contractures, Atlanta, 1983, Stokesville Publishing.

8. Cummings GS, Tillman LJ: Remodeling of dense connective tissue in normal adult tissues. In Currier P. and Nelson RM editors: *Dynamics of human biologic tissue,* Philadelphia, 1992, FA Davis.

9. Gelberman R et al: Tendon. In Woo Savio L-Y, Buckwalter JA, editors: *Surgery and repair of the musculoskeletal soft tissues,* Park Ridge, Ill 1988, American Academy of Orthopedic Surgeons.

10. Hettinga D: Normal joint structures and their reaction to injury, *J Orthop Sports Phys Ther* 1: 83–88, 1979.

11. Reference omitted in galleys.

12. Knott M, Voss P: *Proprioceptive neuromuscular facilitation,* ed 3, New York, 1985 Harper & Row.

13. Kisner C, Colby LA: *Therapeutic exercise foundations and techniques,* Philadelphia, 1990, FA Davis.

14. Lehman JF et al: Effect of therapeutic temperatures on tendon extensibility, *Arch Phys Med Rehab* 50:481–487, 1970.

15. Lentell G et al: The use of thermal agents to influence the effectiveness of a low-load prolonged stretch, *J Orthop Sports Phys Ther* 16,(5): 200–207, 1992.

16. Light K, et al: Low load prolonged stretch VS high load brief stretch in treating knee contractures, *Phys Ther* 64: 330–333, 1984.

17. Longacre JJ: Scar tissue—It's use and abuse in light of recent biophysical and biochemical studies. In Longacre JJ editor: *The ultra structure of collagen,* Springfield, Ill., 1976, Charles C Thomas, Publisher.

18. Louden KL et al: Effects of two stretching methods on the flexibility and retention of flexibility at the ankle joint in runners, *Phys Ther* 65:698, 1988.

19. Markos PD: Ipsilateral and contralateral effects of proprioceptive neuromuscular facilitation techniques on hip motion and electromyographic activity, *Phys Ther* 59: 1366, 1979.

20. Moore M, Hutton R: Electromyographic investigation of muscle stretching techniques, *Med Sci Sports* 12: 322, 1980.

21. Prentice W: A comparison of static and PNF stretching for improvement of hip joint flexibility, *Athletic Training* 18 (1): 56, 1983.

22. Sapega A et al: Biophysical factors in range of motion exercise, *Phys Sports Med* 9: 57–65, 1981.

23. Taylor DC et al: Viscoelastic properties of muscle-tendon units: the biomechanical effects of stretching, *Am J Sports Med* 18(3):300–309, 1990.

24. Tillman LJ, Cummings GS: Biologic mechanisms of connective tissue mutability. In Currier DP, Nelson M, editors: *Dynamics of human biologic tissue,* Philadelphia, 1992, FA Davis.

25. Van Brocklin JD, Ellis DG: A study of the mechanical behavior of toe extensor tendons under applied stress, *Arch Phys Med Rehabil* 46: 369-370, 1965.

26. Warren CG, Lehman, JF, Koblanski JN: Heat and stretch procedures: an evaluation using rat tail tendon, *Arch Phys Med Rehab* 57: 122–126, 1976.

27. Warren CG, Lehman, JF, Koblanski JN: Elongation of rat tail tendon: effect of load and temperature, *Arch Phys Med Rehabil* 52:465–484, 1971.

28. Woo SL-Y et al: Connective tissue response to immobility, *Arthritis Rheum* 18: 257–264, 1975.

29. Zachazewski JE: Improving flexibility. In Scully RM and Barnes MR editors: *Physical therapy,* Philadelphia, 1989, JB Lippincott.

30. Zebas CJ, Rivera ML: Retention of flexibility in selected joints after cessation of a stretching exercise program. In Dotson CO, Humphrey JH editors: *Exercise physiology: current selected research,* New York, 1985, AMS Press.

Strength

KEY TERMS

Epimysium
Fasciculus
Perimysium
Endomysium
Myofibrils
Actin
Myosin
Slow twitch (ST) (type
   I-red-oxidative)
   muscle fiber
Fast twitch (FT) (type
   II-white-glycolytic)
   muscle fiber
Concentric
Eccentric
Isometric
Strength
Tension
Work
Power
Hypertrophy
Atrophy
SAID principle
Delayed onset muscle
   soreness (DOMS)
Progressive resistance
   exercise (PRE)
Plyometrics
Closed kinetic chain
   exercise (CKC)

Maintaining, enhancing, and regaining strength are critical for improving body function during all phases of recovery after surgery, injury, or disease affecting the musculoskeletal system. The physical therapist assistant must understand the basic foundations of strength development and, most importantly, how to apply strength-gaining principles during recovery after immobilization, surgery, or musculoskeletal injury. In this chapter, the physical therapist assistant will be introduced to basic concepts and universally accepted principles that can be applied in numerous clinical situations with various orthopedic pathologies.

The response of human skeletal muscle to intense exercise leads to increased functional performance and morphologic changes, such as hypertrophy, within the muscle. A muscle's angle of attachment to a tendon, its fiber length, its muscle mass, and its cross-sectional area are the primary determinants of its strength and power potential.[18] A basic understanding of muscular composition and gross structure will help clarify concepts of therapeutic exercise and provide a foundation for developing advanced principles and applications of strength.

GENERAL MUSCLE BIOLOGY

The body of an individual muscle is surrounded by noncontractile connective tissue called the **epimysium.** Within the muscle are bundles of fibers called **fasciculi,** which are surrounded by another noncontractile connective tissue called the **perimysium.** The **endomysium** is a noncontractile connective tissue that surrounds each individual muscle fiber. The individual muscle fibers are composed of **myofibrils** that lie parallel to each other and to the muscle fiber itself (Fig. 3-1). The structural

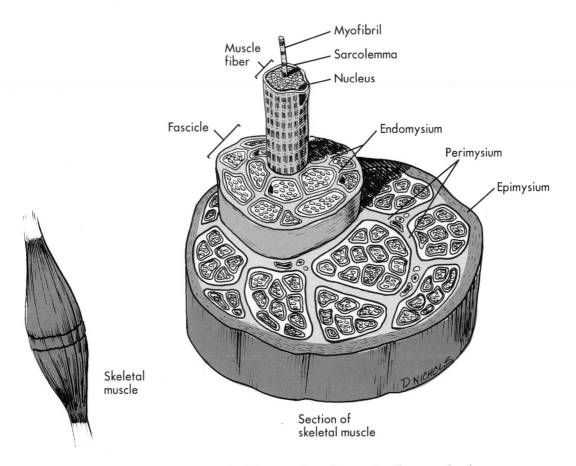

FIG. 3-1 Section of skeletal muscle with contractile and noncontractile connective tissue.

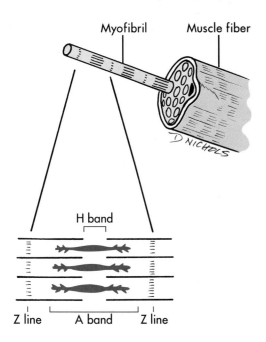

Myofibril   Muscle fiber

H band

Z line   A band   Z line

Sarcomere
(portion of myofibril between z lines)

FIG. 3-2 Functional or contractile unit of skeletal muscle fiber cell.

components of the myofibrils are called myofilaments, and they comprise two predominant proteins, **actin** and **myosin.** The functional, or contractile, unit of a muscle fiber cell is called the sarcomere (Fig. 3-2). Myosin (a thick protein) and actin (a thin protein) are actively involved with the mechanics of muscular contraction, which involves a complex and highly structured series of chemical and mechanical events. The extraordinarily complex biochemical excitation-contraction coupling and mechanical actions of muscular contraction are described in physiology textbooks. In simple terms, the neurologic stimulus to contract a muscle causes the release of acetycholine, which initiates the release of calcium. The calcium ions bond with troponin and tropomyosin, two proteins within the actin filaments. This allows actin–adenosine triphosphate (ATP) to react with myosin–adenosine triphosphatase (ATPase), producing energy so the thick myosin and thin actin filaments can "slide" past each other, generating tension and producing contraction of the muscle.

MUSCLE FIBER TYPES

Generally, two types of muscle fiber have been identified in humans. **Slow twitch (ST) (type I—red oxidative) muscle fibers** possess more mitochondria, triglycerides, and oxidative enzymes (succinic dehydrogenase or SDH), which allow for aerobic work. This type of fiber is specialized for muscular endurance activities. These fatigue-resistant fibers contract slowly, but are highly efficient for prolonged aerobic events.

Fast twitch (FT) (type II—white glycolytic) muscle fibers are, by contrast, anaerobic. These fibers are not as vascular as type I fibers, but they "fire," or contract, at a higher speed than type I fibers and with more force. These fibers have a very high level of myosin-ATPase, which provides energy for speed of contraction and tension; they also have a low myoglobin content and very few mitochondria. However, they are larger in diameter than red fibers. These fibers are used mainly in activities that require speed, strength, and power. Type II fibers can be further broken down into three distinct subclassifications: type II-A, type II-AB, and type II-B.[38,56]

These fiber types differ mainly in terms of endurance and are classified as intermediate fiber types with both aerobic and anaerobic capacities; they are occasionally referred to as fast-oxidative-glycolytic fibers.

The recruitment of muscle fiber types during strength training programs is determined in part by the size of the motor neuron and the intensity of force production. In general, slow twitch fibers are innervated by smaller neurons. Therefore the orderly recruitment of muscle fibers during contraction proceeds according to increased force requirements, as follows:

Slow twitch (ST) → fast twitch (FT) → fast twitch A (FTA) → fast twitch AB (FTAB) → fast twitch B (FTB)

TYPES OF MUSCLE CONTRACTIONS

The three true types of muscle contractions are **concentric, eccentric,** and **isometric.** In a concentric contraction, tension is produced and shortening of the muscle takes place. The action produced by a concentric contraction brings together or approximates the origin and insertion of the contracting muscle (Fig. 3-3).

An eccentric muscle contraction is sometimes referred to as a "negative contraction" or "negative work." In an eccentric contraction, tension is actually produced, but lengthening of the muscle occurs so that the net action is opposite that produced by a concentric contraction. The origin and insertion of the contracting muscle will move farther apart during the contraction (Fig. 3-4). For example, in moving from a standing position to a seated position, you slowly descend to sit in a chair; the quadriceps muscles must eccentrically contract to control the rate of descent (Fig. 3-5), or you would simply fall suddenly to the chair.

In an isometric contraction, tension is produced but no joint movement or action takes place. An example is a quadriceps "set" or "quad set." (The word "set" is used to describe an isometric contraction.) As a knee is held straight and if the quadriceps contracts, tension is produced within the muscle, but no change in joint angle takes place. Clinically, isometric contractions can take place at any joint angle. If the knee is placed at a 90 degree angle and contracts against an object that cannot be moved, then tension is produced but no joint motion or change in joint angle occurs.

Two other terms have been used to describe muscle contractions, *isokinetic* and *isotonic*. These are not types of contractions but rather terms used to describe events. In an isokinetic contraction, the speed, or velocity, of movement is held constant regardless of the magnitude of force applied to the resistance. Examples of isokinetic equipment are Cybex, Biodex, Lido, and Kin-Com.

An isotonic muscle contraction is not an accurate name for what happens physiologically. The name implies that the resistance, force, load, or tension remains constant, but actually the tension or force created in a muscle during this type of action must change as the joint angle changes. For example, when lifting a barbell (constant resistance), the amount of force generated by the contracting muscle varies at different angles during the movement even though the weight itself remains constant. Therefore a more precise and descriptive term, *isoinertial*,[43] can be used in place of *isotonic*. The term *isotonic* will be used in this book to describe the action of variable velocities of movement with a constant load. Examples of isotonic resistance equipment are barbells, dumbbells, and ankle weights, which are collectively referred to as "free weights."

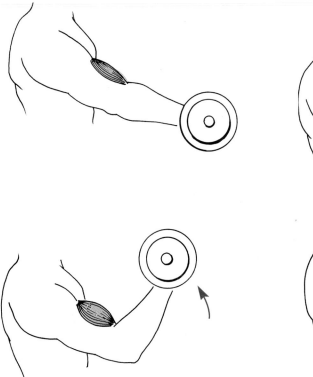

FIG. 3-3 Concentric muscle contraction.

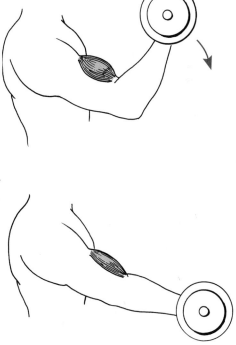

FIG. 3-4 Eccentric muscle contraction.

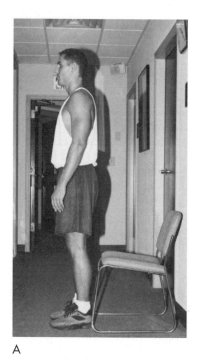 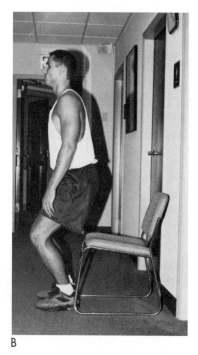 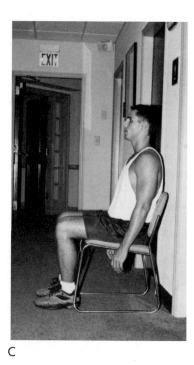

A   B   C

FIG. 3-5 Example of eccentric muscle contraction of the quadriceps. **A,** Starting position. **B,** Midportion of descent. The quadriceps are eccentrically contracting (elongating) to control the velocity of descent. **C,** End phase of descent. Without eccentric muscle contraction of the quadriceps, you would fall suddenly to the chair.

DEFINITIONS OF STRENGTH AND POWER

Strength is a notoriously ambiguous term. Generally strength is the ability of a muscle to generate force. And **tension** is described by Soderberg[50] as "A type of force that tends to pull things apart, it is the only type of force a muscle can generate." In Webster's dictionary,[59] strength is defined as "The capacity for exertion or endurance." *Exertion* and *endurance* are seemingly contrasting terms that do not clearly relate to strength. Harman[28] defines strength as "The ability to exert force under a given set of conditions defined by body position, the body movement by which force is applied, movement type and movement speed." Knuttgen and Kramer[35] offer this definition of strength, "The maximal force a muscle or muscle group can generate at a specified velocity." Without a clear scientific consensus that accurately describes strength, confusion will continue to surround this term.

To help clarify strength clinically, it is perhaps most useful to consider strength in terms that describe performance. **Work** is used to describe the result or product of

a force exerted on an object and the distance the object moves.[28] This term is expressed as Work = Force × Distance. *Force* can be described as either *linear* or *rotary.*[50] Linear force is described as Force = Mass × Acceleration, whereas rotary force is expressed as Force = Mass × Angular acceleration. *Torque* is clearly defined as Torque = Force × Perpendicular distance from the axis of rotation.

Power is defined as the time rate of doing work, which can be expressed in several ways:[43]

$$\text{Power} = \frac{\text{Work}}{\text{Time}} = \frac{\text{Force} \times \text{Distance}}{\text{Time}}$$

or

$$\text{Power} = \text{Force} \times \frac{\text{Distance}}{\text{Time}}$$

or

$$\text{Power} = \text{Force} \times \text{Velocity}$$

Velocity is defined as a vector that describes displacement. Overall, these terms help describe resultant muscular performance as they relate to the development of strength.

MEASURING STRENGTH

Strength can be measured by five methods: (1) manual muscle testing, (2) cable tensiometry, (3) dynamometry, (4) isotonic one-repetition maximum lift, and (5) isokinetics.

Manual muscle testing describes a muscle or muscle group's ability to isometrically "hold" or resist a force applied by the tester. Therefore it is used to generally grade a muscle's isometric contraction capacity at a specific joint angle against an applied force and/or gravity. The grading scale for this test is clinically easy to use (Box 3-1). However, the tester must have a comprehensive and detailed understanding of kinesiology to accurately and consistently reproduce manual grading of muscle strength (performance). The results of manual muscle testing cannot be inferred to relate to anything other than a muscle's ability to isometrically resist an applied force.

Cable tensiometry is used to isometrically measure a muscle's strength (Fig. 3-6). Essentially this tool is a mechanical form of manual muscle testing. Clinically, this form of testing is inappropriate for many acute, chronic, or postsurgical orthopedic patients. This method is primarily used to measure strength in normal subjects in research projects. Many tests were developed in the 1950s to describe static force or isometric strength using the cable tension method.[11,12]

Dynamometry is used extensively in physical therapy. Hand-held dynamometers (Fig. 3-7) are used to quantify grip strength, and the standing back dynamometer is used to evaluate back extension strength. In this latter example, many factors contribute to the subject's ability to generate tension or force during the back pull, including the patient's motivation, degree of pain (if any), arm length, leg length, height, weight, and the obvious contribution from other muscle groups. These variables make dynamometry an unreliable, nonspecific testing tool.

Isotonic one-repetition maximum lift is used to test strength using commercially available exercise equipment or barbells and dumbbells. In this method the patient performs a single, full range of motion (ROM) lift, such as a bench press (Fig. 3-8), shoulder press, or arm curl, for a particular muscle group. Applying this method is difficult because (1) the tester and patient must first establish a reasonable starting weight through trial and error, and fatigue becomes a factor if many trials are needed, and (2) precise performance or execution of the proper lift is determined subjectively by the tester. This method is best used for normal subjects, in a sports medicine environment, or with uninvolved body parts not required for stabilization of a disabled joint.

Perhaps the most widely used and clinically relevant method of objective, reproducible strength testing is through *isokinetics*. The data collected with isokinetic testing document strength (force production), torque,

---

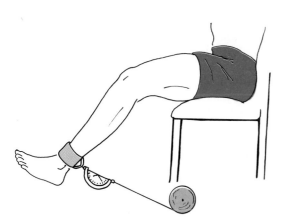

FIG. 3-6 Seated cable tensiometer for quantifying isometric quadriceps strength.

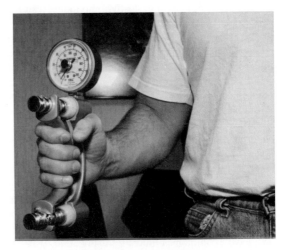

FIG. 3-7 Hand-held grip dynamometer for measuring grip strength.

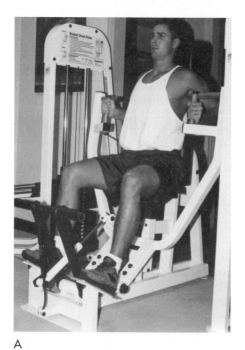 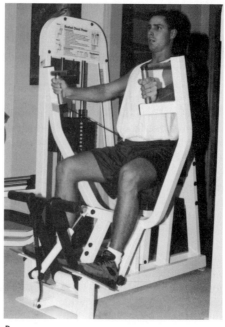

A   B

FIG. 3-8 Concentric and eccentric one-repetition maximum lift test. This is a very generalized nonspecific method to determine strength with commercial isotonic equipment. **A,** Starting position. **B,** End position.

power, and work.[47] As stated earlier, isokinetics employs a fixed speed, or velocity, of movement that allows for maximum loading throughout the full ROM. If a patient experiences pain during any part of the test, or does not apply a maximum force throughout the entire ROM, the velocity remains constant with a variable resistance that is totally "accommodating" to the individual.[15] To test for strength, slow speeds (30 to 60 degrees per second) are generally used.[37] Because isokinetic equipment can be interfaced with computers, a hard-copy graph of the data can be used for evaluation and exercise prescription. In addition to being a valid and reliable tool for strength testing, isokinetics can also evaluate neuromuscular endurance, speed of muscle contraction, and muscular power.[31]

COMPARISON OF MUSCLE CONTRACTION TYPES

Generally, muscle contractions are characterized by the amount of tension the contraction produces and the amount of energy liberated (ATP use) by the contraction. The most common clinically applicable way to strengthen muscle is with concentric and eccentric con-

tractions using isotonic (isoinertial[43]) progressive resistive exercise (PRE). Ankle or cuff weights, hand-held weights (dumbbells), and weight machines are examples of isotonic equipment used in physical therapy practice.* Elftman[19] has demonstrated that the production of maximal force of contraction by various methods occurs in a predictable fashion, as follows: Eccentrics > Isometrics > Concentric exercises. The force of contraction is expressed as the amount of tension developed per unit of contractile tissue. In terms of energy liberated (ATP use), eccentric muscle contractions use the least ATP, and concentric contractions use the most,[3] so Concentric exercises > Isometrics > Eccentrics.

Based on this information, it appears that eccentric muscle contractions are more energy efficient and produce greater tension per contractile unit than both concentric and isometric contractions. However, Davies[15] points out that much of the tension produced by eccentric muscle contraction results from stress imposed on the noncontractile serial elastic components (perimysium, epimysium, endomysium) of the muscle.

---

*Cybex, Nautilus, Rehab Systems, Body Masters, Universal, Paramount.

Therefore eccentric muscle contractions stimulate both contractile and noncontractile elements, whereas concentric contractions and isometrics focus on the contractile elements.[47]

The physical therapist assistant must consider the context in which each muscle contraction type is used clinically. Fundamentally, implementing multiple muscle contraction types during all phases of rehabilitation is well supported.[4,27,52] In comparing muscle contraction types, it is best to view the decision concerning which type to use, when to use it, and in what pathologic conditions it should be used as a progression or continuum rather than a choice of one type over another. Davies[15] has described a classic model of exercise progression (Box 3-2), which can be used as a general guide. Certain criteria must be established for the progression from one type of contraction to another.

First, exercise variables and parameters must be understood so that necessary adjustments can be made in a patient's exercise prescription (Box 3-3).

The criteria established for progressing from one exercise mode to another is based on many factors and is patient specific. In general, pain usually dictates the time frame for progression, although swelling also does to a lesser degree. The sequence proceeds from the least intense to more challenging exercises with increased joint forces and metabolic demands.

Some of the advantages and disadvantages of concentric and eccentric isotonic exercise and isokinetic exercise equipment are outlined for general comparison in Box 3-4.

BOX 3-2	Davies Model of Exercise Progression (1985)

Isometric/eccentric contractions, multiple angle isometrics (sub-max effort)
Multiple angle isometrics (max effort)
Short arc concentric–isokinetics (sub-max effort)
Short arc isotonics–concentric /eccentric
Short arc concentric isokinetics–(max effort)
Full ROM concentric isokinetics (sub-max effort)
Full ROM isotonics–concentric /eccentric
Full ROM concentric isokinetics (max effort)
Full ROM eccentric isokinetics (sub-max effort)
Full ROM eccentric isokinetics (max effort)

From Davies G: *A compendium of isokinetics in clinical usage and rehabilitation techniques*, Onalaska, Wis., 1987, S & S.

BOX 3-3	Therapeutic Exercise Parameters

Frequency

Daily, 3 days a wk, 2 days a wk (QD=once daily, bid=twice daily)

Intensity

Amount of resistance, full range of motion, short arc of motion, velocity of contraction (slow, moderate, fast)

Duration

6 weeks, 8 weeks, 10 weeks

Type of resistance

Isotonic, isokinetic

Muscle contraction type

Concentric, eccentric, isometric

Degree of resistance

Total amount of weight or force applied

Number of repetitions

1-15

Number of sets

1-5

Length of rest between sets

Short rest for aerobic-metabolic pathway, long rest (2-3 min) for anaerobic pathways

Order of exercise

Exercise large muscle groups first, progress to smaller muscle groups.

Degrees of effort

Low intensity (sub-max effort), high intensity (max effort)

MUSCLE RESPONSE TO EXERCISE

Muscle tissue morphology is mutable, that is, it has the ability to change. Muscle mutability has two distinct categories, **hypertrophy** and **atrophy.**

Various stimuli are required to affect muscle mutability. The **SAID principle** (specific adaptations to imposed demands)[20] is the precursor to overload, specificity, and reversibility as related to strength and reconditioning after injury. In part, the SAID principle defines specific adaptations and alterations in response to highly specific demands. After injury, muscle reeducation helps the patient adapt and prepare for return to function.

BOX 3-4 Comparison of Isotonics vs Isokinetics

Commercially available machines and free weights		Isokinetics
Advantages	• Low cost (relative) • Has both concentric and eccentric components • Easy to instruct patients • Objective increase in MS performance by increasing weight • Can perform static or isometric contractions	• Can exercise over a wide velocity (0°-300°) • Accommodates to pain and fatigue • Low compressive forces at high speeds • Provides objective permanent record of data • Valid and reliable
Disadvantages	• Cannot exercise at high speeds (functional) • Momentum is involved • Not safe if patient has pain during the motion of lifting	• Very expensive • Some models do not provide eccentrics • Takes time to switch machine for other body parts (time consuming)

Strength training must be individually tailored to meet the goals of recovery. As stated by DeLee et al,[16] "Function increases with use; functions we do not use, we lose. The intensity, duration, and frequency of activity are all related to the functional capacity that is developed."

The stimuli for adaptive changes in skeletal muscle are described as frequency, intensity, and duration.[8] Human skeletal muscle responds and adapts to these stimuli and is characterized by the nature, rate, magnitude, and duration of the stimulus.[4] In a clinical situation, the stimulus provided to human muscle is the conditioning or training program. These programs are based on certain principles that lead to the needed adaptive changes, which in turn affect function. The principles of overload, specificity, and reversibility[20] provide the foundation for the strength training programs used in physical therapy and are as follows:

Overload principle: For performance and morphologic changes to occur, a stimulus (load, tension) must progress and exceed the normal functional capabilities of the muscles being trained.

Specificity: The specific and predictable adaptations a muscle goes through in response to specific training.

Reversibility: Adaptive changes in response to specific training are reversible;[20] if the stimulus used to elicit morphologic changes is removed, the changes revert to the pretraining state.

In general, type I muscle fibers (red [high myoglobin content] and oxidative) respond more favorably to low-intensity (low tension), high-volume (sets and repetitions) exercise than type II (white [low myoglobin content] and glycolytic) muscle fibers. High-volume, low-intensity exercise is repetitive, and gross muscle movements occur (as in bicycling, running, swimming, and rowing). In this type of training, oxidative capabilities increase and relative percent increases in type I muscle fibers occur in the specific muscle or muscle groups used.

In strength training programs, a desirable and predictable morphologic adaptive change is *hypertrophy,* which is the compensatory increase in individual muscle fiber size as a result of increases in and synthesis of the contractile proteins actin and myosin.[25] Type II muscle fibers increase more than type I fibers do. This can be observed in comparing the body types of long-distance runners with the larger, more muscular physiques of sprinters. The physiques of long-distance runners and most aerobic athletes are thinner, possess less body fat, and have smaller muscles that are more adapted to endurance activities. Highly specific, or "absolute strength," programs use a high-tension (heavy loads) and low-volume protocol. This type of training program requires relatively short bouts of progressive overload to stimulate the type II muscle fibers.

Biochemical adaptations of muscle occur in specifically applied strength training programs. After intense strength training, significant increases appear in glycogen, ATP, and creatine phosphate; increased activity and quantity of enzymes involved with anaerobic glycolysis, creatine kinase, and myokinase are also seen.[13]

Hyperplasia (the development of new muscle fibers) or longitudinal fiber splitting may occur in response to high-intensity strength-training programs. Gonyea et al[26] reported in animal studies that an increase of 19% of the total number of muscle fibers occurred in cat forelimb muscles after weight lifting. This phenomena has not been proved in humans. The predominant change in response to high-intensity strength-training programs is hypertrophy of existing skeletal muscle fibers. The relative contribution (if any) of hyperplasia or muscle fiber splitting has not been determined.[8] Induced hypertrophy in injured or postoperative muscle tissue is important because hypertrophy relates to a potential to generate greater tension.

Interestingly, passive stretching of innervated muscle tissue creates tension and also results in fiber hypertrophy. The change in fiber size associated with this stretch-induced hypertrophy results from increased protein turnover.[8] This feature has clinical relevance in muscle recovery during immobilization.

DELAYED ONSET MUSCLE SORENESS (DOMS)

The clinical features of exercise-induced muscle soreness are diffuse and general, occurring in the absence of specific, intense injury.[45] Acute muscle strain can be differentiated from exercise-induced soreness primarily by the history leading to the injury. With an acute strain, the patient will be able to relate a specific event or episode that can be identified as causing the injury.[45]

Based on this distinction, the physical therapist assistant will be able to identify complaints of diffuse muscle soreness resulting from new or unaccustomed exercise.[45] However, if the patient can describe a history of local, intense pain after a specific episode, an acute muscle strain must be considered.[45]

Although the physical therapist assistant does not interpret and define complaints of pain without consulting with the physical therapist, the assistant must be able to accurately identify and describe the nature and disposition of any pain based on the patient's complaints and relevant history and be able to communicate this information to the physical therapist.

After a specific exercise program muscle soreness is an anticipated byproduct of intense eccentric exercise.* The degree and presence of post-exercise muscle soreness appear to be greater with these eccentric programs than with concentric exercise programs.[7,31,40,49,55]

Symptoms of **delayed onset muscle soreness (DOMS)** include pain, swelling, tenderness, reduced ROM, and stiffness.[3,31,40,49] Albert[3] reports five general theories concerning the process of DOMS:

1. Lactic acid theory
2. Torn tissue theory

3. Tonic muscle spasms
4. Connective tissue damage
5. Tissue fluid theory

The lactic acid theory and tonic muscle spasms do not appear to be related to DOMS.[1,2,48,58] Recent studies[38,39] show evidence that the primary cause of muscle soreness after exercise is skeletal muscle damage. Greater tensions produced by eccentric exercise contribute to the initial muscle damage, although isometric and concentric contractions are not absolved of producing latent muscle soreness. In fact, isometric exercise and concentric exercise can produce DOMS even in well-trained athletes. The treatment of DOMS is outlined in Table 3-1.

VELOCITY OF MUSCLE CONTRACTIONS

Muscle contraction velocity and speed of limb movement are not the same. If two arms are bending at the same speed, but one arm is holding a weight, the muscle bending the arm with more weight must produce a greater speed of contraction to overcome the resistance. Therefore more tension is developed in the muscle lifting the heavier arm, even though the speed of limb movment is the same.

Slower speeds of muscle contraction can produce greater force and tension than the same muscle moving at a higher rate of speed. A slower contracting muscle moving a heavy resistance can produce greater tension than a faster contracting muscle lifting a lighter resistance.[41] When slow speeds of full arc resistance exercise

TABLE 3-1

Suggested Treatment Techniques for Delayed Onset Muscle Soreness

Type	Efficacy
Rest	None
Nonsteroidal antiinflammatory	Highly successful
Steroidal antiinflammatory	Moderately successful
Electrical stimulation	Proposed only
Exercise	Highly successful
TENS	Highly successful
Stretching	Mixed success
Iontophoresis	Not successful
Cryotherapy	Not successful
Calcium antagonists	Proposed only

From Albert M: *Eccentric muscle training in sports and orthopaedics,* New York, 1991, Churchill Livingstone.

---

*References 22, 31, 40, 42, 49, 51.

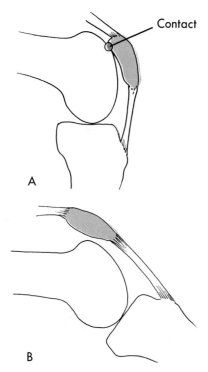

FIG. 3-9 A, With the knee flexed to 90° there are resultant increases in patellofemoral compression with excursion of the knee (leg) into extension. **B,** With the knee in extension there is less patellofemoral compression.

are used to generate greater tension and strength, greater joint compression forces and torque are increased as well. Therefore, to minimize the negative or unwanted effects of joint compression (Fig. 3-9), a program of isometric exercise may be more appropriate in some instances.

Initially, strength programs focus on using slow-speed tension to produce isometric contractions and spare the negative effects of excessive joint motion, torque, and compressive forces found in full ROM slow-speed isotonic (concentric and eccentric) exercises. Fast and slow contraction speeds can be distinguished with isokinetic exercise. By controlling the speed of limb movement with an isokinetic apparatus, better control of joint compression forces can be achieved. (*Speed* is defined isokinetically as control of limb movement, not necessarily the actual speed of muscle contraction.) A slow speed of limb movement using an isokinetic apparatus may be 60 degrees per second, and a fast speed may be 300 degrees per second.

Higher speeds of limb movement require the resistance to be lighter than in a slower moving limb with greater resistance. Isokinetic testing and exercise use the concept of velocity spectrum training, which is the ability to control limb speeds within a range of slow to fast speeds. Higher speeds of limb movement produce less joint compression and lower forces relative to slow-speed, high-resistance training.

Functionally, human limbs move at various speeds and with various degrees of motion. Velocity spectrum training allows a patient to train at speeds of motion that more closely approximate normal human limb speeds.[6,46,61] For example, a training program using the velocity spectrum concept may include submaximal contractions at slow speeds (60 to 90 degrees per second) for two sets of eight to twelve repetitions, then contractions at incrementally increasing speeds up to 240 degrees per second or higher for two or three sets of fifteen repetitions.

In comparing isokinetic to isotonic exercise, most isotonic exercise is performed at approximately 60 degrees per second,[15] whereas isokinetic exercise can be specifically adjusted to train the affected area at speeds more closely duplicating normal functional speeds of movement. Higher velocity contractions using isokinetic exercise allow for:

- Improved functional speeds of contraction
- Reduced joint compression forces
- Accommodation of patient's pain (the patient will not undergo more force than he or she can safely produce)

Using velocity spectrum training with isokinetics allows the progression from multiangle isometrics (0 degrees per second) to slow speeds (60 degrees per second) for greater tension and torque, to higher speeds (240 degrees per second and faster) for functional activities and lower compressive forces.

CLINICALLY RELEVANT EXERCISE PROGRAMS

Three broad fundamental strength protocols are used extensively in physical therapy. The DeLorme[17] **progressive resistance exercise (PRE)** protocol is still used widely for strength training programs after injury to the musculoskeletal system. This program uses the classic and well-recognized exercise of 3 sets of 10 repetitions of resistance. Its protocol states that the patient must establish a maximum weight that can be lifted for 10 repetitions. This is termed the *10 RM* (repetitions maximum). To initiate the program, the patient performs ten repetitions at half (50%) of the predetermined 10 RM. The next set of exercise is performed at three fourths (75%) of the 10 RM. Finally, the third set is performed for ten repetitions at the established 10 RM (100%).

The DeLorme protocol calls for an arbitrary increase in resistance each week. It allows for a systematic and gradual progression during each exercise session by providing a warm-up period using submaximal contractions before the 10 RM.

The Oxford program[62] is the opposite of the De-Lorme protocol. Although it begins by establishing the individual's 10 RM, the second set is performed at three fourths (75%) of the 10 RM and the following set at half (50%) of the established 10 RM. Each set involves ten repetitions. The method reportedly takes advantage of the muscle's fatigue during exercise.

There are fundamental differences in philosophy between the DeLorme PRE protocol and the Oxford technique. The DeLorme program calls for a progressive overload during each session by *adding* resistance while the muscle fatigues. The Oxford technique calls for *reducing* resistance as the muscle fatigues. Both programs were developed in the 1950s, and since then many variations and combinations have been used to discover the most effective and efficient means to regain strength after an injury.

To objectively control the progression or resistance with exercise programs, Knight[34] established the daily adjustable progressive resistance exercise technique (DAPRE). Instead of using three sets of ten repetitions like DeLorme and Oxford, Knight's program calls for four sets with variable repetitions. The protocol calls for establishing the patient's 6 RM instead of 10 RM, with the number six based on research by Berger[5] as the optimum number of repetitions for developing strength.

The first set is performed at half (50%) of the established working weight for ten repetitions. The second set is performed at three fourths (75%) of the 6 RM for six repetitions. The third set is performed at the full previously established maximum weight, but the patient is asked to perform as many repetitions as possible with this weight. The number of repetitions performed in this set is used to determine the weight used in the fourth set. The goal of this technique is to establish a maximum resistance that can be performed for six repetitions.

As the individual's strength increases, the number of repetitions in the third set will increase, which will increase the weight in the fourth set. The hallmark of this program is understanding the guidelines used to adjust the working weight of the third and fourth sets.[16]

The DAPRE adjusted working weight guide is as follows:

Third Set Number of Repititions	Fourth Set Change
0-2	Reduce weight 5-10 pounds
3-4	Reduce weight 5-10 pounds
5-7	Keep weight the same
8-12	Increase weight 5-10 pounds
13 or more	Increase weight 10-15 pounds

The rationale for the weight adjustments described above is to modify resistance during the fourth set in order to maintain the goal of keeping repetitions between five and seven, while encouraging maximum resistance to influence strength increases and morphologic changes, such as hypertrophy.

In this protocol, the exact amount of weight used by the patient will be highly specific and tailored to the individual and the goals of recovery. Adjustments in weight are made to accommodate the specific healing constraints of the injury as well as the individual tolerance level of the patient. Thus extremely close communication and supervision of the patient are required. With the PRE program and Oxford program the patient works with a percentage of an established weight each session and advances in resistance once each week. The DAPRE protocol requires daily adjustments. It takes advantage of the fact that submaximal work does not provide the necessary stimulus for maximal gains in strength. By reducing the volume of repetitions to six and adjusting the weight so that a maximal load is used for six repetitions, the intensity of work is increased.

Other protocols have suggested[53] that by initially focusing on muscular hypertrophy, a greater potential for strength would exist. Because the cross-sectional area of muscle would be increased by a program of higher volume, the potential to develop greater amounts of tension is increased by reducing the volume of exercise and increasing the loads used.

Isometric exercise protocols are commonly used in rehabilitation following the rule of tens.[47] This states that the patient must perform 10-second contractions for ten repetitions with a 10-second rest between each repetition.[15] The patient is taught to perform isometric contractions by gradually developing tension for 2 seconds, maintaining a maximal contraction for 6 seconds, then gradually decreasing tension for 2 seconds (Fig. 3-10).

While performing isometric exercise, an "overflow" of strength occurs approximately 10 degrees above and below the angle (Fig. 3-11) at which the exercise is occurring.[33] Multiple-angle isometrics are taught at

10-degree increments to achieve strength gains throughout a described range of motion.

A circuit training program is a predetermined, organized sequence of exercise. Traditionally this type of program is used for general body conditioning and total fitness. A general circuit program calls for the performance of one or two exercises for each body part in sequence (Table 3-2). Usually a rest period of 30 seconds to 1 minute is allowed between sets. If resistance exercise equipment is used, circuit weight-training programs also tax the aerobic metabolic pathway to a degree. The movement from one station to another does not allow for maximum recovery and high-intensity loads, but it does provide an adequate stimulus for both aerobic and anaerobic work.

The clinical delivery of specific exercise protocols depends on many factors. The patient's pathologic condition, time constraints for healing of specific tissues, and degree of swelling, pain, function, and motivation all play a role in determining the most appropriate program to use and when to use it. Making an organized, systematic progression from one program to another, following specific guidelines, is a responsible and appropriate plan for strength training programs for a wide variety of musculoskeletal system injuries.

Plyometrics

Plyometric exercises are intense power-generating exercises that are traditionally confined to sport-specific functional training near the end of a rehabilitation program. *Plyo* comes from the Greek word *plythein*,

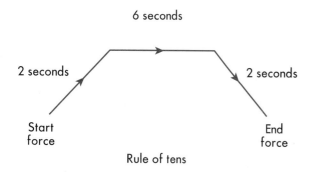

FIG. 3-10 Isometric contractions by rule of tens. (From Davies G: *A compendium of isokinetics in clinical usage and rehabilitation techniques,* Onalaska, Wis., 1987, S & S.

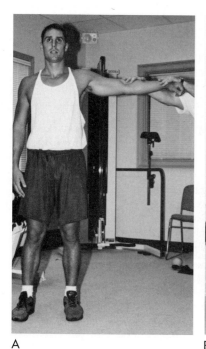 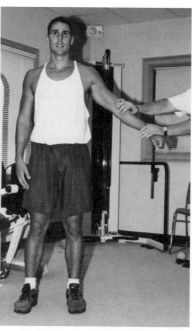 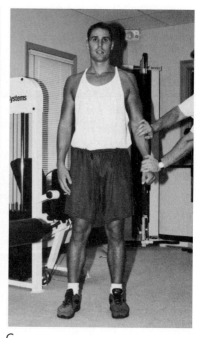

A   B   C

FIG. 3-11 Multiangle isometric shoulder abduction. **A,** Isometric hold in approximately 90° of abduction. **B,** Midrange isometric shoulder abduction. **C,** Isometric "set" in zero degrees of abduction.

meaning to increase, and *metric* refers to measure. **Plyometrics** are a system of exercising that use the stretch reflex to develop muscle contraction speed.[60]

Plyometric exercises are also highly adaptable for use with the general orthopedic patient population. However, the inherent nature of plyometrics requires the patient to be prepared for high-intensity, task-specific, dynamic exercise.

The principles behind plyometrics are based on the neurophysiologic responses from the golgi tendon organs (GTOs) and muscle spindles.[60] The most rudimentary example of plyometrics is the depth jump (Fig. 3-12). In this example, as the foot of the patient contacts the ground (amortization phase), the muscle spindles respond by causing a reflex muscular contraction. Albert[3] states, "The greater and more quickly a load is

TABLE 3-2

Sample Circuit Weight Training Program

Exercise	Repetitions	Sets	Rest
Leg press	10	2	30 sec between each set
Leg extensions	10	2	30 sec between each set
Leg curls	10	2	30 sec between each set
Bench press	10	2	30 sec between each set
Supine flys	10	2	30 sec between each set
Shoulder press	10	2	30 sec between each set
Lat pull-down	10	2	30 sec between each set
Bent over rows	10	2	30 sec between each set
Bicep curls	10	2	30 sec between each set
Tricep press-downs	10	2	30 sec between each set

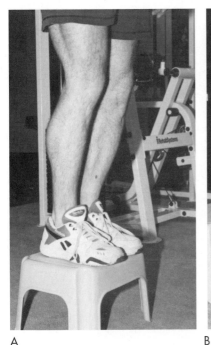
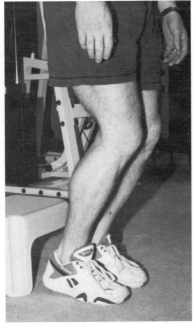
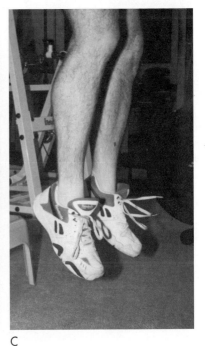

A   B   C

FIG. 3-12 Plyometric "depth jump." **A,** Starting position on a short stool. **B,** Without jumping up, off of the stool, the patient steps down to the ground with both feet simultaneously. The time spent on the ground is called the amortization phase. **C,** Rapid concentric contraction follows the amortization phase, which results in a powerful leap.

applied to a muscle, the greater the firing frequency of the muscle spindle with a corresponding stronger muscle contraction." The fundamental goal of plyometric exercise is to minimize the amortization phase of the exercise, which, in this example, would be contact with the ground.

All forms of jumping, skipping, and hopping can be used in a plyometric exercise program.[60] Upper body exercises, such as throwing and catching a weighted object, are examples of plyometrics. An isotonic supine leg press "hop" is an example of plyometrics used to develop rapid, eccentric loading with a corresponding rapid, concentric contraction.

Plyometrics must be used judiciously and principally as an end component in a phase progression program. The fundamental concept of plyometrics involves ballistic, high-velocity movement patterns, which cannot be used during early rehabilitation when tissues are still healing. As the patient progresses from one program or phase to another, plyometrics can be added to increase function.

Many isotonic strength training programs involve lifting a load from a seated, supine or standing position. These exercises are meant to isolate and strengthen specific muscle groups throughout a single plane of motion. Plyometrics, on the other hand, focus on weight-bearing functional activities that duplicate high-velocity, multiplane, normal human movement.[60] Therefore the physical therapist assistant must recognize the value of plyometrics as primarily preparing the patient to return to function. Naturally, not all patients recovering from an orthopedic injury will require an intense plyometric exercise program. If, however, the patient desires to return to dynamic sporting activities, or his or her job requires dynamic or ballistic physical labor, then plyometrics are appropriate conditioning to withstand high levels of both eccentric and concentric loads.

CLOSED KINETIC CHAIN EXERCISE

During any exercise, if the distal portion of the exercising segment is weight bearing or "fixed," it is termed a **closed kinetic chain exercise (CKC)**. An open kinetic chain exercise (OKC) involves the distal segment moving freely in space, such as a seated knee extension. A CKC is best described as a system of interdependent articulated links. For example, with a weight-bearing leg (Fig. 3-13), as the knee is flexed, the entire chain or link system joining the ankle to the knee and to the hip is

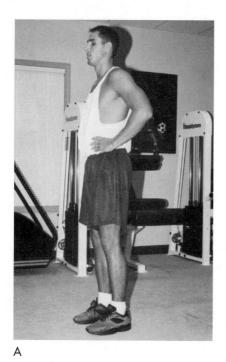
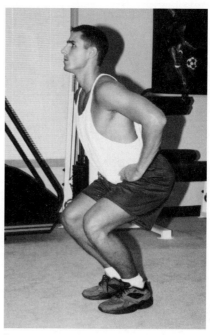

A   B

FIG. 3-13 A closed kinetic chain. **A,** Starting position of a standing squat or leg bend maneuver. **B,** Motion of the knee will produce predictable motion in all joints within the kinetic chain. With knee flexion notice the resultant change in joint position of the ankle, hip, and spine.

affected. In an OKC system, such as the arm (Fig. 3-14), the shoulder and elbow are fixed, while the distal wrist segment moves freely in space. Davies[14] states, "In a closed kinetic chain, motion at one joint will produce motion at all of the other joints in the system in a predictable manner."

The human body functions as a combination of both open and closed-chain activities such as walking and stairclimbing. The primary advantage of CKC exercises is the highly functional nature of the exercises, which use concentric and eccentric muscle contractions synchronously to produce functional movement. In a strength-training program, combinations of OKC and CKC exercises should be used to condition the patient to perform purposeful, functional activities.

In knee rehabilitation programs,[10,44] for example, quadriceps strengthening can be achieved through knee extension exercises (which are open chain), or through leg press exercises or squats (which are closed chain). In many cases, patients are introduced to therapeutic exercises by way of submaximal isometric muscle contractions. As pain, strength, and function allow, more intense and demanding exercises are added. OKC resistance exercises can be employed to further stimulate growth in strength. In some cases, the physical therapist will institute CKC exercises early in the recovery phase of reha-

bilitation. For example, CKC exercises are frequently used within the first few weeks after anterior cruciate ligament reconstructive surgery. In addition, select opened-chain exercises (those that do not place unwanted forces on the newly repaired tissues) are used. Closed-chain exercises may not be appropriate for some patients with osteoarthritis or other conditions where vertical, compressive loads would exacerbate the condition.

The general rationale for using closed-chain exercises in rehabilitation programs are as follows:

- CKC exercises are more functional than OKC exercises
- Loading of the affected joint(s) produces an increase in kinesthetic awareness
- Improved neuromuscular coordination is achieved
- CKC exercises are nonisolation exercises that produce muscular co-contractions

Caution must be used when prescribing CKC activities during rehabilitation when pain, swelling, dysfunction, or muscle weakness is present.[14] Because an articulated joint system is being exercised under these conditions (limited ROM, pain, swelling, and so on), unpredictable compensation may occur in the joint(s) superior and inferior to the affected joint.[14] Therefore OKC exercise must be used to isolate and strengthen the weakened area before progressing to CKC exercises.

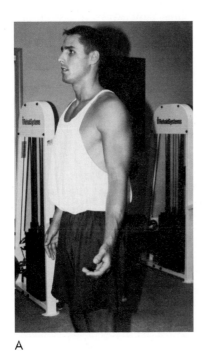
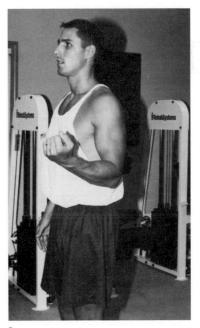

A   B

FIG. 3-14 An open kinetic chain. **A,** Beginning position of elbow flexion. **B,** The distal arm and wrist segments move freely in space.

PERIODIZATION OF STRENGTH TRAINING PROGRAMS

Periodization involves a predictable pattern of exercise volume, intensity, and rest periods that enhance strength-developing capabilities.[54] Its main components are "cycles" or periods of strength training. Many fundamental strength programs call for a progressive resistance exercise system without consideration for variations in frequency, intensity, duration, and recovery. The periodization model takes into consideration progressive cycles of various training loads and degrees of intensity during strength programs.[54]

Periodization can involve any of three cycles: microcycle, mesocycle, or macrocycle. The *microcycle* is the smallest unit of time (usually weeks), and accumulated microcycles form a mesocycle. The *mesocycle* is traditionally a few months long and consists of multiple microcycles that vary in volume, frequency, and intensity. The *macrocycle* is the largest segment of time (it can be a year long) and involves a collection of mesocycles.

Periodization of strength training programs in the clinical rehabilitation setting was originally designed for and used extensively in athletics and is justified by following a series of defined protocols directed specifically at developing strength, while minimizing fatigue and overtraining of the recovering orthopaedic patient.

The fundamental goals and objectives of a classic periodization program are outlined in Fig. 3-15. This is only a basic example, which must be modified to meet the specific rehabilitation goals for recovering patients. It can be adapted for many patients who require strength as part of their rehabilitation program.

In a periodization program, instead of constantly striving to increase resistance during each treatment or each week using the same system of sets and repetitions for a recovering patient, an attempt should be made to cycle the program into specific phases. In general, the first phase (microcycle) would strive to develop basic strength and muscular hypertrophy. There would be small alterations in sets (between 3 and 6 sets) and repetitions (between 8 and 12) in each week of rehabilitation, and a high volume of exercise is used, dictating a lower intensity level (approximately 65% to 70% of the 1 RM). This phase can be called the preparatory phase, or initial rehabilitation protocol. The second phase (mesocycle) is designed to enhance strength by increasing the loads used (85% of 1 RM) and decreasing the volume of exercise to 3 to 5 sets of 4 to 6 repetitions. This mesocycle, as well as the first, may last for 2 or 3 months. It is important to remember that during each mesocycle there are numerous microcycles (weeks) where various changes are made to reduce chronic overwork. The second phase of this basic example is called the first transition phase, or active rehabilitation phase.

The traditional athletic model for this modified periodization program is described in Fig. 3-16. The

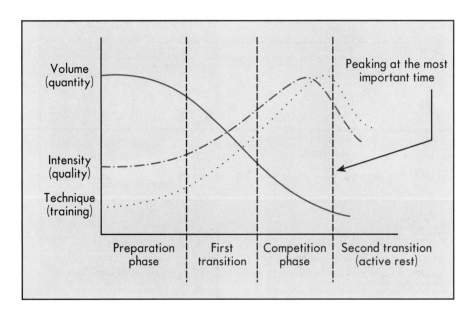

FIG. 3-15 Classic periodization model. (From the *National Strength and Conditioning Association Journal* 15:64-66, 1993).

Phase	Hypertrophy	Basic strength	Strength & power	Peaking or maintaining
Sets	3 - 10	3 - 5	3 - 5	1 - 3
Reps	8 - 12	4 - 6	2 - 3	1 - 3
Days/wk	3 - 4	3 - 5	3 - 5	1 - 5
Times/day	1 - 3	1 - 3	1 - 2	1
Intensity cycle (weeks)	2 - 3/1	2 - 4/1	2 - 3/1	—
Intensity	low	high	high	very high to low
Volume	high	moderate to high	low	very low

Preparation → Transition 1 → Competition → Transition 2 (active rest)

FIG. 3-16 Traditional athletic model of a modified periodization program. (From the *National Strength and Conditioning Association Journal* 15:64-66, 1993).

strength protocol should be modified to fit the specific needs of each individual.

STRENGTH TRAINING FOR OLDER POPULATIONS

Strength training programs for the geriatric population include special considerations. In an elderly population, declines in muscle performance, force-generating capabilities, and concomitant muscle mass are well documented.[30,36] Therefore strength training programs for the elderly are focused on delaying muscle atrophy, improving function, and increasing force-generating capabilities by stimulating muscle hypertrophy. It is important to note that resistance exercise programs for healthy, older populations show rather significant improvements in muscle strength, muscle volume (hypertrophy), and other parameters of muscle structure and function.[57] Thompson[57] reports that studies show, "Given an adequate training stimulus, older men and women show similar gains compared to young individuals after resistive training." In addition, McCartney et al[39] report, "That long term resistance training in older people is feasible and results in increases in dynamic muscle strength, muscle size, and functional capacity."

In addition, multiple conditions and degenerative joint disease must be considered in strength training programs for the disabled elderly. Unstable, chronic, and complex medical problems may preclude certain types of strength-training programs. For example, in cardiovascular disease, chronic obstructive pulmonary disease, and other conditions, a protocol of general, very low-intensity gross body movement may be more beneficial and safer than isometric or isotonic resistance exercise. In advanced cases of osteoarthritis of the knee and hip, it is prudent to avoid vertical compression loads and full ROM-heavy isotonic exercise. Pain and swelling from osteoarthritic lesions, bone spurs, and osteophytes (Fig. 3-17) can be exacerbated by the tibiofemoral vertical compressive loads involved in leg press or squatting exercises.

In general, studies support the fact that high-intensity resistance training promotes force-generating capabilities in aged muscle[32] and that resistance training enhances muscle hypertrophy in the elderly.[9,24] In one study[21], a very small population of very old (89 to 90 years old) men and women showed the beneficial effects of isotonic resistance exercise for this age group. When they trained for 8 weeks, 3 times per week, the force-generating capacity of the trained muscles increased 174% ± 31%. Muscle mass of this group increased

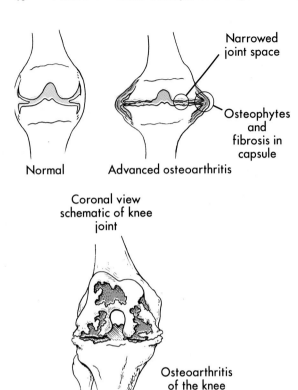

Narrowed
joint space

Osteophytes
and
fibrosis in
capsule

Normal   Advanced osteoarthritis

Coronal view
schematic of knee
joint

Osteoarthritis
of the knee
joint

FIG. 3-17 Advanced osteoarthritis of the knee. Joint space narrowing and osteophytic bone spurs. Vertical compressive loads may not be indicated with osteoarthritic lesions.

$9.0\% \pm 4.5\%$. In addition, two subjects improved in ambulation, no longer requiring the use of a cane. A hypothesis drawn from these findings suggests that increased force-generating capacity can be correlated to increased function.[29]

The previously outlined resistance exercise protocols (DeLorme, Oxford, and Knights DAPRE protocols) may be inappropriate for disabled elderly persons. However, modifications of these programs have provided some guidance in developing strength programs for elderly persons.[29] Frontera[24] states, "The isotonic resistance protocol that produced the greatest increases in force-generation capacity and attenuated atrophy to the greatest extent in older human muscle was three sets of eight repetitions of exercise performed at an intensity of 80% of a muscle's one RM, 3 days a week for 12 weeks."[24] Studies also support the need to closely monitor heart rate, blood pressure, respirations, and subtle signs of distress during any exercise program for elderly persons.[29]

As with any resistance program to elicit strength, intensity of effort is the key element in the magnitude of functional or morphologic change in muscle tissue.[9,24] In the elderly population, intensity of effort must take into account age, history of cardiovascular or pulmonary disease, history of orthopedic pathologic conditions, present disease states, osteoarthritis, and multiple medical conditions present.

THERAPEUTIC EXERCISE EQUIPMENT USED IN STRENGTH TRAINING

The most commonly used strength training tools are ankle or cuff weights. These extremely versatile pieces of equipment are easily adapted to many programs, body parts, and age groups. Theraband, surgical tubing, or latex rubber bands are popular, inexpensive, highly adaptable, very portable (for home use), and effective tools. They allow for diagonal patterns of resistance as well as those involving a single plane. Some manufacturers have added handles to ends of thick rubber cords to enhance the versatility of this equipment.

Dumbbells are also used extensively in physical therapy. Inexpensive, portable, and versatile, dumbbells can also be used to develop excellent ROM as well as unilateral or bilateral motions. Barbells can also be used, but are cumbersome; barbells are effective in sports medicine practices where young athletes need to develop overall strength and fitness, not usually in acute rehabilitation environments or hospital physical therapy departments.

Wall pulleys or cable column systems are also used in most rehabilitation departments. The amount of resistance used with pulleys can vary from a few to over 100 pounds. Cable columns are extremely useful for both upper extremity and lower extremity strength training and can be used for many age groups and conditions.

There are many commercially available isotonic exercise systems.* Generally, isotonic exercise machines are fairly adaptable, provide a wide range of resistance (from 5 to 500 pounds for some leg machines), and are mechanically adjustable to accommodate different body types. Individual pieces can be quite expensive ($3000 or more for a single leg press machine), and a full system may cost $20,000 or more. Various types of muscle contractions can be used with isotonic exercise machines, including concentric and eccentric contractions, isometric static holds, and unilateral or bilateral movements; these can be done over a wide degree of

---

*Some of the more common systems are the Universal, Paramount, Nautilus, Body Masters, and Cybex systems.

contraction velocities. As discussed previously, 1 RM testing can also be performed on isotonic systems.

Space availability is also a consideration when acquiring exercise equipment. While the "footprint" of many of these machines is small, a space of several hundred square feet to a few thousand feet may be needed for complete systems. Most of these systems use weight stacks, cables, straps, cams, and chains, but some use pneumatic (air), hydraulic, or electromagnetic resistance.

Isokinetic exercise systems are used extensively in physical therapy practices for testing, documentation, medico-legal presentations, rehabilitation, and velocity spectrum training. These systems are generally very expensive, with a single multijoint system costing $40,000 or more.*

These systems are extremely adaptable to most major body parts (knee, ankle, hip, wrist, elbow, shoulder, and back attachments are available with most systems), and therapeutically these systems are perhaps the most versatile of all strength training tools. Protocols and training modes that are generally available with most isokinetic systems are as follows:

Passive
    Continuous passive motion
    Active assistive range of motion
Isometric
    Multiangle isometrics
Isotonic
    Types of contraction modes:
        Concentric/eccentric
        Concentric/concentric
        Eccentric/concentric
        Eccentric/eccentric
Isokinetic
    Types of contraction modes:
        Concentric/eccentric
        Concentric/concentric
        Eccentric/concentric
        Eccentric/eccentric

Isokinetic systems typically function from 0 degrees per second to 350 to 400 degrees per second. These systems are designed to isolate, test, and rehabilitate single joints. Unfortunately it is very time consuming to change from one leg to another or from one joint (knee) to another (ankle). Their versatility is presented in Box 3-5.

The impulse inertial exercise apparatus is a system used for submaximal plyometric training. The impulse system provides limited ROM (by design), high-velocity, low-intensity, concentric, and eccentric load-

ing. The application of inertial exercise involves rapid, coordinated, cyclic, and dynamic motions with reduced loads or resistance. The impulse system can be used for upper and lower extremity exercise. Extremely adaptive components with various handles allow for the duplication of sports such as tennis, racquetball, and golf. Clinically, this system is used mainly for neuromuscular coordination and strength in limited degrees of motion. The clinical delivery of inertial exercise is shown in Box 3-6.[3]

BOX 3-5   Example of Knee Rehabilitation

PROTOCOL VERSATILITY USING ISOKINETIC TECHNOLOGY

To gain knee motion

Continuous passive motion (CPM).

To initiate muscle contractions

Use isometric mode. Progress to multiangle isometric—from 0° to 120° of knee motion at 20° increments.

To progress strength

Use isotonic modes. For example, knee extension (concentric)
Quads followed by knee flexion (eccentric)
Quads from 60°/sec to 180°/sec (5 sets: 60°, 90°, 120°, 150°, 180°).

Progress to

Isokinetics.
Knee extension (concentric)
Quads followed by concentric hamstrings velocity spectrum training: (8 sets: 30°, 60°, 90°, 120°, 150°, 180°, 210°, 240°).

BOX 3-6   Application for Inertial Training

Conditions

Submaximal plyometrics
Neuromuscular training
Training of tendon tissue
Alteration of electromechanical delay
Physiologic crossover effects

Indications

Painful arc remediation
Mechanical, reproducible joint pain
Capsular afference/coordination
Proposed prevention of bone loss

From Albert M: Eccentric muscle training in sports and orthopaedics, New York, 1991, Churchill Livingstone.

---

*Some common multijoint systems are the Cybex, Lido, Kin-Com, Biodex, Isotechnologies, and Ariel systems.

REFERENCES

1. Abraham WM: Exercise induced muscle soreness, *Phys Sports Med* 7:57, 1979.
2. Abraham WM: Factors in delayed muscle soreness, *Med Sci Sports Exer* 9:11, 1977.
3. Albert M: *Eccentric muscle training in sports and orthopaedics,* New York, 1991, Churchill Livingstone.
4. Belka D: Comparison of dynamic, static, and combination training on dominant wrist flexor muscles, *Res Exerc Sport* 39:244, 1968.
5. Berger RA: Optimum repetitions for the development of strength, *Res Q Exerc Sport* 33:334-338, 1962.
6. Brinkman JR et al: Rate and range of knee motion in ambulation, *Phys Ther* 62(5):632, 1982 (abstract).
7. Byrnes WC et al: Delayed onset muscle soreness following repeated bouts of downhill running, *J Appl Physiol* 59:7109, 1985.
8. Caplan A et al: Skeletal Muscle. In Woo SL-Y, Buckwalter J, editors: *Injury and repair of the musculoskeletal soft tissues,* Rosemont, Ill., 1988, American Academy of Orthopaedic Surgeons.
9. Charette SL et al: Muscle hypertrophy response to resistance training in older women, *J Appl Physiol* 70:1912-1916, 1991.
10. Chu DA: Rehabilitation of the lower extremity, *Clin Sports Med* 14(1):205-222, 1995.
11. Clarke HH et al: New objective strength tests of muscle groups by cable tension methods, *Res Quart* 23:136, 1952.
12. Clarke HH: Improvements of objective strength tests of muscle groups by cable tension methods, *Res Quart* 21:399, 1950.
13. Conroy BP, Earle RW: Bone, muscle and connective tissue adaptations to physical activity. In Baechle TR, editor: *Essentials of strength training and conditioning,* Champaign, Ill., 1994, Human Kinetics.
14. Davies GJ: *Open and closed kinetic chain exercises and their application to testing and rehabilitation:* Advances on the knee and shoulder, Cincinnati Sports Medicine and Orthopaedic Center, 1993, Course notes.
15. Davies, GJ: *A compendium of isokinetics in clinical usage and rehabilitation techniques,* ed 3, Onalaska, Wis., 1987, S & S Publishers.
16. DeLee J et al: Therapeutic exercise modalities. In Drez D, editor: *Therapeutic modalities for sports injuries: Amer Ortho Society Sports Med,* St. Louis, 1989, Mosby.
17. DeLorme TL, Watkins A: *Progressive resistance exercise,* New York, 1951, Appleton-Century.
18. Edgerton VR et al: Morphological basis of skeletal muscle power output. In Jones NL, McCartney N, McComas AJ, editors: *Human muscle power,* Champaign, Ill., 1986, Human Kinetics.
19. Elftman H: Biomechanics of muscle, *J Bone Joint Surg* 48:363, 1966.
20. Faulkner JA: New perspectives in training for maximum performance, *JAMA* 205:741-746, 1986.
21. Fiatarone MA et al: High intensity strength training in nonagenarians: effects on skeletal muscle, *JAMA* 263:3029-3034, 1990.
22. Francis KT: Delayed muscle soreness: a review *J Orthop Sports Phys Ther* 5:10, 1983.
23. Friden J, Sjostrom M, Ekblom B: Myofibrillar damage following intensive eccentric exercise in man, *Int J of Sport Med* 4:170-176, 1983.
24. Frontera WR et al: Strength conditioning in older men: skeletal muscle hypertrophy and improved function, *J Appl Physiol* 64:1038-1044, 1988.
25. Gollnick PD: Fiber number and size in overloaded chicken anterior latissimus dorsi muscle, *J Appl Physiol* 54:1292, 1983.
26. Gonyea W, Ericson GC, Bonde-Peterson F: Skeletal muscle fiber splitting induced by weight-lifting exercise in cats, *Acta Physiol Scand* 99:105-109, 1977.
27. Hakkinen K, Komi PV: Effect of different combined concentric and eccentric muscle work regimes on maximal strength development, *J Hum Mov Stud* 7:33, 1981.
28. Harman E: Strength and power: a definition of terms, *J NSCA* 15(6):18-20, 1993.
29. Hopp JF: Effects of age and resistance training on skeletal muscle: a review, *Phys Ther* 73(6):361-373, 1993.
30. Jzankoff SP, Norris AH: Effect of muscle mass decreases on age-related BMR changes, *J Appl Physiol* 43:1001-1006, 1977.
31. Kellis E, Baltzopoulos V: Isokinetic eccentric exercise, *Sports Med* 19(3):202-222, 1995.
32. Klitgaard H et al: Function, morphology and protein expression of aging skeletal muscle: a cross-sectional study of elderly men with different training backgrounds, *Acta Physiol Scand Suppl* 140:41-54, 1990.
33. Knapik JJ et al: Angular specificity and test mode specificity of isometric and isokinetic strength training, *J Orthop Sports Phys Ther 5(2)58-65,* 1983.
34. Knight KL: Quadriceps strengthening with the DAPRE technique: case studies with neurological implications, *Med Sci Sport Exerc* 17(6):646-650, 1985.
35. Knuttgen H, Kramer W: Terminology and measurement in exercise performance, *J Appl Sports Sci Res* 1:1-10, 1987.
36. Kuta I, Parizkova J, Dycka J: Muscle strength and lean body mass in old men of different physical activity, *J Appl Physiol* 29:168-171, 1970.
37. Mangine R, Heckman TP, Eldridge VL: Improving strength, endurance and power. In Scully RM, Barnes, MR, editors: *Physical therapy,* Philadelphia, 1989, JB Lippincott.
38. McAllister RM, Amann JF, Laughlin MH: Skeletal muscle fiber types and their vascular support, *J Reconstruc Microsurg* 9(4):313-7, 1993.
39. McCartney N et al: Long-term resistance training in the elderly: effects on dynamic strength, exercise capacity, muscle, and bone, *J Gerontol Appl Biol Sci Med Sci* 50(2):97-104, 1995.

40. Miles MP, Clarkson PM: Exercise-induced muscle pain, soreness, and cramps, *J Sports Med Phys Fitness* 34(3) 203-216, 1994.

41. Newham DJ et al: Ultrastructural changes after concentric and eccentric contractions of human muscle, *J Neuro Sci* 61:109-122, 1983.

42. Newham DJ et al: Pain and fatigue after concentric and eccentric muscle contractions, *Clin Sci* 64:55, 1983.

43. Norkin CC, Levangie PK: *Joint Structure and function: a comprehensive analysis*, ed 2, 1992, FA Davis.

44. Nyland J et al: Review of the afferent neural system of the knee and its contribution to motor learning, *J Ortho Sports Phys Ther* 19(1):2-11, 1994.

45. Page P: Pathophysiology of acute exercise induced muscular injury: clinical implications, *J Ath Train,* 30(1):29-34, 1995.

46. Palmieri G: Weight training and repetition speed, *J Appl Sport Sci Res* 1(2):36-38, 1987.

47. Rothstein JM, Lamb RL, Mayhew TP: Clinical uses of isokinetic measurements: critical issues, *Phys Ther* 67:1840, 1988.

48. Schwane J et al: Blood markers of delayed onset muscle soreness with downhill treadmill running, *Med Sci Sports Exer* 13:80, 1981.

49. Smith LL et al: Impact of a repeated bout of eccentric exercise on muscular strength, muscle soreness and creatine kinase, *Br J Sports Med* 28(4):267-271, 1994.

50. Soderberg G: *Kinesiology: application to pathological motion,* Biltmore, Md., 1986, Williams & Wilkins.

51. Stauber WT: Eccentric action of muscles: physiology, injury and adaptation, *Exerc Sport Sci Rev* 19:157, 1989.

52. Steadman JR: Rehabilitation of athletic injury, *Am J Sports Med* 7:147, 1979.

53. Stone M: Literature review: explosive exercise and training, *NSCA J* 15(3):6-19, 1993.

54. Stone MH et al: Periodization, *NSCA J* Part I reprinted 15(1): 1993.

55. Talag TS: Residual muscular soreness as influenced by concentric, eccentric and static contractions, *Res Q Exerc Sport* 44:458, 1973.

56. Talmadge RJ, Roy RR, Edgerton VR: Muscle fiber types and function, *Curr Opin Rheumatol* 5(6):695-705, 1993.

57. Thompson LV: Aging muscle: characteristics and strength training, *Issues on Aging* 18(1)25-30, 1995.

58. Waltrous B, Armstrong R, Schwane J: The role of lactic acid in delayed onset muscular distress, *Med Sci Sports Exer* 13:80, 1981.

59. *Webster's new collegiate dictionary,* Springfield, Mass., 1981, G & C Merriam Co.

60. Wilk KE et al: Stretch-shortening drills for the upper extremities: theory and clinical application, *J Ortho Sports Phys Ther* 17(5):225-239, 1993.

61. Wyatt MP, Edwards AM: Comparison of quadriceps and hamstring torque values during isokinetic exercise, *J Orthop Sports Phys Ther* 3(2):48-56, 1981.

62. Zinowieff AN: Heavy resistance exercise: the oxford technique, *Br J Phys Med* 14:129, 1951.

Endurance

Endurance activities can be classified as either those affecting the muscular system or those affecting the cardiovascular system. During endurance exercises the body relies on aerobic activity, which involves those metabolic pathways that use oxygen to provide energy for muscle contractions.[14,24] Aerobic metabolism takes place in structures called mitochondria. In this metabolic process the breakdown of protein, fats, and carbohydrates forms energy-rich adenosine triphosphate (ATP), a process known as oxidative phosphorylation.[14,24] This aerobic energy system (oxidative capacity) can produce approximately 19 times the ATP produced by the anaerobic adenosine triphosphate-phosphocreatine (ATP-PC) energy system.[15,24]

The degree of aerobic fitness, or the ability to do work (see definition of work in Chapter 3), one possesses is expressed as **aerobic capacity, cardiovascular endurance,** cardiovascular fitness, or cardiorespiratory fitness. The efficiency of the aerobic system is measured by the maximum volume of oxygen consumed during exercise, termed **maximal oxygen uptake (Vo_2 max).**[14,24] Activities that stress long-duration, low-intensity exercise enhance aerobic fitness. The main rationale for aerobic conditioning is to improve the body's aerobic capacity. Researchers have established guidelines for prescribing aerobic exercise for untrained, moderately trained, trained, and highly trained individuals (Box 4-1).[8,21] In general, long-term aerobic training can improve aerobic fitness approximately 10% to 20%.[1,2]

BOX 4-1 Exercise Prescription Recommendations for Untrained, Moderately Trained, Trained, and Highly Trained Individuals

Frequency

3-5 days per week for untrained to moderately trained; 5-7 days per week for highly trained

Intensity

60% to 90% of maximum heart rate (MHR)—Untrained, 60%; Highly trained, 90%

Duration

15 to 60 minutes or more (continuous)

ADAPTIVE PHYSIOLOGIC CHANGES WITH AEROBIC EXERCISE

The most notable changes in the oxygen transport system after long-term aerobic exercise training are as follows:[3,12,24]

- Increased size and number of mitochondria
- Increased myoglobin content
- Improved mobilization and use of fat and carbohydrates
- Selective hypertrophy of type I slow-twitch oxidative muscle fibers
- Decreased resting heart rate and submaximal heart rate
- Increased blood volume and hemoglobin
- Reduced systolic and diastolic blood pressure
- Significantly improved oxygen extraction rates from the blood

MEASURING AND PRESCRIBING AEROBIC EXERCISE

Perhaps the most clinically relevant and practical way to prescribe aerobic fitness programs for healthy adults (those without chronic or unstable complicated medical conditions) involves the **age-adjusted maximum heart rate (AAMHR).** The American College of Sports Medicine (ACSM)[22] defines the minimal training intensity threshold for improved Vo_2 max as approximately 60% of the maximum heart rate (MHR). An individual's MHR is determined by the following equation:

$$220 - Age = MHR$$

The recommended intensity level (ACSM)[22] range is 60% to 90% of MHR. The individual's target or training heart rate (THR) is established as follows:

$$THR = MHR \times Intensity\ level\ range\ (60\%\ to\ 90\%)$$

For example, if the MHR is 180, THR = 180 × 70% (.70) = 126 or 180 × 80% (.80) = 144.

Another method for establishing a THR is with the **Karvonen formula.** The training intensity range for this formula is 50% to 85% of Vo_2 max. The Karvonen method uses the difference between the MHR and the resting heart rate (RHR), which is called the maximum heart rate reserve (MHR reserve). The following are examples of the Karvonen formula:

$$MHR\ (in\ beats\ per\ minute) = 180$$

$$RHR = 180 - 60 = 120$$

$$Intensity\ level = 70\%$$

$$120 \times .70 = 84$$

$$RHR = 60$$

$$RHR + Intensity\ level = Maximum\ training\ heart\ rate$$

$$60 + 84 = 144$$

BOX 4-2 . Borg Scale of Relative Perceived Exertion

6
7 Very, very light
8
9 Very light
10
11
12
13 Somewhat hard
14
15 Hard
16
17 Very hard
18
19 Very, very hard

The range of intensity using the Karvonen method is expressed as follows:

$$\text{Low THR} = (50\% - \text{MHR reserve}) + \text{RHR}$$

$$\text{High THR} = (85\% - \text{MHR reserve}) + \text{RHR}$$

Clinically, the intensity of exercise can be monitored using a subjective estimate of exercise stress. The relative perceived exertion scale is used to prescribe exercise intensity based on an individual's perception of exertion. The classic **Borg Scale**[4] is used to describe perceived exertion (Box 4-2).

The **frequency, intensity, duration,** and mode of activity recommended by the ACSM[22] are as follows:

Frequency of training: 3 to 5 days per week
Intensity of training: 60% to 90% of age-adjusted MHR or 50% to 85% of MHR
Duration of training: 20 to 60 minutes of continuous aerobic activity

The mode of activity is any activity that uses large muscle groups, can be maintained continuously, and is rhythmic and aerobic. Examples include walking, bicycling, jogging, stairclimbing, rowing, and swimming.

When initiating or intensifying an aerobic conditioning program with any patient, it is important to recognize that greater levels of intensity have been associated with higher cardiovascular risk,[23] increased rates of orthopedic injury[19,20] and reduced compliance with exercise as compared with lower levels of intensity.[7,19]

METHODS OF AEROBIC TRAINING

Aerobic conditioning programs are either continuous or discontinuous. **Continuous aerobic activities** provide no rest interval during the entire bout of exercise, and generally little variation in heart rate occurs. Examples of continuous activities are jogging, walking, running,

cycling, and stairclimbing. As with all forms of exercise, the benefits obtained are specific to the type, quality, and quantity of exercise undertaken.

For clinical puposes, stationary bicycle ergometers and treadmills are commonly used (Fig. 4-1). Continuous

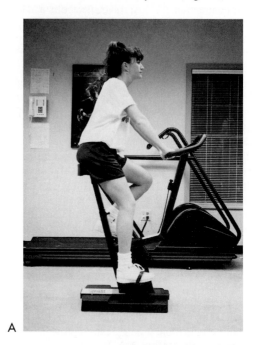

A

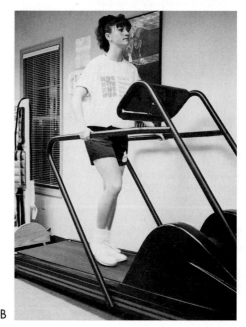

B

FIG. 4-1 A, Seated stationary bicycle ergometer. **B,** Standard treadmill.

aerobic activities that use more muscles burn more calories and consume more oxygen than continuous activities that use fewer muscles. For example, jogging on a treadmill burns more calories and uses more muscle than pedaling a seated bicycle ergometer.

Discontinuous aerobic activities are also called interval training activities. They can involve the same activities as continuous aerobic programs, but in interval training, repeated exercise bouts are interspersed with rest intervals. One advantage of interval training over continuous aerobic activities is that interval training provides large amounts of high-intensity work in a relatively short amount of time. However, interval training tends to develop strength and power more than endurance.[5]

Adjusting the ratio of work (aerobic) to rest (recovery) is the foundation of interval training.[14] For aerobic fitness, a work-to-rest ratio of 1:1 or 1:1.5 is advised. The rest or recovery interval can be passive (total rest) or active (active recovery). Active recovery involves reducing the intensity of work, which allows the individual to continue the activity for long periods of time. It is most appropriate for stressing the aerobic metabolic pathways and minimizing the capacity to develop strength and power using high-intensity interval training.

ORTHOPEDIC CONSIDERATIONS DURING AEROBIC EXERCISE

The use of endurance activities for orthopedic patients is challenging. Acute injury or surgery requires a period of rest so that the injured part can heal properly.

After a back injury, aerobic endurance activities are essential.[26] However, sitting on the saddle seat of a stationary ergometer may not be appropriate for many patients with back problems. A recumbent cycle has a large bucket car seat (Fig. 4-2) to provide lumbar support so that the patient can comfortably perform the aerobic exercise. In some cases, back patients may tolerate treadmill activities more than seated aerobic activities. If treadmill walking is not tolerated, an underwater treadmill can provide enough buoyancy during walking to allow patients to do aerobic activity (Fig. 4-3).

Patients having a lower extremity injury or surgery can maintain or improve cardiorespiratory fitness using an upper body ergometer (UBE) (Fig. 4-4). This is an effective tool for continuous or interval training when patients cannot perform lower body endurance activities. Older patients with hip, knee, or ankle osteoarthritis (degenerative joint disease) may not tolerate the vertical compressive loads developed during treadmill walking,

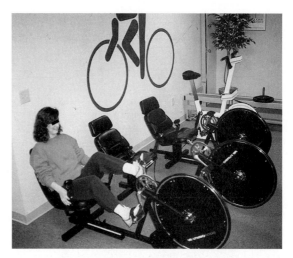

FIG. 4-2 Recumbent bicycle ergometer. Large bucket seat used in a recumbent position may allow some patients to tolerate seated aerobic activities.

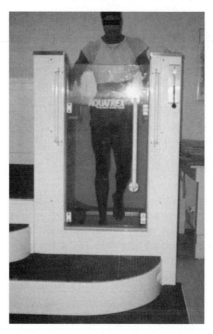

FIG. 4-3 Underwater treadmill. The buoyancy of the water may allow early vertical loading and the initiation of normalized gait mechanics.

stairclimbing, or even stationary cycling; therefore, a UBE may provide an effective aerobic activity for these individuals. Patients who have a lower extremity injury can be instructed in how to do a single-leg stationary bicycle ergometer exercise (Fig. 4-5).

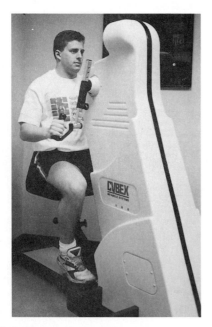

FIG. 4-4 For patients with lower extremity injuries, an upper body ergometer (UBE) will allow for continued aerobic activities during periods of immobilization.

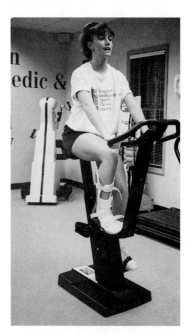

FIG. 4-5 In some cases, a single-leg stationary cycle ergometer can be used for cardiovascular fitness during periods of immobilization.

Patients with upper extremity conditions can use a stationary cycle or treadmill for endurance training. Patients can also be instructed to use one-arm cycling on a UBE (Fig. 4-6) to maintain upper-body aerobic fitness.

Many throwing athletes and industrial workers require specific aerobic fitness, strength, and power in their shoulders and arms. During recovery after injury or surgery to the shoulder, elbow, arm, or hand, the patient can maintain a certain level of specific fitness by using a one-arm aerobic activity.

Modifications can be made on stationary cycles to allow for continued aerobic conditioning after an ankle injury or surgery. Typically, the seat height should allow for slight knee flexion (approximately 10 degrees) at the end of the pedal stroke. With the seat in normal position, the foot generally plantar flexes toward the end of the pedal stroke, causing stress to the anterior talofibular ligament. Therefore, with a severe ankle sprain, the seat height is lowered to allow for a complete pedal stroke and to keep the ankle joint in neutral (Fig. 4-7).

Stairclimbing, seated rowing, and cross country ski machines are popular aerobic tools, but must be used judiciously. Stairclimbers require the patient to be correctly positioned vertically and maintain balance (holding the handrails) to perform the exercise the right way. Therefore stairclimbers are difficult for many patients in

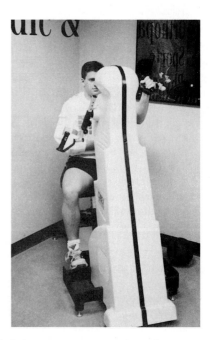

FIG. 4-6 A one-arm, upper body cycling activity with a UBE is also an effective aerobic exercise activity.

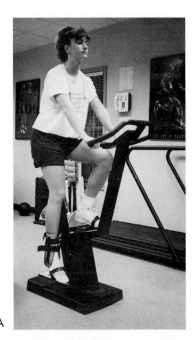

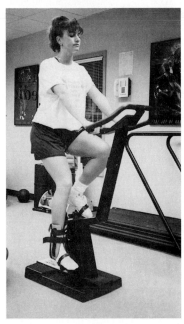

FIG. 4-7 A, Normal seat elevation for the performance of a seated bicycle ergometer allows for greater plantar flexion motion. Plantar flexion may be contraindicated with acute and subacute sprains of the lateral ligament complex of the ankle. **B,** With the saddle seat lowered, the affected ankle can be maintained in a more appropriate neutral position during periods of aerobic activity on the cycle ergometer.

the acute or immediate postorthopedic surgery period to use. Rowing machines require both a pulling motion with the arms and hip and knee flexion and extension. These simultaneous motions make modifications for use with specific orthopedic problems quite difficult. Cross-country ski machines require bilateral, reciprocal leg and arm motions and are also difficult to modify for orthopedic patients with acute disorders. However, stair-climbers, rowing machines, and cross-country ski machines can be effective tools in aerobic conditioning programs after the acute phase of recovery from injury or surgery.

MUSCLE FATIGUE AND LOCAL MUSCULAR ENDURANCE

Two hypotheses attempt to clarify peripheral neuromuscular fatigue as a result of prolonged or strenuous muscle activity.[9,16] One states that **muscle fatigue** results from decreasing amounts of the energy substrates ATP, glycogen, and phosphocreatine. The other states that muscle fatigue occurs when noxious metabolites (hydrogen ions and ammonia) accumulate. Either of these events may occur as a result of high-intensity or prolonged muscular effort.

Being able to perform repeated submaximal bouts of physical activity is a vital and critical component of recovery after injury or surgery.[26]

Circuit training is, in effect, a combination of resistance exercise and aerobic exercise. Its goal is to improve **local muscular endurance,** cardiorespiratory fitness, and muscular strength. The intensity of **circuit training** directly affects the specific adaptations desired. Intensity can be increased by decreasing the amount of time allowed to perform the exercise, by keeping the time constant but increasing the repetitions or sets of desired exercise, or by decreasing the time allowed for rest between exercises.

Generally a circuit may contain 12 to 15 exercise stations offering various levels of resistance. Typically the resistance is 40% to 50% of the predetermined 1 RM (maximum repetition). The patient performs each exercise in sequence.

The two types of circuits are fixed load circuits and target circuits.[25] In a fixed load circuit, the load or resistance remains constant. Improved fitness occurs as the individual completes the circuit in less time. In a target circuit, the time required to complete the program is constant, and the individual is required to complete as many repetitions as possible during the prescribed time. Generally, the exercises are performed in 15-second to 20-second bouts in a nonstop sequence. Another way to structure a target circuit is to perform each exercise in 30-second sets with a short 15-second rest between sets.

An important metabolic adaptation that occurs with muscular endurance exercise is a significant increase in oxidative enzyme levels. High-volume aerobic exercise increases the oxidative enzymes succinate dehydrogenase (SDH) and malate dehydrogenase (MDH).[6,11]

COMBINING ENDURANCE AND STRENGTH TRAINING

Recovering from orthopedic trauma or disease frequently involves rehabilitation programs that stress endurance, strength, and flexibility. Strength may be inhibited to some degree during simultaneous endurance training[10] because of the intensity of each program.[13,18] If the major goal of training is to improve strength, a program of strength training should be combined with a moderate, long-duration endurance program. Conversely, if the rehabilitation goal is to primarily improve endurance, then a program of strength and high-intensity interval training should be used.[10,18]

The adaptations to specific training modes are highly selective and related to the metabolic pathways stressed and the muscle groups used as well as the intensity of the prescribed programs. Modest gains in both strength and endurance can occur during combined programs.[17] The key of the therapeutic exercise program is to emphasize the intensity of the specific mode of training to obtain the desired physiologic adaptation.

REFERENCES

1. Astrand PO, Rodahl K: *Textbook of work physiology,* ed 2, New York, 1977, McGraw-Hill.
2. Astrand PO: Physical performance as a function of age, *JAMA* 205:105-109, 1968.
3. Barnard RJ et al: Effects of exercise of skeletal muscle. I. Biochemical and histochemical properties, *J Appl Physiol* 28:762, 1970.
4. Borg GAV: Psychophysical bases of perceived exertion, *Med Sci Sports Exerc* 14:377, 1982.
5. Burnett CN: Principles of aerobic exercise. In Kisner C, Colby LA, editors: *Therapeutic exercise: foundations and techniques,* ed 2, Philadelphia, 1990 FA Davis.
6. Costill DL et al: Adaptation in skeletal muscle following strength training, *J Appl Physiol,* 46:96-99, 1979.
7. Dishman RK, Sallis J, Orenstein D: The determinants of physical activity and exercise, *Public Health Rep* 100:158-180, 1985.
8. Fardy PS: Training for aerobic power. In Burke E, editor: *Toward an understanding of human performance,* New York, 1977, Movement Publications.
9. Fitts RH, Metzger JM: Mechanisms of muscular fatigue. In Poortmans JR, editor: Principle of exercise biochemistry, *Med Sport Sci* 27:212-229, 1988.
10. Hickson RC: Interference of strength development by simultaneous training for strength and endurance, *Eur J Appl Physiol* 45:255-263, 1980.
11. Holloszy JO: Biochemical adaptations to exercise: aerobic metabolism, *Exerc Sport Sci Rev* 1:45-71, 1973.
12. Kiessling K: Effects of physical training on ultra structural features in human skeletal muscle. In Pernow B, Saltin B, editors: *Muscle metabolism during exercise,* New York, 1971, Plenum Press.
13. Kraemer WJ et al: Compatability of high-intensity and endurance training on hormonal and skeletal muscle adaptations, *J Appl Physiol* 78(3):976-989, 1995.
14. Kraemer WJ: General adaptations to resistance and endurance training programs. In Baechle TR editor: *Essentials of strength training and conditioning,* 1994, Human Kinetics Books.
15. Lamb DR: *Physiology of exercise: responses and adaptations,* Indianapolis, 1978, MacMillan.
16. Maclaren DPM et al: A review of metabolic and physiological factors in fatigue, *Exerc Sport Sci Rev* 17:29-66, 1989.
17. McCarthy JP et al: Compatability of adaptive responses with combining strength and endurance training, *Med Sci Sports Exerc* 27(3):429-436, 1995.
18. Nelson AG et al: Consequences of combining strength and endurance regimens, *Phys Ther* 70(5): 287-294, 1990.
19. Pollock ML: Prescribing exercise for fitness and adherence. In Dishman RK, editor: *Exercise adherence: its impact on public health,* Champaign, Ill., 1988, Human Kinetics Books.
20. Pollock ML, Wilmore JH: *Exercise in health and disease: evaluation and prescription for prevention and rehabilitation,* ed 2, Philadelphia, 1990, WB Saunders.
21. Pollock ML, Wilmore JH, Fox III SM: *Health and fitness through physical activity,* New York, 1978, John Wiley & Sons.
22. The recommended quantity and quality of exercise for developing and maintaining cardiorespiratory and muscular fitness in healthy adults. Position stand, Indianapolis, 1990, American College of Sports Medicine.
23. Siscovick DS et al: The incidence of primary cardiac arrest during vigorous exercise, *N Engl J Med* 311:874-877, 1984.
24. Stone MH, Conley MS: Bioenergetics. In Baechle TR editor: *Essentials of strength training and conditioning,* Champaign, Ill., 1994, Human Kinetics Books.
25. Totten L: General physical training for the weightlifter. In *United states weightlifting federation coaching manual,* vol 2, Colorado Springs, 1986, United States Weightlifting Federation.
26. Trafimow JH et al: The effects of quadriceps fatigue on the technique of lifting, *Spine* 18(3):364-367, 1993.

Balance and Coordination

EXERCISE IN ORTHOPEDIC DISORDERS

Rehabilitation after an acute injury, surgery, immobilization, or a chronic orthopedic condition must address all the components of normal function. Regaining lost strength, reducing pain and swelling, improving flexibility, enhancing local muscular endurance, and building cardiovascular fitness are obvious and vital areas requiring specific therapeutic interventions. Optimal recovery from orthopedic injury requires normalized sequencing and patterns of movement that produce synchronous, fluid, and stable motor function.

The interdependence of gait, posture, and coordinated functional movements must be restored for complete recovery from injury. Long-term convalescence reduces strength, flexibility, and cardiorespiratory fitness, as well as the vestibular and afferent neural input needed for balance and coordination.

DEFINITION OF BALANCE AND COORDINATION

Balance is "the ability to maintain equilibrium; that is, it is the ability to maintain the center of body mass over the base of support."[6] *Static balance* refers to the ability to maintain posture during nonmovement activities,[10] whereas *dynamic balance* relates to the ability to maintain body mass over the base of support while the body is in motion.[6,10] Balance is one component of **coordination,**[6] which is the ability to perform fine motor skills, tasks requiring postural control, and reciprocal motions, such as walking and performing functional activities.[6]

Terms related to balance and coordination are *position sense, kinesthesia* or *kinesthetic sense,* and *proprioception.* Brunnstrom[4] classifies position sense as static balance or "awareness of static position." **Kinesthesia** deals with sensory receptor signals from muscle, tendons, and joints, and relates to an awareness of joint motion.[4] **Proprioception** is the function of joint receptors (sensory and mechanoreceptors) to deliver input concerning joint position, movement, direction, speed, and amplitude.[4]

The mechanoreceptor system

In addition to muscle spindles and Golgi tendon organs, joints are innervated with various types of specific mechanoreceptors that provide the central nervous system with information concerning **joint displacement, velocity and amplitude of joint motion, pressure,** and **stretch and pain.** Four types of mechanoreceptors have been classified.[8,17] Type I mechanoreceptors, or **ruffini mechanoreceptors,** respond slowly to static joint position.[17] **Pacinian mechanoreceptors,** type II, adapt very

quickly to changes in joint position. These highly sensitive receptors detect ligament tension and velocity of motion.[13] Type III mechanoreceptors are active at "extremes of joint motion, such as motions that produce joint injury."[12] **Free nerve endings** are type IV mechanoreceptors and transmit information related to pain and inflammation.[12]

The mechanoreceptor feedback system (**afferent neural input**) is vital in regulating adaptive changes related to joint movement and body position.[9]

Balance and coordination tests

To prescribe appropriate balance and coordination exercises, it is essential to have data related to present balance and coordination status. Various simple, clinically applicable coordination tests are used to assess a patient's ability to replicate accurate reciprocal motions. Box 5-1 outlines common coordination tests.

Interestingly, balance tests and specific balance treatment activities are rarely separated, with the same movements used for fundamental balance exercises and clinically relevant balance tests. The double-leg stance

BOX 5-1 Coordination Tests	
Finger to nose:	A reciprocal motion test in which the patient touches the tip of the index finger to the tip of the nose.
Finger opposition:	A reciprocal motion test in which the patient alternately touches the tip of each finger with the tip of the thumb.
Fixation-position hold:	A static position test in which the arms are held horizontal or the knees extended.
Pronation-supination:	A reciprocal motion test in which the palms are rotated up and down.
Tapping foot or hand:	A reciprocal motion test in which the patient is asked to repeatedly tap the ball of one foot while keeping the heal in contact with the floor. With the hand, the patient is asked to tap his hand on his knee.
Heel on shin:	A reciprocal motion and accuracy test. in which the patient is supine and is asked to slide the heel of one leg from the ankle to the knee of the opposite leg.
Throwing / catching a ball:	A reciprocal motion test in which the patient is asked to receive and deliver a ball.

test (DLST), for example, is a static test first performed with the eyes open. The amount of postural sway and the amount of time the patient can maintain static equilibrium are recorded. This very simple test is made more challenging by having the patient maintain balance on both legs with his or her eyes closed. Obviously, this test can easily be used as a static balance training drill, with visual, vestibular, and proprioceptive afferent neural input all contributing to the maintenance of balance.[5] Balance tests frequently call for a progressive battery of specific tasks of incremental difficulty that attempt to eliminate visual input.

Another progressive test also used as an exercise is the single-leg stance test (SLST) (Fig. 5-1). Functionally, this test is perhaps more practical to administer because walking, turning, climbing stairs, etc., all have components of single-leg standing. To master single-leg stance equilibrium, progressive training is needed. The SLST can be made more difficult by asking the patient to close his or her eyes while documenting the degree of postural sway and the amount of time equilibrium is maintained, then providing a manual external force to stimulate a quick-balance response.

Another balance test is tandem walking (straight line, heel-to-toe sequencing). This test is graded in distance (feet). The patient is asked to maintain equilibrium for a prescribed distance while walking heel-to-toe, first with the eyes open, then with the eyes closed. In the foam test, the patient is asked to maintain equilibrium while standing on unstable foam padding. First, high-density padding is used to provide a relatively stable, unyielding surface. Then the surface is progressively changed until it is a low-density, unstable foam padding, creating a task demanding a high level of balance.

A very critical component of all balance tests and training activities is close observation of the patient's protective reactions during loss of balance. Immediate corrective action by the patient to maintain balance is needed to move the patient from low-level balance activities to more challenging, complex maneuvers.

Automatic activities, such as catching a ball, can be performed in sequence from a seated position to a standing position. The velocity, angle, and direction of throwing the ball to the patient challenge the patient's ability to rapidly move arms and trunk out of a static balance state, then back to equilibrium.

Other tests use pulley systems and sophisticated computerized machinery. Wolfson et al[16] designed the postural stress test (PST) to help quantify static balance. This test measures a patient's ability to maintain balance during a series of progressive "graded destabilizing forces."[5] It is clinically cumbersome in that it involves applying a belt to the patient's waist and attaching a weight-pulley system behind the patient. Without the patient's knowledge, a weight is applied to the pulley system, which provides a sudden posterior force necessitating rapid correction of the postural interference. The test is graded on a scale from 0 to 9, with 0 representing a total inability to correct balance, while 9 represents no loss of balance. Sophisticated computer systems such as NeuroCom's Balance Master (Clackamas, Oregon) manipulate visual, vestibular, and proprioceptive input, specifically, by grading postural sway as the patient stands on a force plate.

The reach test (Fig. 5-2) is a very practical and functional test that determines a patient's ability to perform simple daily tasks. The test can be performed with the patient seated or standing. The patient is offered a target that is slightly out of reach to test the diagonal component of reaching.

Dynamic balance tests require the patient to maintain a base of support, to negotiate a single plane or multidirectional movement, and to keep the body in motion. Walking in a straight line for a prescribed functional distance (i.e., from a chair to the bathroom) is a simple test to administer. Adding directional changes, like turning a corner or negotiating a random series of obstacles, provides information concerning the patient's dynamic balance.

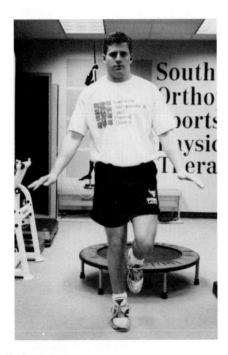

FIG. 5-1 Single-leg stance test.

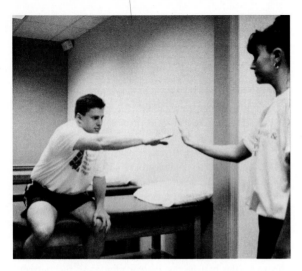

FIG. 5-2 Seated reach test. The clinician offers the patient a target to reach for, which tests the patient's margin of support while seated.

Functional balance training in orthopedics

In concert with regaining strength and motion, specific functional tasks must be incorporated into the rehabilitation plan to accentuate muscular coordination, equilibrium, and dynamic stability. Progressive static and dynamic balance exercises exploit the proprioceptive-afferent neural input system to improve static and dynamic task-specific equilibrium. Duncan* has identified several factors that may significantly contribute to balance dysfunction:

   a. Perception
   b. Behavior
   c. Range of motion
   d. Biomechanical alignment
   e. Weakness
   f. Sensory
   g. Synergistic organization strategy
   h. Coordination
   i. Adaptability

Many unique studies[1-3,7,11] have demonstrated how injury, surgery, immobilization, and rehabilitation programs without specific proprioceptive training can have a profound negative effect on joint receptors. One study shows that patients with anterior cruciate ligament injuries suffer from a significantly lower perception of joint position compared with healthy subjects.[2] Other studies report that patients complain of perceived joint instabil-

---

*From Duncan PW: Balance dysfunction: Implications for geriatric and neurological rehabilitation, Course Notes, Nov. 1994, Advanced Educational Seminars, Inc.

ity, weakness, and specific fatigue after rehabilitation programs devoid of balance training.[1,3,11]

It can be concluded from these studies that the physical therapist assistant must clearly recognize that injury, surgery, and nonweight bearing immobilization negatively affect the proprioceptive feedback system, and that when balance training to improve proprioception is neglected, function is affected and reinjury is likely. Therefore functional balance and coordination training combined with closed kinetic chain (CKC) resistive exercises allows for afferent neural input from peripheral joint mechanoreceptors, which may enhance the perception of joint stability, joint position, and proprioception.

Specific balance tasks in orthopedics

In cases of lower extremity injury with long-term, bed-bound convalescence, manual resistive hip and knee extension may be appropriate to initiate CKC proprioceptive feedback. Progressive balance training is initiated by vertical weight bearing (double-leg standing) or by seated weight bearing. For proper gait mechanics, weight shifting (changing base of support from one leg to another) is critical.

After the patient masters double-leg standing static balance, the physical therapist assistant should begin training the patient to shift balance from one leg to the other. Progressing along an increasingly difficult sequence, the patient can begin single-leg static balance training. Generally, the length of time the patient can maintain equilibrium on one leg is recorded. As balance and strength improve, the time the patient is able to maintain equilibrium increases.

Because considerable perceptual awareness is gained by visual input, progressive balance training involves eliminating this sensory input system. Single-leg standing with eyes closed is a challenging task. Progressively more difficult tasks can be initiated in which the clinician applies sudden force to the patient while the patient is standing on one leg with the eyes closed (Fig. 5-3). For teaching and safety purposes, all balance drills should be initiated on the uninvolved limb. As confidence and motor learning progress, the patient then performs the balance activity on the involved limb. In all cases of balance training, manual support is provided as required.

Static balance drills can be initiated with the patient seated. Similar progressive sequencing can be used, with the patient first attempting to maintain balance with the eyes open, then with the eyes closed. Manually applied external force can be applied while the patient's eyes are closed. Standing or seated, manual postural stress applied in different directions and with varying degrees of

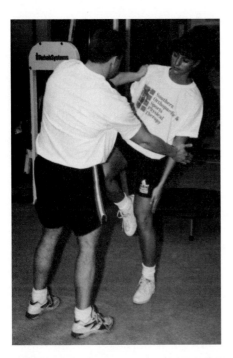

FIG. 5-3 To test and challenge a patient's protective reactions, the clinician can apply a sudden external force while the patient's eyes are closed. Close protection and support must be provided by the clinician during this activity.

BOX 5-2	Progressive Balancing Exercises
Seated:	Eyes open, eyes closed, manually applied postural stress. Throwing and catching a ball.
Seated:	Uneven surface, physioball (swissball). Eyes open, eyes closed.
Standing:	Double leg standing—eyes open, eyes closed, manually applied postural stress, weight shifting. Single leg standing—eyes open, eyes closed, postural stress.
Surface changes:	All standing drills can be advanced by changing the inclination and type of surface: • Concrete • Carpet (short dense, thick) • Asphalt • Tile (slick), linoleum • Grass, loose gravel, dirt
Minitrampoline:	Double leg standing—eyes open, eyes closed, hopping. Single leg standing—eyes open, eyes closed, hopping.
Foam padding:	Double and single leg standing, ambulation, eyes open, eyes closed.
Balancing devices:	BAPS board, KAT, balance board, seated position, standing position, double-leg and single-leg standing—eyes open, eyes closed.

force can enhance the patient's ability to "right" or correct balance. Box 5-2 describes various static and dynamic balance activities.

Dynamic balance activities involve progressively challenging tasks that stimulate the patient's ability to safely and accurately negotiate obstacles and make multidirectional changes while in motion. Forward and backward gait, sidestepping (lateral steps), and braiding steps (carioca) are examples of dynamic gait exercises.

Other functional CKC proprioceptive exercises can replicate the specific demands of daily activities or athletic skills. Frequently, progressively demanding tasks are omitted from rehabilitation programs, with reliance put on increased clinical strength tests, greater range-of-motion grades, and reduced pain and swelling, as objective data leading to discharge from formal therapy. Functional balance drills, such as hopping, increase muscle strength, power, coordination, and balance. Hopping drills can be rather simple vertical leaps or quite challenging combinations of vertical and horizontal patterns. Hopping is useful with an athletic population and can be done on a flat, hard surface or on a **minitrampoline** (Fig. 5-4).

Using the minitrampoline after hip, knee, or ankle injury for static standing balance and for dynamic single-leg or double-leg hopping is unique and challenging for many patients. As with other balance drills, single-leg or double-leg standing or hopping can progress from eyes open to eyes closed. The forgiving, uneven rebound surface of the minitrampoline adds an appropriate challenge for progressive balance training.

Various training devices have been developed to assist with proprioceptive training, including the **biomechanical ankle platform system (BAPS).** The name is misleading because this unit can be used for a wide variety of lower extremity conditions. The generic names for this tool are **wobble board** and balance board (Fig. 5-5). This device is very adaptable, portable, and affordable for many physical therapy environments. Initially, double-leg support progresses to single-leg standing. One of the most challenging balance drills is to perform single-leg standing on a balance board with the eyes closed.

Another device used for balance training is the **kinesthetic ability training device (KAT)** (Breg, Vista, Cal.). This tool is similar to the BAPS board or balance boards. The KAT is unique (Fig. 5-6) in that an air-filled

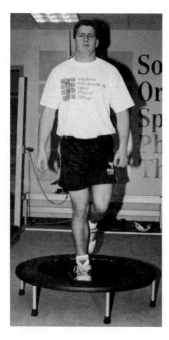

FIG. 5-4 A minitrampoline provides a unique, challenging, and "forgiving" surface to encourage balance and proprioception while hopping or standing.

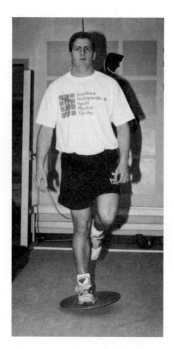

FIG. 5-5 A wobble board or BAPS (biomechanical ankle platform system) board can be used to challenge single or double leg proprioception and balance.

bladder under the standing platform provides various degrees of stability under manual control of the inflation and deflation of the bladder. When the bladder is fully inflated, the balancing surface is stable. As the bladder deflates, the standing surface becomes unstable, requiring greater degrees of balance. Measurements are taken by documenting the pounds-per-square inch (PSI) the patient is able to deflate the bladder while maintaining equilibrium. Specific manual control of incremental degrees of surface stability can be used to document subjective and objective data for patients on a firm stable surface versus a highly random unstable surface.

A rehabilitation protocol rarely suggests a comprehensive, specific sequence using each balance activity just described. Generally, drills are initiated and progressed according to the abilities of the patient and the desired goals of the patient and clinician. For example, one patient may progress from double-leg standing to single-leg hopping on a minitrampoline, while another patient may progress from single-leg balancing with eyes closed to braiding steps. No particular sequence of balancing is used for every patient.

Often balance training begins with the patient in a seated position as mentioned previously. A large **physioball** or swissball can be used as part of a static and dynamic trunk-balancing program (Fig. 5-7). The phys-

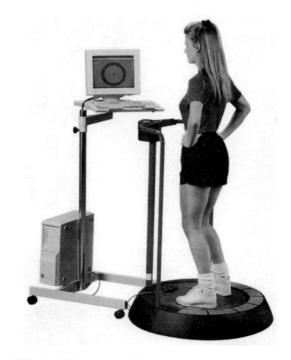

FIG. 5-6 Kinesthetic ability trainer. (Courtesy of Breg, Inc., Vista, Calif.).

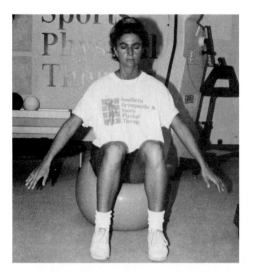

FIG. 5-7 Sitting trunk balance can be progressed using a physioball (plyoball) to challenge and test a patient's ability to demonstrate protective reactions and appropriate muscular corrective action while seated.

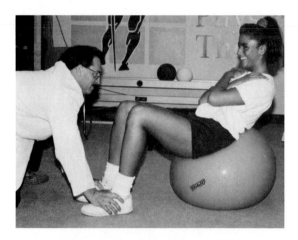

FIG. 5-8 Supported partial direct sit ups for improving trunk balance and strength on a large diameter physioball (plyoball).

ioball, which is a rather demanding exercise apparatus, has many applicable and creative uses in balancing and strengthening programs for various orthopedic patients. One very challenging test is the performance of support situps on the physioball (Fig. 5-8). Obviously, this particular exercise is for a rather active population, not for all patients.

Very generally, adaptive balance changes and improvements in equilibrium occur with consistent and practiced bouts of CKC, proprioceptive training drills.

Proprioceptive training for the upper extremity

Many household chores involve the repetitive use of the arms and shoulders to lift, pull, and carry. Industrial workers, manual laborers, and assembly line workers all use their arms and shoulders in vigorous weight-bearing positions (weight bearing in these instances refers to overhead lifting, pulling, and climbing maneuvers). Athletes in particular use their arms and shoulders to perform sports skills. Gymnasts require extraordinary flexibility, strength, and glenohumeral stability during demanding upper-body, weight-bearing activities.

As previously mentioned, injury, surgery, and immobilization lead to significant loss of proprioceptive awareness. Specific proprioceptive exercises have been proposed that, when used in conjunction with proprioceptive neuromuscular facilitation exercises, rhythmic stabilization strengthening exercises, and general range of motion, may contribute to improved proprioception in the upper extremity.[14,15]

The upper extremities can be progressed in much the same way as with the lower extremities. Using the balance board, the patient balances with both arms and with eyes open (Fig. 5-9). This exercise can be intensified

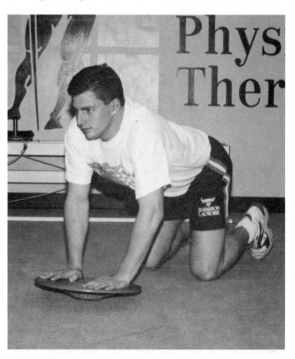

FIG. 5-9 For upper extremity proprioception and balance training, a wobble board can be used; initially, both arms are involved. As the patient gains strength, balance, and confidence, one arm can be used.

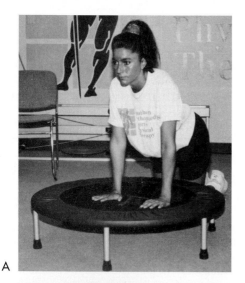

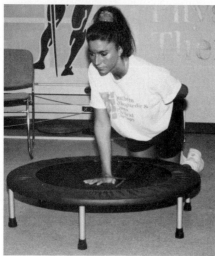

FIG. 5-10 A, The minitrampoline can also be used to encourage closed chain proprioception for the upper extremities; **B,** Progressing this activity will have the patient perform one arm balancing, push ups, and hopping maneuvers on the "forgiving" surface of the minitrampoline.

by having the patient use one arm with the eyes closed. The minitrampoline can also be used as a balance training device for upper extremity injuries (Fig. 5-10). The patient begins the exercise using both arms with eyes open and progresses to single-arm balancing with eyes closed. Global stability of the glenohumeral joint can effectively be enhanced with the use of a physioball (Fig. 5-11). The patient begins the progression of this exercise by kneeling in front of the ball and placing

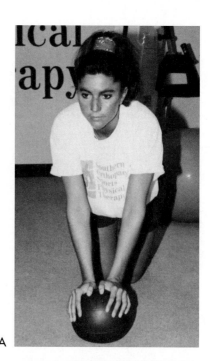

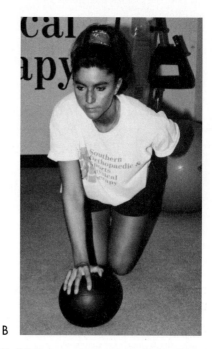

FIG. 5-11 A, A small physioball (plyoball) can also be used to encourage dynamic closed chain proprioception for the upper extremities; **B,** Closed-chain, weight-bearing activities can be progressed by having the patient balance and support on one arm on a plyoball.

both hands on the ball. As the exercise progresses, extraordinary joint stability, strength, and balance are required to maintain equilibrium. Stone et al[14] proposed these exercises specifically for an athletic population. However, they can be adapted to the general orthopedic population who must rely on dynamic vigorous weight-bearing shoulder and arm activities to accomplish tasks of daily living.

REFERENCES

1. Barber S et al: Quantitative accessment of functional limitations in normal and anterior cruciate deficient knees, *Clin Orthop* 255:204-214, 1990.
2. Barrack R, Skinner H, Buckley S: Proprioception in the anterior cruciate deficient knee, *Am J Sports Med* 17 (1):1-6, 1989.
3. Bonamo J, Fay C, Firestone T: The conservative treatment of the anterior cruciate deficient knee, *Am J Sports Med* 18 (6):618-623, 1990.
4. Lemkuhl DL, Smith LK: *Brunnstrom's clinical kinesiology,* ed 4, Philadelphia 1983, FA Davis Co.
5. Chandler JM, Duncan PW, Studenski SA: Balance performance on the postural stress test: comparison of young adults, healthy elderly, and fallers, *Phys Ther* 70 (7): 410-415, 1990.
6. Crutchfield CA, Shumway - Cook A, Horak FB: Balance and coordination training. In Scully RM, Barnes MR, editors: *Physical therapy,* Philadelphia, 1989, JB Lippincott
7. Freeman MAR, Dean MRE, Hanham WF: The etiology and prevention of functional instability of the foot, *J Bone Joint Surg* 473:678-685, 1985.
8. Freeman MAR, Wyke BD: The innervation of the knee joint: an anatomical and histological study, *J Anat Cat* 101:505-532, 1967.
9. Gentile A: Skill acquisition: action, movement, and neuromotor processes. In Carr JH, Shepherd RB, Gordon J, editors: *Movement science; foundations for physical therapy in rehabilitation,* Gaithersburg, Md., 1987, Aspen.
10. Meyer TJ: Coordination. In *Review book for the physical therapist assistant,* Herman, Mo., 1993, Midwest Hi-Tech Pub.
11. Noyes F, Barber S, Mooar L: A rationale for assessing sports activity levels and limitations in knee disorders, *Clin Orthop* 246:238 - 249, 1989.
12. Nyland J: Review of the afferent neural system of the knee and its contribution to motor learning, *J Orthop Sports Phys Ther,* 19: 2-11, 1994.
13. Schutte M et al: Neural anatomy of the human anterior cruciate ligament, *J Bone Joint Surg* 69A(2):243-247, 1987.
14. Stone, JA et al: Upper extremity proprioceptive training, *J Ath Train* 29:15-18, 1994.
15. Wilk KE et al: Stretch-shortening drills for the upper extremities: theory and clinical application, *J Orthop Sports Phys Ther,* 17(5): 225-239, 1993.
16. Wolfson LI et al: Stressing the postural response: quantitative method for testing balance, *J Am Geriatr Soc* 34:845-850, 1986.
17. Wyke BD: Articular neurology: a review, *Physio Ther* 58:94-99, 1972.

Review of Tissue Healing

The physical therapist assistant must understand the general healing mechanisms of specific tissues to make sound clinical recommendations, develop a progression of rehabilitation exercises, and readily identify problems associated with immobilization, surgery, or injury. Trauma and immobilization (usually longer than 4 weeks) profoundly affect bone and soft tissues. To understand the events and factors that negatively influence healing, the physical therapist assistant must be aware of the tissue response to injury, surgery, and immobilization. Different tissues (ligament, tendon, bone, muscle, and cartilage) heal or remodel at different rates.[2]

When beginning therapeutic exercises after ligament surgery, cast removal, or an acute traumatic injury, initial clinical information must include which specific tissues are involved, length of time immobilized, weight-bearing status during immobilization, and which surgical procedure, if any, was performed. These points will help the clinician recognize healing constraints of specific tissues, as well as indications and contraindications for modifying therapeutic interventions and functional activities. This section will provide information concerning immobilization, stress, exercise, joint protection, inflammation, repair, and remodeling, as well as outline the clinical foundations for specific exercises and progressions.

Three overlapping, interrelated series of events initiate healing: phase I, the inflammatory response; phase II, the repair sequence; and phase III, connective tissue formation or remodeling (Fig. II-1).[3]

The five cardinal signs of **inflammation** are: redness, swelling, pain, heat, and loss of function (these are all present with acute inflammatory reactions). The acute phase of inflammation lasts 24 to 48 hours, with the entire inflammatory response generally complete after 2 weeks.[3,8]

Immediately after injury, vasoconstriction, stimulated by serotonin,[1,7] limits blood and fluid loss for a few minutes. A platelet plug occludes small vessels surrounding the injury site, blocking the flow of blood and fluids away from the site. Other strong chemical mediators responsible for vascular constriction and later tissue permeability are histamine (permeability), serotonin (vasoconstrictor), bradykinin (permeability), and prostaglandins (inflammatory regulators, permeability, and pain) (Fig. II-2).[2]

A principal feature of the inflammatory response to injury is the process of ridding the injured area of tissue debris (autolytic wound debridement). This occurs via neutrophils that migrate to the injury site.[3] Other phagocytic cells, macrophages, and lymphocytes help produce enzymes that foster this process.[4]

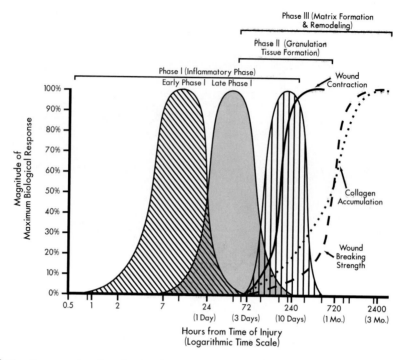

FIG. II-1 The three overlapping phases of wound repair. (From Kloth, McCulloch, Feedar: *Wound healing: alternatives in management,* Philadelphia, 1990, FA Davis).

The repair phase is characterized by fibroplasia, myofibroblast activity, and the organization and production of **collagen** (Fig. II-3).[3] Collagen formation begins about 5 days after injury.[3] Type III immature collagen predominates, providing very limited structural strength to the injury site. The synthesis, orientation, and deposition of new collagen is random, which reduces scar formation strength. After about 21 days, the strength of the new collagen is only 20% of its original strength.[5]

Phase III, the remodeling phase, begins about 2 weeks after injury and can last from a few months to as long as a year or more.[1] As the name implies, in remodeling, new collagen and connective tissue gradually reorient along the lines of physical stress imposed on the injured site (Fig. II-4).[1] If tissues are immobilized for prolonged periods, new collagen becomes highly disorganized and is laid down randomly. Active stress, or muscular contractions with progressive joint motion, promote longitudinally organized, stronger, more functional collagen arrangements.[1]

Box II-1 outlines basic healing mechanisms.

The inflammatory process

After bleeding is stopped, cellular and vascular responses to the injury are initiated. This is the body's natural damage-control mechanism: it protects the body from foreign objects at the wound site, cleans the site and brings cells necessary for directing healing in the next stage to the site.

Definition:

Inflammation is part of the reaction phase and consists of a cellular and vascular response. Normally, this phase lasts 2-5 days.

Collagen's work

Collagen's role during the reaction phase is to help mediate some of the activities of the inflammation process.

Attracts plasma components, absorbs fluids and stops bleeding.

Cleans the wound, removes bacteria, and debris by absorbtion.

Attracts white cells. Provides environment for macrophages.

How the body reacts to injury

Three steps are characteristic of the inflammation phase:

step 1

Vasodilation

Swollen vessel brings more blood and plasma components to the wound site.

step 2

Increased permeability

Allows more white cells to travel through the vessel wall to combat foreign bodies.

step 3

Cellular response

White cells ingest bacteria, debris and dead cells. Exhausted white cells build up in plasma, forming pus.

Evolution of cellular response

PMNs are the first cells to the injury site but must be replaced by larger cells and macrophages for wound healing to progress normally.

PMN

Polymorphonuclear leukocytes (PMN) are white cells responsible for cleaning the wound site. They provide resistance to microorganisms and are scavengers of tissue debris and foreign materials.

Monocytes

These intermediary white cells replace PMNs and eventually become macrophages. Monocytes function similarly to PMNs.

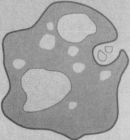

Macrophage

Toward the end of the reaction phase, the macrophage is the most common white cell present in the tissue and is the major mediator of inflammation and repair in wound healing.

Signs of inflammation

The classic four clinical signs of inflammation are: rubor (redness), tumor (swelling), calor (heat or warmth) and dolor (pain).

Rubor

The injury turns red because more blood is present in the area (a result of vasodilation).

Tumor

Swelling is caused by increased fluid mobility and accumulation of body fluids in the tissue.

Calor

The wounded area is heated by warm blood flowing into the region.

Dolor

Pain is caused by the pressure from the swelling of nearby tissue and the accumulation of white cell by products.

FIG. II-2 The inflammatory process and cellular response to injury. (Courtesy of © BioCore, Inc., Topeka, Kan.)

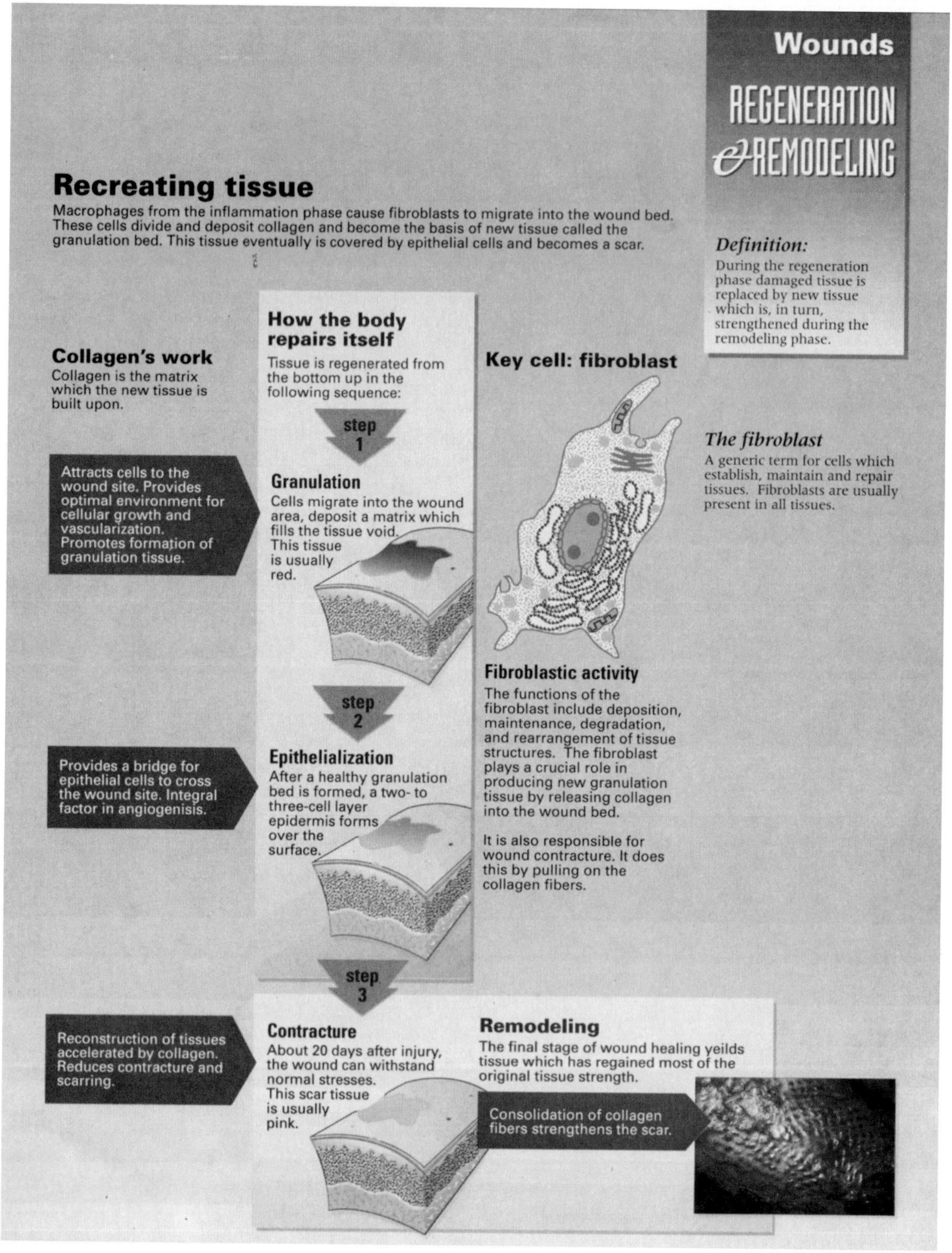

Recreating tissue

Macrophages from the inflammation phase cause fibroblasts to migrate into the wound bed. These cells divide and deposit collagen and become the basis of new tissue called the granulation bed. This tissue eventually is covered by epithelial cells and becomes a scar.

Definition:
During the regeneration phase damaged tissue is replaced by new tissue which is, in turn, strengthened during the remodeling phase.

Collagen's work
Collagen is the matrix which the new tissue is built upon.

How the body repairs itself
Tissue is regenerated from the bottom up in the following sequence:

Key cell: fibroblast

The fibroblast
A generic term for cells which establish, maintain and repair tissues. Fibroblasts are usually present in all tissues.

step 1

Attracts cells to the wound site. Provides optimal environment for cellular growth and vascularization. Promotes formation of granulation tissue.

Granulation
Cells migrate into the wound area, deposit a matrix which fills the tissue void. This tissue is usually red.

step 2

Fibroblastic activity
The functions of the fibroblast include deposition, maintenance, degradation, and rearrangement of tissue structures. The fibroblast plays a crucial role in producing new granulation tissue by releasing collagen into the wound bed.

It is also responsible for wound contracture. It does this by pulling on the collagen fibers.

Provides a bridge for epithelial cells to cross the wound site. Integral factor in angiogenisis.

Epithelialization
After a healthy granulation bed is formed, a two- to three-cell layer epidermis forms over the surface.

step 3

Reconstruction of tissues accelerated by collagen. Reduces contracture and scarring.

Contracture
About 20 days after injury, the wound can withstand normal stresses. This scar tissue is usually pink.

Remodeling
The final stage of wound healing yeilds tissue which has regained most of the original tissue strength.

Consolidation of collagen fibers strengthens the scar.

FIG. II-3 Remodeling and regeneration. Collagen and fibroplasia provide key functions that characterize this phase of tissue healing. (Courtesy of © BioCore, Inc., Topeka, Kan.)

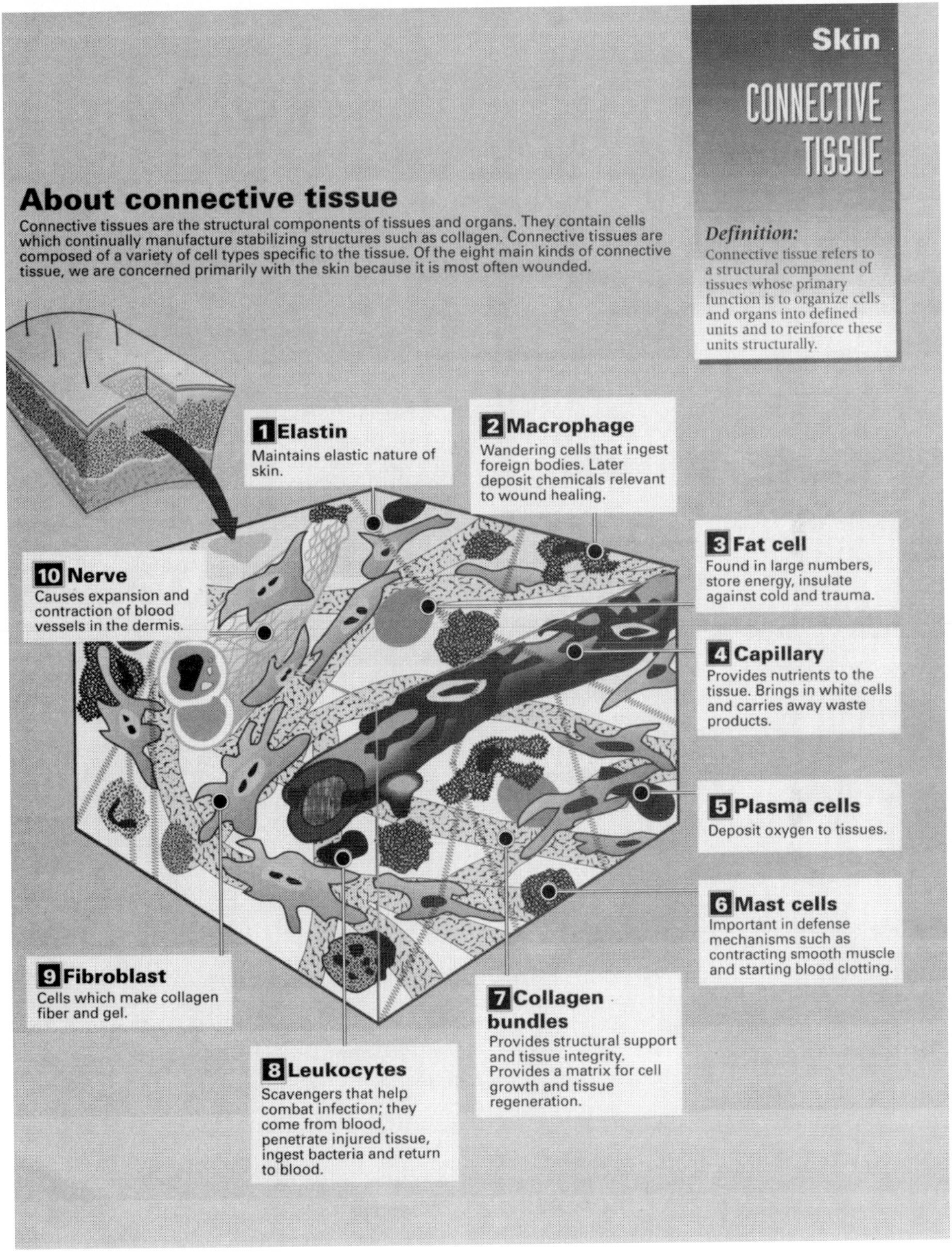

About connective tissue

Connective tissues are the structural components of tissues and organs. They contain cells which continually manufacture stabilizing structures such as collagen. Connective tissues are composed of a variety of cell types specific to the tissue. Of the eight main kinds of connective tissue, we are concerned primarily with the skin because it is most often wounded.

Definition:
Connective tissue refers to a structural component of tissues whose primary function is to organize cells and organs into defined units and to reinforce these units structurally.

1 Elastin
Maintains elastic nature of skin.

2 Macrophage
Wandering cells that ingest foreign bodies. Later deposit chemicals relevant to wound healing.

3 Fat cell
Found in large numbers, store energy, insulate against cold and trauma.

4 Capillary
Provides nutrients to the tissue. Brings in white cells and carries away waste products.

5 Plasma cells
Deposit oxygen to tissues.

6 Mast cells
Important in defense mechanisms such as contracting smooth muscle and starting blood clotting.

10 Nerve
Causes expansion and contraction of blood vessels in the dermis.

9 Fibroblast
Cells which make collagen fiber and gel.

8 Leukocytes
Scavengers that help combat infection; they come from blood, penetrate injured tissue, ingest bacteria and return to blood.

7 Collagen bundles
Provides structural support and tissue integrity. Provides a matrix for cell growth and tissue regeneration.

FIG. II-4 Components of connective tissue. (Courtesy of © BioCore, Inc., Topeka, Kan.)

BOX II-1   Review of Basic Healing Mechanisms

Day 2-4

Scar tissue composition: A clot forms in the wound. Connective tissue cells infiltrate the area, with macrophages attracting fibroblasts. In this initial stage of scarring, the tissue is very fragile and easily disrupted because of the predominance of weak and unstable type III collagen. Adhesion is by cellular attachments, and stretching of the scar causes tearing of the cells.

Day 5-21

Fibroplasia and contraction: This stage is very cellular. The scar increases in bulk because of fibroplasia, with an increase in the quantity of collagen fibers. This is a highly active stage of collagen synthesis and degradation. Treatment to increase range of motion and function of a joint can be very effective during this stage because of the collagen remodeling process.

Day 21-60

Consolidation: The scar contains well-organized collagen. The tissue gradually changes from predominantly cellular to fibrous, with a large amount of collagen fibers. There is a gradual increase in strength of the scar because of an increased stable covalent bonding. During this time, there will be a continuous decrease in the ability of the scar to respond to treatment.

Day 60-360

Maturation: Type I collagen fibers are compact and large. The fully mature scar is only 3% cellular and almost totally collagenous. Response to treatment is poor, and hypertrophic and keloid scar tissue increases when stretched in multiple directions.

From Currier D, Nelson R: Mechanisms of connective tissue. In Currier D, Nelson R, editors: *Dynamics of human biologic tissues,* Philadelphia, 1992, FA Davis.

REFERENCES

1. Bushbacher R: Tissue injury and healing. In *Musculoskeletal disorders: a practical guide for diagnosis and rehabilitation,* Boston, 1994, Andover Medical Publishers.
2. Cummings GS, Tillman LJ: Remodelling of dense connective tissue in normal adult tissues. In Currier DP, Nelson RM, editors: *Dynamics of human biologic tissues,* Philadelphia, 1992, FA Davis.
3. Kloth LC, Miller KH: The inflammatory response to wounding. In Kloth LC, McCulloch JM, Feedar JA, editors: *Wound healing: alternatives in management, contemporary perspectives in rehabilitation,* Philadelphia, 1990, FA Davis.
4. Laub R et al: Degradation of collagen and proteoglycan by macrophages and fibroblasts, *ACTA Biochem Biophys* 721:425, 1982.
5. Levenson SM et al: The healing of rat skin wounds, *Ann Surg* 161:293-303, 1965.
6. Tillman LJ, Cummings GS: Biologic mechanisms of connective tissue mutability. In Currier DP, Nelson RM, editors: *Dynamics of human biologic tissues,* Philadelphia, 1992, FA Davis.
7. Vander AJ, Sherman JH, Luciano DS: *Human physiology: the mechanisms of body function,* ed 3, Minneapolis, 1980, McGraw-Hill.
8. Zarro V: Mechanisms of inflammation and repair. In Michlovitz S, editor: *Thermal agents in rehabilitation,* Philadelphia, 1986, FA Davis.

Ligament Healing

The most common injury of joints are **sprains,** which are injuries involving **ligaments.** The knee and ankle joints are common areas of ligament sprains, with the incidence of knee ligament sprains, particularly those of the medical collateral ligament (MCL), occurring in as many as 25% to 40% of all knee injuries.[6,17]

Not all ligaments heal at the same rate or to the same degree.[2] For example, the anterior cruciate ligament (ACL) does not appear to heal as well as the MCL of the knee.[21] Factors affecting ligament healing include blood supply and function.[10,21]

Ligaments heal through the three phases of inflammatory response, with phase I lasting approximately 48 hours after injury; phase II lasting 48 to 72 hours or more after injury; and phase III lasting a year or more. It is estimated that ligament-tensile strength is only 50% to 70% of its original strength 1 year after injury.[15]

Three key conditions must be present for ligaments to properly remodel or heal:[2]
1. Torn ligament ends must be in contact with each other.
2. Progressive, controlled stress must be applied to the healing tissues to orient scar tissue formation.
3. The ligament must be protected against excessive forces during the remodeling process.

The continuum of the healing process outlined here is ligament specific, and healing is related to blood supply, degree of injury, and mechanical stresses applied to the ligament.[2]

Nonsurgical Repair Versus Surgical Repair

Ligaments can be surgically repaired or allowed to heal without surgery depending on the degree of injury and the involvement of supporting tissues. In addition, investigators have shown that untreated ligaments heal by way of scar tissue proliferation rather than by true ligament regeneration.[7] Untreated ligament tears are biochemically inferior, possessing a large portion of type III immature collagen, and are generally not healed even at 40 weeks after injury.[7]

The following is a list of **grades of injury** occurring to ligament tissue. They are graded as to severity:

Grade I   Microscopic tearing of the ligament without producing joint laxity

Grade II   Tearing of some ligament fibers with moderate laxity

Grade III   Complete rupture of the ligament with profound instability and laxity

Grade I and II ligament sprains are most common, with only 15% of all knee ligament sprains classified as grade III.[3] Generally, grade I and II ligament sprains can be treated with protective bracing and comprehensive and progressive rehabilitation with appropriate strengthening to provide dynamic muscular support. With grades I and II ligament sprains of the knee (ACL, MCL, posterior cruciate ligament [PCL], and lateral collateral ligament [LCL]), good to excellent results can be anticipated in 90% of those cases treated nonsurgically.[2]

Surgical repair of a grade III ligament injury frequently involves repair of associated tissues. Cartilage (meniscus) and MCL, LCL, or PCL-related injury is often seen with primary ACL grade III injury.

Effects of Immobilization

Immobilization, surgery, injury, and rehabilitation of ligaments must take into consideration not only the healing response of the ligament itself but also that of the ligament-bone interface. Stress deprivation of the ligament and ligament-bone complexes resulting from prolonged **immobilization** after injury or surgery can have significant and profound negative effects. Joint stiffness after immobilization is related to adhesion formation, active shortening of dense connective tissue (ligament),[2] and decreases in water content. Studies show a gradual deterioration in ligament strength, loss of bone, weakening of cartilage and tendons, significant muscle atrophy, and negative effects on joint mechanics[1] after periods of immobilization (Box 6-1). Immobilization also affects ligament bone complexes. Studies report that loss of bone directly beneath the junction of ligament and bone reduced the strength of both the insertion site and the entire ligament-bone complex.[13]

BOX 6-1   Effects of Immobilization on Ligament Tissue and Associated Structures

Reduced physiologic motion
Decreased afferent neural input
Muscular atrophy
Ligament shortening
Reduction of water content, proteoglycans and glycosaminoglycans
Bone loss—periosteal bone reabsorption
Articular (hyaline cartilage) erosion
Reduced ligament weight
Reduced ligament size
Reduced ligament strength
Adhesion formation
Increased ligament laxity
Joint stiffness related to synovial membrane adherence

From Kloth, McCulloch, Feedar: *Wound healing: alternatives in management,* Philadelphia, 1990, FA Davis.

Rigidly immobilized joints produce chemical and morphologic changes in ligaments 2 and 4 weeks after injury, respectively.[8] After 8 weeks of immobilization, ligaments lose 20% of their weight, significant atrophy results, and marked infiltration of connective tissue is observed surrounding the ligament.[8] Although immobilization may be needed to promote healing of damaged tissues, the extended use of rigid cast immobilization should be limited. As an alternative, limited range of motion braces (Fig. 6-1) can be used to protect healing structures and decrease unwanted external forces, as well as allow for progressive motion of involved joints to minimize the negative effects of immobilization.

Exercise

As stated, stress deprivation of the ligaments because of immobilization results in atrophy.* Conversely, motion, stress, and general physical activity prescribed for healing ligaments produce hypertrophy and increased tensile strength.[2,8] Research shows that ligament and ligament-bone complex strength is related to the type and duration of exercise used during rehabilitation.[2] Tipton[20] has shown that endurance-type exercise is more effective in producing larger diameter collagen than nonendurance-type exercise. In addition, the long-term detrimental effects of prolonged immobilization on ligament-bone insertion sites are reversible.[2] The effects of mobilization and exercise are seen between 4 months and 1 year after immobilization.[2]

Continuous Passive Motion

Motion, exercise, and protected-progressive stress can influence and determine the degree and type of healing occurring after trauma and subsequent immobilization.[14] Studies have demonstrated that healing is dramatically different in immobilized joints compared to those moved passively through limited motion.[9] Gelberman et al[9] have shown that joints moved passively have well-organized, longitudinally oriented collagen fibers in which no adhesions are present. Conversely, joints that were immobilized demonstrated scar tissue and adhesions.

The concept of early protected motion applied to healing soft tissues has resulted in the development of a technique termed **continuous passive motion (CPM)** (Fig. 6-2). CPM is used in the treatment of the following: knee joint contractures, postoperative ACL reconstructions, joint effusions, knee, elbow, and ankle fractures (after immobilization), joint arthrosis, and in total knee arthroplasty.[12] Early motion after surgery or immobilization acts to enhance and facilitate connective tissue strength, size, and shape; evacuate joint hemarthrosis (bloody effusion within the joint space); improve joint nutrition; inhibit adhesions; initiate normal joint

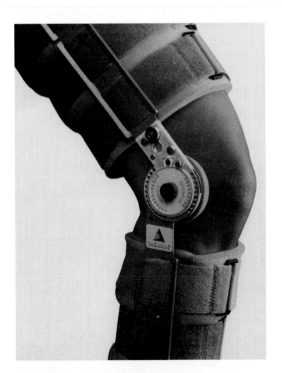

FIG. 6-1 Limited range of motion long leg brace. (Courtesy of Thera-Kinetics, Inc., Mount Laurel, N.J.).

*References 2,7,8,15,16,21.

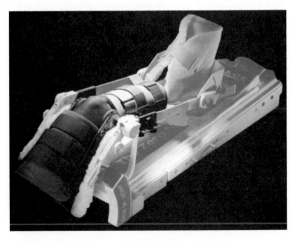

FIG. 6-2 Continuous passive motion (CPM) machine. (Courtesy of Thera-Kinetics, Inc., Mount Laurel, N.J.).

kinematics; reduce articular surface changes; and minimize other deleterious effects of prolonged immobilization.[12] Many studies report that the use of CPM can significantly improve joint range of motion, reduce joint swelling, allow patients to ambulate and perform straight leg raises earlier, and promote the healing of hyaline articular cartilage. With postoperative ACL reconstruction, no stretching out of the graft occurs when CPM is used.[4,5,14,18] CPM can be used postoperatively, applied in the operating room, or done a few days after surgery, immediately upon cast removal, or during the early phases of rehabilitation.

CPM devices have been designed for use on many body parts.[12] The knee is the most common, with the ankle, shoulder, elbow, wrist, hand, and hip joints also benefitting from CPM. The CPM machine is calibrated in cycles per minute and degrees of motion. Progressive increases in the cycle mode and degrees of motion are made gradually so as not to initiate pain or increase the time required for healing.

The clinical applications of CPM vary greatly. Protocols range from 24 hours a day for as long as a month, to as little as 6 hours a day after surgery. The speed of movement, cycles (rate), and total volume of repetitions depend on patient comfort, surgical procedure, and structures involved. Generally, one cycle (flexion and extension) per minute is well tolerated. The degree of motion should allow for the greatest amount of pain-free or tolerable motion. If the degree of motion, or speed, causes distress, a reduction is needed; pain inhibits relaxation and causes reflexive muscle guarding or splinting.

CPM is generally used in conjunction with other agents to reduce swelling and pain. Among these are ice packs, oral or intravenous analgesics, antiinflammatory medications, transcutaneous electric nerve stimulators (TENS), and joint compression bandages.

When not using the CPM, the patient performs active and passive range of motion exercises, as well as active assisted exercises to gain motion. Gentle, progressive strengthening exercises, functional electrical stimulation, scar massage, and joint mobilization are also used.

Practical Considerations

The time constraints and healing mechanics of ligaments are well documented.* Careful consideration must be given to the progression of therapeutic exercises and functional activities for patients with ligament injuries. Usually the absence of pain and swelling is an exceedingly poor indicator of healing tissue. With an ACL

---

*References 2,3,7,11,13,15,19,21,22.

reconstruction, pain and swelling generally subside within a few weeks, but return of functional joint motion requires a couple of months. Strength values gradually increase, with muscle hypertrophy following slowly.

As the outward clinical signs point to healing, the ligament, being a dynamic tissue, continues to remodel and mature for up to a year. Protection of the joint is critical during healing. Functional knee braces with range-limiting devices protect healing ligaments during the various phases of rehabilitation. Initiating progressive resistance exercises after knee ligament injury or surgery, while maintaining joint protection, can be challenging. Placing the resistance (weight) above the joint line during straight leg raises (Fig. 6-3) after ACL surgery can be the first phase of progressive resistance while protecting the healing ligament.

To strengthen hip adduction with an MCL sprain, resistance is initially applied above the joint line so as not to stress the MCL (Fig. 6-4). As the time constraints of healing allow, progressive strengthening of the adductors can involve loading the joint more distally, provided joint protection is applied. Awareness of the time required for healing as well as the duration of immobilization after trauma, weight-bearing status, and degree of injury will guide the physical therapist assistant in making clinical recommendations regarding the progression of exercise and the placement of force during rehabilitation.

Developing a progressive therapeutic exercise and functional activities program with ankle sprains is similarly challenging. Generally a grade II anterior talofibu-

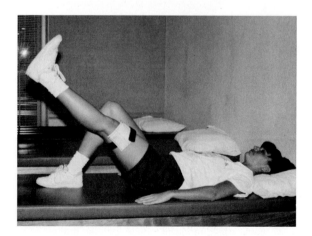

FIG. 6-3 Supine straight leg raises (SLR) with the resistance placed proximal to the knee joint in order to reduce anterior translatory forces following anterior cruciate ligament (ACL) reconstructive surgery.

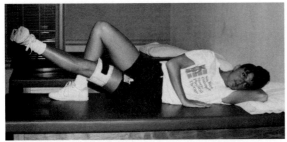

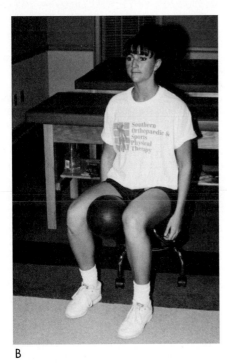

FIG. 6-4 A, Sidelying hip adduction exercise with the resistance placed proximal to the knee joint in order to protect the healing medial collateral ligament MCL; **B,** Isometric hip adduction with the use of a ball placed proximal to the joint line.

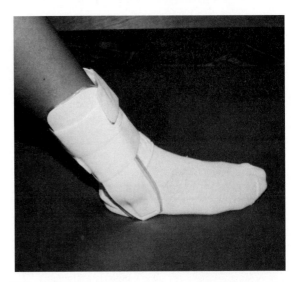

FIG. 6-5 Joint protection from unwanted forces must be considered essential for many weeks following ligament injuries. Air-stirrup brace for lateral ligament complex sprain of the ankle.

as soon as tolerated, while protecting the joint, helps in establishing normal joint kinematics and gait.

Protecting the ligaments from further stress not only involves external bracing but also avoidance of motions that place unwanted force on the healing ligaments. For example, the anterior talofibular ligament of the ankle is stressed with plantar flexion and inversion. To protect the ligaments, these two motions should be avoided during the early (postacute) and middle phases of rehabilitation.

After ligament injury, repair, or immobilization, early protected motion is encouraged, taking great caution to avoid overstressing the ligament or duplicating motions that place unwanted strain on the ligament too soon after injury. The acute and postacute phases of rehabilitation after ligament injury or repair usually involve pain management techniques, swelling reduction, muscle re-education (isometric muscle contraction, functional muscle stimulation), CPM, active range of motion, ligament protection devices via range-adjustable bracing, and weight-bearing gait maneuvers with crutches as needed. During this early phase of recovery, it is particularly important to avoid excessive motions that may disrupt the intentional scar formation needed for joint stability. The degree of motion, direction of forces, and velocity of joint movement applied during this early postacute phase must be joint specific, functional, and *protected.* For example, with a cruciate ligament sprain, movements that are allowed include knee flexion and extension (within limits), but no rotary or torque-producing

lar ligament sprain does not produce significant pain or functional limitations after a few weeks of conservative treatment involving splinting, crutch walking (non-weight-bearing progressing to full weight-bearing), ice, compression, and elevation. Thus because the process of ligament healing occurs slowly, the physical therapist assistant will need to protect the ligament for many weeks after injury (Fig. 6-5).

As pain subsides, the patient may begin to stress the injured ligaments too soon. Encouraging weight bearing

TABLE 6-1

Therapeutic Considerations During Stages of Ligament Healing

DAY 2-4	DAY 5-21	DAY 21-60	DAY 60-360
Acute fibroblast stage. Weak, fragile tissue. Unstable type III collagen.[19]	Highly cellular stage. Scar formation. Active collagen synthesis and remodeling process.	Consolidation. Very gradual changes in collagen strength. Tissue changes from cellular to fibrous.[19]	Maturation.
TREATMENT Rest, ice, compression, elevation, pain management techniques (TENS, Oral-IV analgesics). Nonweight bearing or weight bearing as tolerated. Can initiate CPM (within limited range of motion) *Protection of Ligaments* from unwanted stress—usually adjustable range braces or hinged casts. Strict, rigid, long-term cast immobilization should be minimized. Isometric muscle contractions. Contralateral limb exercise as tolerated.	**TREATMENT** Continue RICE treatment. Progressive CPM. Active-progressive motion. Continued *ligament protection.* Progressive weight bearing. Protected, controlled, active resisted exercise. Cycling (for motion). Isometric exercise progression. Electrical muscle stimulation. Initiate gentle multiangle static holds (isometrics). Avoid excessive motion.	**TREATMENT** Continue RICE as needed. Begin low-load static stretch if needed. Preheating tissues if needed. Continue CPM. Full weight bearing. Isokinetic exercise with continued *ligament protection* with *bracing.* Eccentric isotonic exercise. Progressive concentric isotonic exercise. Hydrotherapy-swimming. Progressive cycling. Initiate closed kinetic chain exercise.	**TREATMENT** Prolonged low load static stretching. Thermal modalities (heat, US), ice as necessary. Progressive advanced isokinetic and isotonic exercise. Cycling—stairclimbs. Proprioception—balance—coordination exercise. Advanced CKC exercise, progressing to plyometric exercise. Jogging, running, jumping, *maintain joint protection* with functional bracing as needed.

motions. After an MCL sprain, knee flexion and extension motion can be initiated in the postacute phase (within limits); however, no valgus stress should be applied. As stated earlier, the reason for ligament protection, maintenance of joint stability, and improved motion is that collagen fiber growth and parallel alignment are stimulated by early tensile loading within the normal physiologic range of the healing ligament.

Table 6-1 outlines the stages of ligament healing and subsequent therapeutic interventions that enhance the healing of ligament tissues.

REFERENCES

1. Akeson WH: An experimental study of joint stiffness, *J Bone Joint Surg* 43A:1,022-1,034, 1961.
2. Andriacchi T et al: Ligament: injury and repair. In Woo SL-Y, Buckwalter J, editors: *Injury and repair of the musculoskeletal soft tissues,* Rosemont, Ill., 1988, American Academy of Orthopaedic Surgeons.
3. Buschbacher R: Tissue injury and healing. In: *Musculoskeletal disorders: a practical guide for diagnosis and rehabilitation,* Boston, 1994, Andover Medical Publishers.
4. Coutts RD, Toth C, Kaita JH: The role of continuous passive motion in the rehabilitation of the total knee patient. In Hungerford DS, Krackow KA, Kenna RV, editors: *Total knee arthroplasty: a comprehensive approach,* Baltimore, Md., 1984, Williams & Wilkins.
5. Davis D: Continuous passive motion for total knee arthroplasty, *Phys Ther* 64:709, 1984.
6. DeHaven KE, Lintner DM: Athletic injuries: comparison by age, sport and gender, *Am J Sports Med* 14:218-224, 1986.
7. Frank C et al: Medial collateral healing: a multidisciplinary assessment in rabbits, *Am J Sports Med* 11:379-389, 1983.
8. Gamble JG, Edwards CC, Max SR: Enzymatic adaption in ligaments during immobilization, *Am J Sports Med* 12:221-228, 1984.
9. Gelberman RH et al: Flexer tendon healing and restoration of the gliding surface: an ultrastructural study in dogs, *J Bone Joint Surg* 65:70-80, 1983.
10. Inoue M et al: Treatment of the medial collateral ligament I: the importance of anterior cruciate ligament

on the varus-valgus knee laxity, *Am J Sports Med* 15:15-21, 1987.

11. Kloth LC, Miller KH: The inflammatory response to wounding. In Kloth LC, McCulloch JM, Feedar JA, editors: *Wound healing: alternatives in management, contemporary perspectives in rehabilitation,* Philadelphia, 1990, FA Davis Co.

12. McCarthy MR et al: The clinical use of continuous passive motion in physical therapy, *J Orthop Sports Phys Ther* 15:132-140, 1992.

13. Noyes FR, DeLucas JL, Torvik PJ: Biomechanics of anterior cruciate ligament failure: an analysis of strain-rate sensitivity and mechanisms of failure in primates, *J Bone Joint Surg* 56A:236-253, 1974.

14. Noyes FR, Mangine RE: Early motion after open arthroscopic anterior cruciate ligament reconstruction, *Am J Sports Med* 15:149-160, 1987.

15. Noyes FR et al: Advances in the understanding of knee ligament injury, repair and rehabilitation, *Med Sci Sports Exerc* 16:427-443, 1984.

16. O'Donoghue DH et al: Repair and reconstruction of the anterior cruciate ligament in dogs: factors influencing long-term results, *J Bone Joint Surg* 53A:710-718, 1971.

17. Powell J: 636,000 injuries annually in high school football, *Athl Train* 22:19-22, 1987.

18. Salter RB et al: The effects of continuous passive motion on the healing of articular cartilage defects: an experimental investigation in rabbits, *J Bone Joint Surg* 57A:570-571, 1975.

19. Tillman LJ, Cummings GS: Biologic mechanisms of connective tissue mutability. In Currier DP, Nelson RM, editors: *Dynamics of human biologic tissues,* Philadelphia, 1992, FA Davis.

20. Tipton CM et al: Influence of exercise on strength of medial collateral knee ligaments of dogs, *Am J Physiol* 218:894-902, 1970.

21. Woo SL-Y et al: New experimental procedures to evaluate the biomechanical properties of healing canine medial collateral ligaments, *J Orthop Res* 5:425-432, 1987.

22. Zarro V: Mechanisms of inflammation and repair. In Michlovitz S, editor: *Thermal agents in rehabilitation,* Philadelphia, 1986, FA Davis.

Bone Healing

LEARNING OBJECTIVES

1. Identify and describe the phases of bone healing.
2. Discuss the objectives that serve as the foundation of fracture management and bone healing.
3. Define osteoblasts, osteoclasts, and osteocytes.
4. Define and discuss Wolff's law.
5. Discuss stress deprivation, immobilization, and normal physiologic stress as they apply to fracture healing.
6. Define three complications of bone healing.
7. Outline and describe six areas of descriptive organization of classifying fractures.
8. Describe the five types of pediatric fractures defined by Salter-Harris.
9. Define pathologic fractures and list four types.
10. Discuss how osteoporosis affects fractures.
11. Define osteomalacia.
12. List common methods of fracture fixation, fixation devices, and fracture classifications.
13. Discuss clinical applications of rehabilitation techniques used during bone healing.

KEY TERMS

Salter-Harris fractures
Pathologic fractures
Osteoporosis
Osteomalacia
Spongy bone
Compact bone
Cancellous bone
Cortical bone
Osteoblasts
Osteocytes
Osteoclasts
Remodeling
Wolff's law
Piezoelectric effect
Bone callus
Immobilization
Delayed union
Nonunion
Malunion
External fixation devices
Internal fixation devices
Open reduction with
  internal fixation
  (ORIF)

CHAPTER OUTLINE

Orthopedic conditions involving bone tissue are extremely common ailments treated in physical therapy. Therefore the physical therapist assistant must appreciate the organized, dynamic nature of bone healing and must recognize the various methods of treating fractures. As with other tissues and injuries, not all fractures heal the same way or to the same degree;[2] bone healing varies greatly, depending largely on which methods of treatment are used.[9] In general, three basic objectives have been identified that serve as the foundation of fracture management and bone healing:

- *Fragment reduction:* The approximation of bone fragments. It is essential to place the bone fragments in anatomic alignment and apposition.
- *Maintenance of alignment:* Securing fracture fragments over time maintains proper anatomic alignment and promotes healing. External fixation devices, traction, or internal fixation may be used.
- *Preservation and restoration of function:* Rehabilitation after the initial phases of fracture management involves regaining lost mobility, improving muscular strength and function, restoring balance and coordination (proprioception and kinesthetic awareness), and teaching proper gait mechanics (for lower extremity injuries).[2]

CLASSIFICATIONS OF FRACTURES

By definition, a fracture is any abnormal disruption in the normal anatomic continuity of bone. Therefore the classification of fractures takes into account the following criteria:[12,13]

- *Site of injury:* The area of insult on the bone itself. An epiphyseal fracture describes the site, as does an intraarticular fracture or diaphyseal (shaft) fracture. Generally, the site is described as the proximal, middle, or distal portion of a bone (Fig. 7-1).
- *Extent of injury:* Complete or incomplete (Fig. 7-2). As the name implies, a complete fracture traverses the bone entirely. Incomplete fractures are commonly described as hairline cracks or green-stick fractures.
- *Configuration or direction of abnormality:* The direction of the fracture. In a traverse fracture, the fracture line goes straight across (horizontally) through the bone; an oblique fracture crosses the bone diagonally. A spiral fracture describes a torsion or rotational injury where the fracture line literally spirals through the bone. An impacted fracture is a long-axis compression injury where the fracture fragments are forced together. Where there are more than two fragments present, the fracture is classified as comminuted.

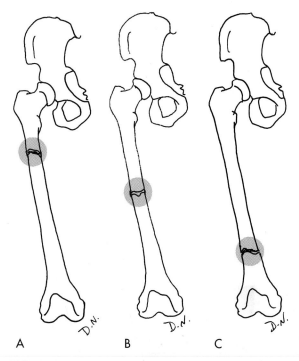

FIG. 7-1 Fracture classification site of injury. **A,** Proximal fracture of the femur; **B,** Middle fracture of the femur; **C,** Distal femur fracture.

- *Relationship of fracture fragments to each other:* Can be displaced, nondisplaced, angulated, twisted, rotated, or overriding. An example is an avulsion fracture where a portion of bone is pulled away as part of a musculotendinous attachment or ligament-bone attachment.
- *Relationship of fracture fragments to the environment:* Whether the injury is open (compound fracture) or closed (simple).
- *Complications:* Resulting in delayed union, nonunion, or malunion of the fracture fragments. An uncomplicated course of healing is called uneventful.

Pediatric fractures have a special classification of injuries involving the epiphysis. Depending on the type of epiphyseal fracture, the eventual growth of the bone can be profoundly affected.

In Fig. 7-3 Salter's fracture classification is outlined. Type I **Salter-Harris fractures,** modified by Rang,[9,11-13] are transverse fractures through the physis. Type II fractures are the same as Type I, but also have a metaphyseal fragment. Type III fractures involve both the physis and the epiphysis. Typically these are intraarticular fractures. Type IV fractures are the same as type III but include the metaphysis. These are significant

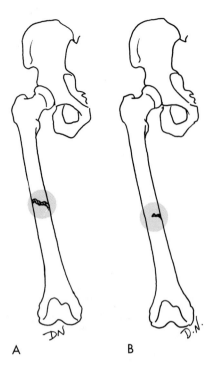

FIG. 7-2 Fracture classification, extent of injury. **A,** Complete fracture of the femur; **B,** Incomplete femur fracture.

injuries that can lead to a reduction in bone growth. Type V fractures are severe injuries classified as crush injuries to the physis. This type of fracture can also lead to the arrest of growth. The physical therapist assistant should also be aware of the AO classification system, which is universally applied to both fracture patterns and the devices used for internal fixation. This system will be discussed later in this chapter.[8]

Pathologic fractures are caused by tumors[9] (malignant or primary bone disease), osteoporosis (most common), microtrauma from repetitive overload (stress fractures), or metastatic bone disease (second most common). These usually occur in the elderly person secondary to osteoporosis and can happen spontaneously or with very minor trauma.[9]

Osteoporosis

Osteoporosis is an age-related heterogeneous bone disease characterized by decreased bone tissue. Osteoporosis occurs when osteoblast (bone formation) activity is surpassed by osteoclast (bone resorption) activity.[7] It involves an overall decrease in the quality of bone, not necessarily the quality of bone tissue.[9] This creates

weaker bones that are subjected to greater rates of fracture. Over 1 million fractures a year can be attributed to osteoporosis;[9] vertebral body compression fractures are the most common.

Women are at greater risk for developing osteoporosis for several reasons. One reason is related to bone loss. Age-related cortical bone loss generally begins at about age 40,[7] with the rate thereafter being approximately 0.5% annually for both men and women. However, because of lowered estrogen during menopause,[7] women lose bone at a rate of 2% to 8% annually, resulting in a much greater total loss.

Poor absorption of calcium that leads to decreased bone mineralization is called **osteomalacia**.[9] Causes include calcium-deficient diet, accelerated calcium loss, and malabsorption of calcium.[7] Femoral neck fractures are common in patients with osteomalacia.[9]

To appreciate the fragile nature of fractures that occur as a result of osteoporosis or osteomalacia, consider this case:

A frail, elderly woman with osteoporosis suffers resultant multilevel thoracic vertebral body compression fractures. Bed rest with relative immobilization is ordered. She suffers further decrease in bone strength caused by immobilization. Obviously, rehabilitation is complicated by osteoporosis and fractures. Then the general overall negative effects of immobilization on the body's systems are added, and the effects of immobilization on the remaining skeletal tissue interfere with exercise, sitting, progressive ambulation, and functional activities.

COMPONENTS OF BONE HEALING

Most of the adult skeleton (80%) is composed of compact, cortical bone. Approximately 20% of the skeleton is cancellous, or **spongy bone. Compact bone** is extremely dense and unyielding to bending, whereas **cancellous bone** is more elastic and less dense than **cortical bone.**[9]

Three types of cells take part in the highly dynamic, reparative process in bone. **Osteoblasts** help form and synthesize bone. **Osteocytes** are mature bone cells that account for approximately 90% of all bone tissue. **Osteoclasts** are active in bone resorption.

The normal, dynamic process of bone synthesis and resorption is termed **remodeling.** Remodeling and *stress* occur together, which profoundly influences bone shape, density, internal architecture, and external configuration.[1,4,6,9] With normal bone remodeling, weight-bearing forces and muscular contractions provide the stress needed for bone formation and adaptation. The absence

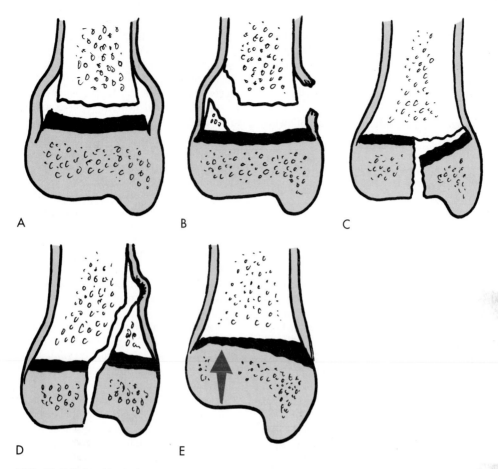

FIG. 7-3 Salter-Harris fracture classification. **A,** Type I—transverse fracture through the physis; **B,** Type II is same as Type I but also has metaphyseal fragment; **C,** Type III—Intraarticular fracture. Involves both the physis and the epiphysis; **D,** Type IV—Same as Type III, also involves the metaphysis; **E,** Type V—crush injury to the physis.

of physiologic loading, or stress, is detrimental to bone, ligament, cartilage, muscle, and tendons as well as the cardiorespiratory systems. **Wolff's law**[1] states that intermittently applied stress,[2] as well as changes in function of bone, cause definite changes.[2,4] After a fracture, treatment may involve rigid cast immobilization and non-weight-bearing over a period of weeks. This decreased stress on the bone causes rapid osteoclast activity (bone resorption) and decreased osteoblast activity.[10] Therefore, while the removal of stress is paramount for healing, the decrease in external force also causes significant bone loss.[9] Bone loss caused by immobilization is reversible after progressive weight bearing, active motion, resistive exercise, and vertical loading (closed

kinetic-chain exercise).[9] It is recommended that strict, long-term, rigid cast immobilization be minimized whenever possible.

Although normal stresses promote bone development, excessive stress can also lead to gradual bone resorption.[4] Stress that is unrelenting and does not allow for osteoblastic repair of bone can lead to pathologic accelerated bone resorption and eventual stress fracture.[1,4,6]

Bone remodeling is also influenced by electrical charges when forces are applied to bone. The **piezoelectric effect** describes a negative electric charge toward the concave, or compression, side of a force applied to a bone. An electropositive charge is seen on the tension, or convex, side of the bone. The negative charge side responds by stimulating osteoblasts, whereas the positive charge side (tension side) responds by increasing osteoclast activity.[9]

PROCESS OF BONE HEALING

Bone healing can be characterized by the following sequence of events:

- Fracture occurs.
- Bleeding occurs, and a hematoma results.
- Granulation tissue is formed by the hematoma (soft callus formation).
- Osteoblasts produce new bone, and a bony or hard callus is formed.
- The callus is gradually reabsorbed, and the anatomic contour of the bone is regained.

As with soft tissue, the immediate inflammatory response lasts 24 to 48 hours and is characterized by the development of granulation tissue, blood clotting, and fibroblast and osteoblast proliferation.[2,9] The repair phase of bone healing signals the development of bone scarring, or callus formation, which is usually detected within the first 2 weeks after injury. The degree of callus formation depends on anatomic alignment of the fragments and the degree and quality of immobilization. If motion occurs through the fracture site during this phase, a soft **bone callus** (primarily of cartilage) will bridge the fragments.[2,9] This type of callus also forms if the union between the fragments is poor, even when immobilization prevents motion.

Primary cortical healing (hard callus) forms with anatomic alignment and fragment apposition, immobilization, and appropriately applied progressive stress. The remodeling phase of bone healing is an extraordinarily long process that can take up to several years to complete and is strongly influenced by Wolff's law.[1]

As with ligament healing, protection of the injury site is vital to a successful outcome. There is an exceedingly narrow line to follow with respect to motion after bone injury. In many cases, a reducing plan of **immobilization** is used to secure the bone fragments and protect the fracture, and provide needed motion for healing. For example, a rigid cast can be applied for a few weeks (2 to 4 weeks), then a limited-range hinge-brace could be used to protect the healing structures and initiate physiologic motion within set limits. Depending on the severity of the insult, some fractures may require secure immobilization for extended periods to allow for proper healing.

EFFECTS OF IMMOBILIZATION ON BONE TISSUE

For bone healing to occur, a major goal is to immobilize the fracture site. However, when bone tissue does not receive physiologic loads (ambulation, vertical loads, muscle contractions), the normal remodeling processes are negatively affected. The rate of normal bone remodeling changes when immobilization lasts slightly longer than 1 week.[3] The "turnover" or remodeling of bone during immobilization is characterized by a loss of calcium, resulting in localized bone loss. Immobilization leads to a reduction in the hardness of bone related to the duration of immobilization.[3] By 3 months, bone strength is only 55% to 60% of normal strength.[15] The relationship between soft tissue structures and bone during periods of immobilization reflects the interdependence of muscular contractions, forces acting on joints, compressive loads, circulation (blood flow affecting nutrition), and motion in maintaining bone remodeling equilibrium.

A definite contrast is seen in the care of healing bone tissue. It is necessary to *immobilize* the fracture fragments so healing can occur, yet *minimize the negative effects of immobilization* through the judicious application of progressive motion, exercise, and weight bearing. The length of time needed to regain bone strength after immobilization is considerably longer than the duration of immobilization. Therefore the length of the immobilization is an important component in the overall process of healing bone tissue.

COMPLICATIONS

Occasionally the process of bone healing leads to three distinct complications:

1. Delayed union
2. Nonunion
3. Malunion

In **delayed union,** the dynamic biologic repair processes of bone healing occur at a slower rate than anticipated. Brashear and Raney[2] describe delayed union as clinically detectable when firm callus is not present at 20 weeks (for fractures of the tibia and femur) and at 10 weeks (for fractures of the humerus). An important cause of delayed union is "inadequate or interrupted immobilization."[2] Rehabilitation can significantly affect the healing process either positively or negatively. If therapeutic interventions are begun too soon or too vigorously, then possible delayed union could occur because of excessive motion occurring at the fracture

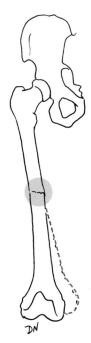

FIG. 7-4 Malunion of the femur. Dotted line indicates normal anatomical alignment.

appreciated. This also allows the physical therapist assistant to understand the degree of tissue healing required before vigorous rehabilitation exercises can be undertaken.

The remarkable sensitivity of bone to normal biologic stress is well known.[1,4,9,13] After fractures, an attempt is made to stabilize the fracture, bring the fragments together by apposition (approximation) and alignment, and remove or minimize forces that may slow the normal healing process. Two general methods of immobilization are used in the treatment of fractures. In one method, the area is immobilized by **external fixation devices.** This method involves the use of casts, traction, splints, and braces and the external fixation devices employed with significant open (compound comminuted) fractures where the risk of infection is present (Fig. 7-5). These rather ominous-looking devices help fix the fracture site while allowing care of the open wounds with skin grafts, tissue flaps, or debridement. These are classified as external fixation devices because the pins used to immobilize the fracture do not contact the fragments directly, but are used to hold the bone segments in rigid alignment and anatomic apposition. With closed (simple) fractures, various rigid lightweight

site. Unfortunately, the trade off when caring for delayed bone union cases is the need to provide extended periods of immobilization for healing. However, cast braces and walking casts can be used to provide the weight bearing (Wolff's law) needed to enhance healing.

In **nonunion,** the healing processes have stopped. Nonunion occurs when there is a significant and severe associated soft tissue trauma, poor blood supply, and infections.

In **malunion,** healing results in a nonanatomic position (Fig. 7-4). Malunion is caused by ineffective immobilization and failure to maintain immobilization for an adequate period of time. For appropriate bone healing to occur, anatomic alignment (apposition) of fragments, adequate fixation (external or internal), and length of time of immobilization must occur in concert. If these factors are not balanced, the chance of complications is increased.

BONE FIXATION DEVICES

When caring for patients who have had fractures, the physical therapist assistant must be aware of various methods used to immobilize or stabilize the fracture so a clear understanding of the extent of trauma can be

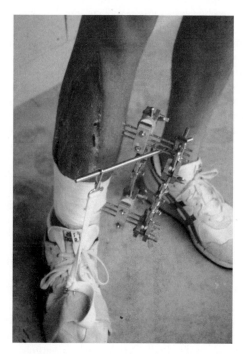

FIG. 7-5 External fixation device (external fixator).

TABLE 7-1

Internal Fixation Devices

TYPE	USE
Compression plate	Diaphyseal fractures
Intramedullary rod	Lower extremity diaphyseal fractures (femur, tibia); removed at 1 or 2 years
Reconstruction plate	Used in pelvis fractures and distal humerus fractures
Tension wires	Patella fractures and olecranon fractures
Sliding hip screws	Intertrochanteric hip fractures
Condylar screws	Distal femur fractures
Cannulated screws	Femoral neck fractures

From Miller M, *Review of orthopaedics*, Philadelphia, 1992, WB Saunders.

fiberglass casts, plaster casts, hinged-plaster casts, and adjustable-range hinged braces are used for immobilization.

The second method of immobilization uses **internal fixation devices** and is best for displaced fractures where external fixation does not provide the degree of immobilization needed to effect healing (See Box 7-1 for the AO classification system). Internal fixation is called **open reduction with internal fixation (ORIF)** and involves surgically exposing the fracture site to reduce, approximate, and align the bone fragments. The materials used for ORIF procedures include metals (stainless steel and metal alloys of cobalt-chromium-molybdenum and titanium) and nonmetals (high-density polyethylene, polymethylmethacrylate, silicones, and ceramics). Metal internal fixation devices are usually combinations of screws, staples, pins, nails, tension-band wires, and various plates. The placement of these materials can affect the delivery of certain therapeutic agents, such as ultrasound. Also, a hole or tunnel defect in a bone with or without a screw in it effectively reduces the overall strength of the bone up to 50%.[9] Even after screw removal, the bone will not regain normal strength for up to a year.[9]

Metal internal fixation devices occasionally loosen and can "back out," as is the case with screws. If the physical therapist assistant notes signs of hardware loosening (pain, swelling, crepitus), he or she must immediately consult with the supervising physical therapist and physician. Many metal fixation devices are designed to be left in place, as with most plates, but these devices may need to be removed if metal allergy reactions occur. Table 7-1 depicts the various internal fixation devices.

CLINICAL APPLICATION OF REHABILITATION TECHNIQUES DURING BONE HEALING

Immobilization after bone injury may not be total. Nonimmobilized structures should be exercised throughout the period of immobilization. For example, a program of lower extremity strengthening and endurance activities (stationary cycle, treadmill, leg extension) should be instituted for patients with upper extremity fractures. The same principle applies for patients with lower extremity fractures. Endurance activities can be either single-leg stationary cycling or upper-body ergometer (UBE) exercises in these cases.

Specific exercises for the injured area frequently involve isometric muscle contractions. Therapeutic exercise programs during bone healing are designed to minimize muscle atrophy while maintaining or improving muscular strength. Muscle contractions provide forces acting to approximate fragments, improve circulation, promote motion to nonimmobilized body parts, and stimulate the piezoelectric effect.

With active range of motion exercises involving the affected limb, the cast or brace serves as resistance in the initial phases. Ankle weights can be applied to the cast or brace for added resistance in later stages. It is best to apply the external resistance superior to the injury site at first, such as in ligament injuries. A more distal application of external force may produce excessive, unwanted shearing, or torque through the fracture site.

Occasionally, electrical muscle stimulation (EMS) is used during cast immobilization to help retard atrophy and maintain strength. A small "window" is cut in the cast to allow the application of the electrodes. The patient is instructed to isometrically contract simultaneously with the electrically evoked muscle contraction. Benefits of electrical stimulation on muscle tissue during immobilization are controversial. The piezoelectric effect is enhanced by applying a negatively charged electrode to stimulate osteoblast activity, which is called *direct current* (any current in which electrons flow in one direction). An externally applied electrode with an external power source is called *inductive coupling*.[9]

In some cases of intraarticular or extraarticular fractures of the tibia and femur, continuous passive motion devices (CPM) are used.[5] Although this appears to conflict with the notion of secure immobilization leading to bone healing, Salter[14] has found positive effects of CPM on the development of chondrocytes and the reduction of intraarticular synovial adhesions when judiciously applied to healing intraarticular fractures.

The goals of rehabilitation programs during immobilization of healing fractures are as follows:

- Improve the overall fitness of the patient
- Promote motion of unaffected, nonimmobilized joints
- Minimize muscle atrophy (isometrics, muscle stimulators)
- Maintain or improve muscular strength
- Protect the healing structures; avoid unwanted, premature, or excessive motion
- Teach safe and effective transfers and gait activities (with cumbersome long-leg plaster casts, or external fixators)

After immobilization, progressive exercise must be directed cautiously. Motion and circulation can be promoted by using various thermal agents. Strengthening exercises should systematically progress through isometrics, concentric and eccentric resistance, isokinetics, and closed kinetic-chain resistance exercises. Balance, coordination, and proprioceptive exercises are also included during the postimmobilization phases of rehabilitation. Stationary cycle ergometers, upper body ergometers, stairclimbers, and treadmills are tools that can enhance cardiorespiratory fitness both during and after immobilization.

REFERENCES

1. Bassett C: Effect of force on skeletal tissue. In Downey JA, Darling RC, editors: *Physiological basis of rehabilitation medicine,* Philadelphia, 1971, WB Saunders.
2. Brashear RH, Raney RB: Fracture principles, fracture healing. In *Handbook of orthopaedic surgery,* St. Louis, 1986, Mosby.
3. Engles M: Tissue Response. In Donatelli R, Wooden MJ, editors: *Orthopedic physical therapy,* New York, 1989, Churchill Livingstone.
4. Guoping L et al: Radiographic and histologic analyses of stress fracture in rabbit tibias, *Am J Sports Med* 13:285-294, 1985.
5. Hamilton HW: Five year's experience with continuous passive motion, *J Bone Joint Surg* 64B(2):259, 1982.
6. Kisner C, Colby LA: *Therapeutic exercise: foundations and techniques,* Philadelphia, 1990, FA Davis.
7. Lewis CB, Bottomley JM: *Geriatric physical therapy: a clinical approach,* New York, 1994, Appleton & Lange.
8. McRae R: *Practical fracture treatment,* New York, 1994, Churchill Livingstone.
9. Miller MD: *Review of orthopaedics,* Philadelphia, 1992, WB Saunders.
10. Morris JM: Fatigue fractures, *Calif Med* 108:268-274, 1968.
11. Rang M: *Children's fractures,* Philadelphia, 1974, JB Lippincott.
12. Rothstein JM, Roy SH, Wolf SL: *The rehabilitation specialists' handbook,* Philadelphia, 1991, FA Davis.
13. Salter RB: *Textbook of disorders and injuries of the musculoskeletal system,* ed 2, Baltimore, 1983, Williams & Wilkins.
14. Salter RB et al: Clinical applications of basic research on continuous passive motion for disorders and injuries of synovial joints. A preliminary report of a feasibility study, *J Orthop Res* 3:325-342, 1983.
15. Steinburg FU: *The immobilized patient: functional pathology and management,* New York, 1980, Plenum Medical Books.

Cartilage Healing

Understanding the mechanisms involved in the healing of articular (**hyaline**) **cartilage** and fibroelastic cartilage promotes the appropriate application of rehabilitation techniques. Therefore rehabilitation techniques are based on the foundation of intrinsic cartilage repair (chondrogenesis), the time required for healing, and extrinsic reparative interventions. **Osteoarthritis** (degenerative joint disease), chondromalacia (softening of hyaline cartilage), meniscal lesions, and many other articular and meniscal pathologic processes are exceedingly common problems the physical therapist assistant will see clinically. Therefore understanding injury and repair of articular cartilage defects and meniscal lesions will help the physical therapist assistant understand the rationale for appropriate rehabilitation techniques.

ARTICULAR CARTILAGE

Composition

Articular cartilage covers the ends of bones with synovial joints. It is composed primarily of water (approximately 65% to 80%),[4,7] which provides for load deformation of the cartilage surface.[8] The tensile strength of articular cartilage depends on type II collagen, which is approximately 20% of the total composition of hyaline cartilage.[11] Proteoglycans contribute 10% to 15% of the structure of articular cartilage. These proteoglycans are made up of glycosaminoglycans, which are in part responsible for bearing the compressive strength of articular cartilage. Finally, **chondrocytes** (mature cartilage cells) make up 5% of the articular cartilage.[8,11]

Function

The viscoelastic structure of articular cartilage, by virtue of its component parts of collagen, water, and proteoglycans, make hyaline cartilage incredibly durable.[8,11] Generally, articular cartilage is only 2 to 4 mm thick, yet it is capable of bearing compressive loads many times greater than body weight.[17] Articular cartilage is extremely resistant to wear, is almost entirely frictionless, and is responsible for influencing and dissipating compression, shear, and tension forces within diarthrodial synovial joints.[8,11,17]

Articular cartilage is also permeable. The chondrocytes within the cartilage must receive nutrition to remain viable. The synovial fluid surrounding the articular cartilage provides the necessary nutrients through joint motion and normal physiologic weight bearing by diffusion, convection, or both.[11] Therefore normal joint motion is needed to maintain the cartilage integrity, fluid movement (lubrication between articulating surfaces), and nutrition of hyaline cartilage.[11]

Injury

Articular cartilage can be damaged in many ways.[11,17] Erosion of the articular surface and degeneration can be seen clinically in patients ranging from young athletes to elderly people. Causes of degenerative joint disease include related joint instability, blunt trauma, repetitive overloading, and immobilization.[17] Articular cartilage degeneration is generally characterized by three progressively overlapping degenerative events (Fig. 8-1).[17] Initially the hyaline cartilage begins to fray or fibrillate. Progressive destruction leads to blistering of the articular surface. Further joint deterioration leads to splitting or clefting (fissuring) of the surface, which affects the deeper layers of cartilage and eventually progresses to denuded bone.[17] Although blunt trauma, progressive friction abrasion, and a sharp concentration of weight-bearing forces mechanically erode articular cartilage causing various degrees of wear, joint immobilization does not cause mechanical changes. However, joint immobilization may lead to loss of the load-bearing structural compression-resistant component proteoglycans (glycosaminoglycans).[11] Such loss is related to decreased normal joint loading (which is needed for cartilage nutrition) and physiologic motion.

Hyaline cartilage erosion can occur after trauma, penetrating injury, infection, or compressive loads, joint immobilization, and reduction of normal joint mechanics. The therapeutic application of exercise and functional activities must be adjusted and modified to minimize the progressive destruction of tissue in patients who have a range of osteoarthritic changes to articular cartilage changes caused by long-term immobilization.

Healing and repair

Articular cartilage defects heal differently, depending on the extent or depth of the injury.[8,11,17] Less serious, more superficial lesions of articular cartilage do not remodel or heal as well as deeper or full-thickness injuries. Healing of these superficial layers occurs through proteoglycans and chondrocyte proliferation, but the strength, composition, and durability of this healing tissue are exceedingly weak and inferior to those of normal articular cartilage.[11]

The reason superficial articular cartilage defects do not heal as well as deeper injuries is that these injuries do not stimulate an inflammatory reaction.[11] The thickness of the articular cartilage (2 to 4 mm) forms a barrier between the superficial layers of the cartilage and subchondral blood vessels, effectively eliminating any contact between fibrin, fibroblasts, and inflammatory response cells (neutrophils, macrophages). In effect, the chondrocytes do not adhere to the defect and they do not fill the injury site with new tissue.

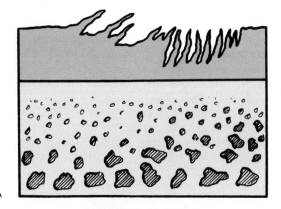

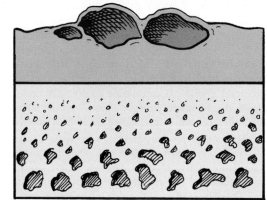

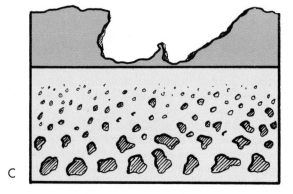

FIG. 8-1 Articular cartilage degeneration is generally characterized by three progressive overlapping stages: **A,** Fibrillation or fraying of articular cartilage; **B,** Blistering of articular surface; **C,** Splitting, clefting, or fissuring of articular surface.

Deeper wounds or full-thickness injuries expose **subchondral bone** blood vessels to the defect site, which stimulates the acute **inflammatory response.** Full-thickness cartilage injuries heal spontaneously with

large amounts of type I collagen (articular cartilage is primarily composed of type II collagen). In fact, 1 year after injury, approximately 20% of the repaired defect remains type I collagen.[11] Although full-thickness injuries heal considerably better than superficial wounds, the quality of the scar formed within the defect remains inferior to normal articular cartilage, and the healed scar does not maintain its integrity over time.[11]

Techniques of stimulating cartilage repair and therapeutic applications. When treating patients recovering from injury, immobilization, or disease of the articular cartilage, appropriate physical therapy measures are those which stimulate cartilage repair.

Arthroscopic surgical shaving of articular cartilage is a common practice in patients with femoral and patellar articular cartilage disease.[5,9] The procedure is designed to remove the loose fibrillated tissue and smooth the articular surface contours. Ideally, removing the irritated tissue lessens the symptoms of pain and dysfunction. Articular cartilage repair is promoted when the injury site can go through the inflammatory process and when factors lead to chondrocyte proliferation. Therefore with some cartilage defects, surgically abrading or drilling multiple small holes (perforating) through the cartilage layers down to bone stimulates bleeding and initiates the healing process.

Noninvasive therapeutic measures are also beneficial in the treatment of articular cartilage injury. Limited weight-bearing activities can arrest symptoms of pain and swelling in some cases of articular cartilage injury. Reducing vertical compressive loads (stairclimbing, squats, walking) is a critical first step in the care of tibiofemoral articular cartilage defects. Patients can maintain strength with isometric exercise or limited open kinetic-chain progressive-resistive exercise.

In cases of patellofemoral articular cartilage disease, vertical compressive loads generally do not negatively affect function. Full range-of-motion knee extension exercises may, however, produce symptoms of pain, swelling, and crepitus (noise, grinding, cracking). With patellofemoral disease, limited range-of-motion exercises that do not produce pain and crepitus, along with isometric exercises, are most appropriate.

As mentioned in Chapter 6 (Ligament healing), **continuous passive motion (CPM)** is used in the care of articular cartilage injury. Again, the benefits from the use of CPM are limited to full-thickness hyaline cartilage defects.[13,14] Salter et al[13,14] demonstrated that CPM used on full-thickness cartilage injury in rabbits showed healing of the defect with tissue resembling hyaline cartilage. Salter and associates,[12-14] who believe that CPM can help stimulate chondrocyte formation, also found that using CPM with full-thickness hyaline cartilage injuries improves articular cartilage nutrition by enhancing fluid mechanics, inhibiting adhesions, and clearing the joint of noxious material.

Maintaining near-normal joint motion through modified exercise regimens and weight-bearing activities (depending on the location and severity of the articular defect) are necessary both for healing of cartilage injuries and for maintenance of hyaline cartilage nutrition.

MENISCUS (FIBROELASTIC CARTILAGE)

Understanding **meniscus injury and repair** is a necessary foundation for the appropriate delivery of rehabilitation programs. The physical therapist assistant must also be aware of the differences in healing between articular cartilage and **fibroelastic** (meniscus) **cartilage.**

Composition

Fibroclastic cartilage is found within the synovial joints of the acromioclavicular joint, sternoclavicular joint, glenohumeral joint, hip, and knee. A large percentage of fibroelastic cartilage is water,[8] whereas a major constituent of meniscal tissue is collagen. Meniscal tissue contains four types of collagen:[1] type I collagen comprises about 90%, whereas types II, V, and VI account for 1% to 2% each in the total collagen in the meniscus. Proteoglycans and elastin (0.6%) complete the components of fibroelastic cartilage.[1]

Function

The menisci of the knee are semilunar (C-shaped) fibroelastic tissues that have several functions. Generally, the meniscus dissipates extreme compressive (vertical) loads. By virtue of its anatomic position within the knee and its collagen make up, the meniscus acts as a mechanical buffer between the load-bearing surfaces of the tibia and the femur. The meniscus of the knee also functions as a shock absorber.[1] Studies have shown that a knee without a meniscus has 20% less shock-absorbing capacity than normal knees.[19] Total **meniscectomy** (complete removal), subtotal meniscectomy (partial removal), and repair (suturing of torn parts) are discussed in the section on orthopedic management beginning on page 166. The concept of partial removal and repair of the meniscus is in part founded on maintaining as much viable tissue as possible to serve in load bearing, shock absorption, joint stability, and lubrication.

The meniscus functions as a secondary restraint in joint stability. Several factors influence its effect, including ligament stability, joint surface congruency, and joint compression loads.[1] With an isolated, total meniscec-

tomy, significant joint instability does not occur. However, a meniscectomy combined with anterior cruciate-ligament injuries produces profound joint instability.[16]

The meniscus also limits knee hyperextension as a passive restraint and functions in joint lubrication and nutrition.[6] Normal physiologic joint motion promotes the lubricating effects of a thin layer of fluid between the joint surfaces. The meniscus may spread this lubrication medium during motion.[10]

Injury

Injuries to the meniscus can either be traumatic or degenerative. Traumatic intraarticular fibrocartilage tears usually occur in a younger population (less than 40) and generally result from a combination of compression, torque, acceleration, or deceleration. These events usually occur during running, jumping, twisting, and dynamic change-of-direction activities.

Degenerative meniscal tears typically occur in an older population (greater than 40). These injuries do not present with a history of sudden trauma, but rather with a minor event that precipitates complaints of pain and dysfunction.[1]

Healing

The vascular anatomy of the meniscus profoundly influences the type of healing that occurs as well as the degree of remodeling, such as with articular cartilage. The peripheral borders of the medial and lateral meniscus of the knee are vascularized between 10% and 30% of the width of the tissue.[1] If an injury occurs within a nonvascular region of the meniscus, spontaneous, intrinsic repair is not possible because no vascular supply communicates with the injury site. If, however, the injury extends to the periphery where the cartilage is vascularized, then healing is possible through the inflammatory-response mechanism.

Surgical repair or excision of meniscal tissue is based on the extent of the injury and whether the injury is located within a vascularized area. If the tear is within the vascularized peripheral border (only 15% to 20% of all meniscal injuries occur within the vascularized bed of the meniscus), then arthroscopic repair can be done by placing sutures in the meniscus to approximate the torn tissue.[1] Surgeons refer to a zone system of evaluating meniscal injuries, as follows:[3]

Zone I   Both portions of the meniscus are torn within the vascularized periphery; **"red-on-red"**

Zone II   One portion of the meniscus is torn within the vascularized periphery, while the other portion is in the avascular region; **"red-on-white"**

Zone III   No blood supply on either side of the injury; **"white-on-white"**

Both red-on-red and red-on-white zones are considered reparable. However, in animal studies,[2] if an injury is present within the white-on-white nonvascularized Zone III area of the meniscus, researchers surgically create a **"vascular access channel"** to connect the blood supply of the periphery to the area of injury without circulation.[1,3] This study shows that the blood vessels migrated to the injury site and provided an avenue for repair.

When injuries occur in an avascular portion of the meniscus, the surgeon must perform either a subtotal (partial removal) or total meniscectomy. After either of these procedures, some studies have shown partial or complete regeneration of fibrocartilaginous tissue.[1] However, for the regeneration of tissue to occur after a meniscectomy, the tissue must be removed to expose the vascular synovium.[1]

Arnoczky et al[1] state, "Thus it appears that the synovial and peripheral meniscal vasculatures are capable of generating a connective tissue replacement for the removed meniscus. It should be noted, however, that this regeneration is not always complete and does not occur in all cases."

Clinical application of rehabilitation techniques after meniscal injury

The mechanics of meniscal injury, surgical repairs, meniscectomies, and criteria-based programs are covered in Chapter 13. However, an understanding of how and why fibroelastic cartilage responds to a repair procedure versus a meniscectomy and how these procedures affect the course of rehabilitation is clinically relevant to the physical therapist assistant.

In general terms, after a subtotal or total meniscectomy, treatment focuses on pain management, reduction in swelling, improved range of motion, normalized gait, increased strength, increased girth of the thigh musculature, development of aerobic fitness, and improved proprioception. With a meniscectomy patient, range-of-motion exercises (active, active assistive) can be instituted immediately and progressed according to the patient's tolerance. Weight bearing should progress in the same manner.[15] Usually full weight-bearing is used within 10 days of surgery.[15] Stationary cycling, isometric exercise progressing to concentric and eccentric resistance exercise, and progressive closed kinetic-chain exercises can be initiated when pain, swelling, and strength allow. Gaining full range of motion and progressive weight bearing does not alter or inhibit the healing processes after a meniscectomy, depending on whether or not there is any associated articular cartilage defect.

The rehabilitation program after meniscal repair has the same long-range goals (reduced pain and swelling, progressive motion, strength, and progressive weight bearing) as for a meniscectomy patient, but its implementation must be altered, taking into account the initiation of weight bearing and range-of-motion exercises in relation to the healing process of a repaired meniscus.[3,15] In a surgically repaired meniscus, if full or even partial weight bearing is progressed too soon, the compressive forces and load bearing mechanics during gait disrupt the healing processes.[2,3] Full weight bearing is generally not allowed until 4 to 6 weeks after surgery.[15] However, toe-touch weight bearing may be allowed at 3 weeks and progressive partial weight bearing 4 to 5 weeks after surgery.

Range of motion can also influence the healing of a repaired meniscus. If full flexion is allowed too early, the motion created within the knee may place "undue stress upon the sutures and the repair site."[3] Therefore range-of-motion activities must progress cautiously until secure healing of the sutured meniscus has occurred.

The contrasts in rehabilitation programs between those used for meniscectomies and those used for repaired (sutured) meniscus are founded on the nature and disposition of healing mechanics related to forces acting on the meniscus (weight bearing and range of motion), time, and the vascular supply supporting the healing tissues. Strengthening exercises can be initiated if they progress gradually from isometrics, to multi-angle isometrics, to open kinetic-chain exercises, to isokinetics, and finally to closed-chain resistance exercises.

Many rehabilitation programs are organized in phases (maximum protection phase, moderate protection phase, minimum protection phase), which are developed in part to minimize unwanted forces on healing tissues.[18] For meniscal injuries, phased programs allow for continued clinical assessment of a patient's progress while restraining unnecessary motion and weight bearing and allowing for proper, secure healing.

REFERENCES

1. Arnoczky SP et al: Meniscus. In Buschbacher JA, Woo SL-Y editors: *Injury and repair of the musculoskeletal soft tissues,* Rosemont, Ill, 1988, American Academy of Orthopaedic Surgeons.
2. Arnoczky SP, Warren RF: The microvasculature of the meniscus and it's response to injury: an experimental study in the dog, *Am J Sports Med* 11:131-141, 1983.
3. Hammesfahr JR: Surgery of the knee. In Donatelli R, Wooden MJ editors: *Orthopaedic physical therapy,* 1989, Churchill Livingston.
4. Jaffe FF et al: Water binding in the articular cartilage of rabbits, *J Bone Joint Surg* 56A: 1031-1039, 1974.
5. Johnson LL: *Diagnostic and surgical arthroscopy,* St. Louis, 1980, Mosby.
6. MacConaill MA: The function of intra-articular fibrocartilages, with special reference to the knee and inferior radio-ulnar joints, *J Anat* 66:210-227, 1932.

7. Mankin HJ: The water of articular cartilage. In Simon WH, editor: *The human joint in health and disease,* Philadelphia, 1978, University of Pennsylvania Press.

8. Miller MD: *Review of orthopaedics,* Philadelphia, 1992, WB Saunders.

9. O'Donoghue DH: Treatment of chondral damage to the patella, *Am J Sports Med* 9:10-12, 1981.

10. Radin EL, Bryan RS: The effect of weight bearing on regrowth of the medial meniscus after meniscectomy, *J Trauma* 12:169, 1970.

11. Rosenberg L et al: Articular cartilage. In Woo SL-Y, Buckwalter JA, editors: *Injury and repair of the musculoskeletal soft tissues,* Rosemont, Ill., 1988, American Academy of Orthopaedic Surgeons.

12. Salter RB et al: Clinical applications of basic research on continuous passive motion for disorders and injuries of synovial joints: a preliminary report of a feasibility study, *J Orthop Res* 3:325-342, 1983.

13. Salter RB et al: Continuous passive motion and the repair of full-thickness articular cartilage defects: a one year follow-up, *Trans Orthop Res Soc* 7: 167, 1982.

14. Salter RB et al: The biological effect of continuous passive motion on healing of full-thickness defects in articular cartilage: an experimental study in the rabbit, *J Bone Joint Surg* 62A:1232-1251, 1980.

15. Seto JL, Brewster CE: Rehabilitation of meniscal injuries. In Greenfield BH, editor: *Rehabilitation of the knee: a problem-solving approach,* Philadelphia, 1993, FA Davis.

16. Shoemaker SC, Markolf KL: The role of the meniscus in the anterior-posterior cruciate-deficient knee, *J Bone Joint Surg* 68A:71-79, 1986.

17. Threlkeld JA: Electrical stimulation of articular cartilage. In Currier DP, Nelson RM, editors: *Dynamics of human biologic tissues,* Philadelphia, 1992, FA Davis.

18. Timm KE: Knee. In Richardson JK, Iglarsch ZA, editors: *Clinical orthopaedic physical therapy,* Philadelphia, 1994, WB Saunders.

19. Voloshin AS, Wosk J: Shock absorption of meniscectomized and painful knees: a comparative in vivo study, *J Biomed Eng* 5:157-161, 1983.

Muscle and Tendon Healing

Injuries to muscle and tendon are common, clinically significant conditions treated with physical therapy procedures. The physical therapist assistant must recognize the different types of injuries that occur to muscle, tendon, and the musculotendinous junction, and must appreciate how these specific tissues respond to injury and immobilization. A general understanding of injury, healing response mechanisms, and the effects of muscle position during immobilization will guide the choice of therapeutic interventions to enhance recovery and minimize the deleterious effects of immobilization.

MUSCLE

Definitions

When treating patients recovering from injury to muscle, it is wise to clarify the exact nature of the original injury. The mechanisms of injury, the specific tissue response to the insult, and the rationale for rehabilitation will become focused and the purpose of rehabilitation techniques will be clarified.

Previously, a **sprain** was defined as an injury to ligament tissue. A **strain** refers to an injury involving muscle and tendon tissue. It may also be referred to as a pulled muscle or a muscle tear.[10] **Microtrauma** injuries resulting in pain and dysfunction are called **overuse** injuries.[18] Although not entirely related to just muscle and tendon tissue, *overuse* is a term frequently used to describe repetitive microtrauma injury to muscle and tendon.

In an **indirect muscle injury** the muscle or, more commonly, the musculotendinous junction[10] becomes injured by a sudden stretch or concentric, or eccentric muscle contraction. Also included in the definition of indirect muscle injury is delayed onset muscle soreness (DOMS) (see Chapter 3). Indirect strains are classified as either complete or incomplete tears.[10] **Direct muscle injury** refers to lacerations, surgical incisions, contusions, or blunt trauma. Clinically, both direct and indirect musculotendinous injuries are seen. Occasionally, severe contusions to muscle result in bone deposits within the muscle tissue, producing myositis ossificans. If the injury extends deeply enough to contuse bone, periosteal or heterotopic bone (bone tissue separate from the underlying contused bone) can form within the muscle.[10]

Injury and healing

Muscle tissue heals by acute, intense inflammatory response. The highly vascular and innervated nature of muscle is very conducive to repair and healing. In addition, with most muscle injuries, the speed at which the tissue is repaired is directly related to the degree of vascularity within the injury site during the repair phase of healing.[17] When a blunt trauma to a muscle (**contusion**) occurs, an acute inflammatory response creates connective tissue scarring; strength loss and dysfunction result.[4] When muscle lacerations and surgical incisions occur, muscle tissue tends to heal with dense connective scar tissue.[11] To minimize this scar tissue and achieve more normal functioning, the muscle tissue must be in near anatomic approximation.

Incomplete muscle tears are clinically much more common than **complete muscle tears.**[10] Sudden stretching, rapid, eccentric muscle loading, running, jumping, and dynamic change-of-direction activities can lead to various muscular strains.

Animal studies have shown that after an incomplete muscle tear, hemorrhage, edema, fibroblasts, and granulation tissue are present within 4 days.[20] Scar tissue forms at 1 week with a resultant decrease in the muscle's ability to generate active force during the initial stages of healing.

Clinically, the musculotendinous junction appears to be much more susceptible to indirect, incomplete muscle strain than the muscle belly is.[10] In addition, eccentric muscle contractions are a frequent cause of indirect muscle strains.

Effects of immobilization

Perhaps the most profound change in human skeletal muscle during **immobilization** is **atrophy.** The degree of atrophy depends on both the duration of immobilization and the position or stretch imposed on the muscle.[4,9,10] When a muscle is immobilized in a shortened position, it may atrophy more than muscle casted in a lengthened position. Sarcomeres decrease up to 40% in muscles immobilized in the shortened position.[22] However, sarcomere numbers are replaced when immobilization is ended.[22] Muscles that are immobilized in a shortened position are also less extensible after cast removal than muscles immobilized in a stretched position. Finally, muscles immobilized in a shortened position undergo far greater rates of protein degradation than muscle casted in a passive tension, or stretched position.[13]

Muscle fiber types are also affected by position during immobilization. When muscles are immobilized in a shortened position, type I muscle fibers (slow twitch—"red"— oxidative) atrophy (decrease in both number of fibers and fiber diameter) far more than type II fibers (fast twitch—white —glycolytic).[16] When a large percentage of type I muscle fibers atrophy during periods of immobilization, the relative number of type II fibers increases.[23]

Conversely, muscles immobilized in a lengthened position demonstrate an increase in sarcomere numbers up to 20% after 4 weeks of immobilization.[22] Protein synthesis also increases. Generally, muscles immobilized in a shortened position experience accelerated atrophy (type I fibers), decreased numbers of sarcomeres, reduced protein synthesis, and decreased oxidative and anaerobic enzyme levels.

Muscle atrophy also results in a decrease in muscle weight.[7] Muscle that has atrophied and lost weight also loses its ability to generate force and tension.[7] The greatest amount of atrophy occurs within 1 week of immobilization, and muscle fiber size decreases by approximately 17% within 3 days of immobilization.[3] Box 9-1 depicts the various physiologic changes that occur in skeletal muscle during immobilization.

Clinical applications of rehabilitation techniques on skeletal muscle during recovery and immobilization

The healing response of muscle is far greater than bone, ligament, or tendon tissue due to the highly vascular makeup of human skeletal muscle.[7] Specific rehabilitation programs directed at maintaining muscular strength and minimizing atrophy during prolonged periods of immobilization attempt to enhance and magnify intrinsic muscular repair.

Typically, isometric muscle contractions are initiated during immobilization. However, Gould et al[15] described a protocol involving 400 maximal isometric contractions with normal healthy subjects casted for 2 weeks. The results of their program showed no attenuating effect on loss of strength. Other studies have shown beneficial effects of isometrics on reducing strength loss during immobilization.[21] Gould et al,[14] in a later study, demonstrated that a protocol of electrical muscle stimulation for 16 hours per day during immobilization reduced the negative effects of atrophy and loss of strength in patients after open meniscectomy.

Combination protocols involving maximal voluntary isometric muscle contractions, with electrically evoked muscle stimulation, appear to provide more consistent results than either isometrics or muscle stimulation alone.[2,8] The effects of electrical muscle stimulation and isometric contractions during immobilization may retard disuse atrophy, reduce strength losses, and minimize the loss of aerobic oxidative enzymes (succinic dehydrogenase).[2,14,15,21]

Concentric and eccentric dynamic muscle contractions can also be used during immobilization, provided a range-limiting hinged cast-brace is used. As previously stated, muscles that are immobilized in a lengthened position increase in muscle weight and protein synthesis. Therefore stretching immobilized muscle along with using hinged cast-braces, combined isometric muscle contractions, and electrically evoked muscle contractions may promote strength while minimizing atrophy during immobilization.[2]

Recovery from muscle injury (direct or indirect) not related to immobilization is directed at reducing pain (oral analgesics), eliminating swelling (nonsteroidal anti-inflammatory drugs, ice, elevation, Ace wraps), and improving function. Once the acute inflammatory phase is controlled, ice packs, elastic compression bandages, elevation, and gentle isometric muscle contractions are applied. Depending on the severity of injury, gentle active range-of-motion activities can be initiated during the early repair phase of healing. With severe muscle contusions, it is wise to avoid progressive motion, massage, heat, or exercise early in the rehabilitation program. Myositis ossificans may develop with vigorous activity. In these cases, rest, ice, elevation, medications, and the delayed judicious use of motion, exercise, and thermal agents are recommended.

Progressive isometric muscle contractions (i.e., weighted straight-leg raises) or isometric static holds with resistance can be initiated soon after many direct and indirect muscle strains. Once pain and motion improve, concentric and eccentric resistance exercise and isokinetics can begin. With most unilateral muscle injuries, the patient is instructed in general aerobic, strength, and flexibility programs that do not compromise the healing processes of the injured structures.

With all direct and indirect muscle strains, the timing for applying motion and resistance exercise, and the intensity of effort, must be specific to each patient. The degree of injury, which structures are involved, repair (intrinsic regeneration, scar formation, or surgical repair), and pain tolerance will strongly influence the rehabilitation protocol. Relatively minor muscle strains heal spontaneously with conservative treatment, consist-

BOX 9-1   Effects of Immobilization on Skeletal Muscle Tissue (Shortened)
Muscle atrophy
(Type I)
Sarcomeres decreased
Increased protein breakdown
Decreased muscle extensibility following immobilization
Decreased muscle weight
Decreased force generating capacity
Increase in connective tissue
Decreased anaerobic glycolytic enzymes
Decreased aerobic oxidative enzymes

ing of ice, compression wraps, elevation, gentle, active motion, isometrics progressing to isotonic and isokinetic exercise, and finally closed chain functional activities.

More severe muscle injuries may require longer periods of rest, ice, compression, and elevation along with delayed yet progressive motion, exercise, gait, and functional activities. Box 9-2 describes various therapeutic techniques used for immobilization and healing skeletal muscle injuries.

TENDON

Because tendon attaches to bone via muscle, the two structures are interrelated and are frequently injured together (i.e., musculotendinous junction muscle strains). However, a number of injuries seen clinically involve isolated tendon pathologic processes (**tendinitis,** Achilles tendon ruptures).

Tendon receives its blood supply generally from the musculotendinous junction, synovium, periosteal attachments, and the length of the tendon itself.[6,19] The tendon-bone interface and musculotendinous junction provide nutrition to the distal third of the tendon.[6] The midportion of the tendon receives its blood supply primarily from the synovial sheath or paratendon.[6]

Response to injury

Tendons heal through three organized stages: inflammation, repair, and remodeling.[12] Inflammation occurs during the 72 hours after injury, whereas collagen synthesis and fibroblasts are arranged in a random, disorganized fashion over the 1 to 4 weeks after injury.[12]

Curwin and Stanish[6] cite Chavapil[5] for further classification and organization of tendon healing into four stages:

1. Cell mobilization
2. Ground substance proliferation
3. Collagen protein formation
4. Final organization

Tendons have both an intrinsic and an extrinsic capacity to heal.[12] Therefore tendons can heal spontaneously from the formation of **tenocytes** (tendon cells) and from fibroblasts and vascular-inflammatory response mechanisms from adjacent tissues.[12]

When tendons are injured to the degree that a gap disrupts the normal anatomic continuity, collagen, granulation tissue, and fibroblasts migrate to the gap and fill it with scar tissue. The process of tendon healing depends largely on the degree of injury, the degree or contribution of vascular-inflammatory response from other structures, the amount of mobilization or immobilization after injury, and whether surgical repair was needed to approximate the torn tissue to obliterate the gap.

Tendon healing is a slow process requiring periods of rest as well as limited, controlled stress to develop strength. Gelbermann et al[12] report that between 21 and 42 days after injury, fibroblasts are vigorously reorienting along the long axis of the tendon to form dense connective tissue. Complete maturation of tendon scar appears 112 days after injury.[12]

Although tendons possess the capacity to heal, ultimately healed tendon is not strong enough to keep the torn tissue together.[12] Thus while minor tendon strains (incomplete) may be able to heal nicely, more severe tendon injury (Achilles tendon rupture) may require surgical repair for increased strength.

The fundamental concept behind suture repair of torn tendon is to minimize scar formation by using sutures to close or repair the gap. In response to surgical repair of the tendon, Miller[19] reports, "Tendon repairs are weakest at 7-10 days, they regain a majority of their original strength at 21 to 28 days, and achieve maximal strength in 6 months."

BOX 9-2 Therapeutic Interventions During Immobilization and Healing of Skeletal Muscle		
Immobilization	**Indirect muscle strains, muscle pulls, or tears**	**Direct muscle injury, lacerations, blunt trauma incisions**
TREATMENT	*TREATMENT*	*TREATMENT*
Isometric muscle contractions (10 sec hold) in combination with electrically evoked muscle contractions. Stretch immobilized muscle if possible. Aerobic, strength, and flexibility programs for general fitness. Perform concentric-eccentric muscle contractions with hinged cast-braces if possible. Weight bearing as tolerated.	Rest. Ice. Compression. Elevation. Gentle, active ROM, progressive exercise. Isometrics, Isotonics, Isokinetics. Stationary cycle. Weight bearing as tolerated. NSAIDs. Do not overstretch muscles too soon after injury. Allow for scar formation—regeneration of muscle tissue. General fitness program.	RICE. Weight bearing as tolerated. Gentle isometrics. Active ROM. General fitness programs. NSAIDs. *CAUTION:* Progress very gradually with severe muscle contusions. Progressive-resistive exercise. Concentric-eccentric isotonic and isokinetic exercise. Allow for scar formation. No vigorous motion during acute phase or early repair phase.

Effects of motion and immobilization

As with other musculoskeletal tissues, long-term negative effects occur with immobilization of the tendon. Overall tensile strength is decreased, proteoglycans (glycosaminoglycans) are significantly reduced, and water content of tendon is severely compromised.[1,24] Conversely, stress and exercise produce increased tensile strength, stiffness, and increased collagen size.[24]

Historically it was felt that early motion after tendon injury and repair produced gap formation, accelerated adhesion formation, delayed collagen maturation, increased scar size, and disorganized collagen and fibroblast formation.[12] Miller[19] suggests that early motion provides increased motion but decreased tendon strength. Conversely, immobilization creates improved strength of the tendon but with less motion. Periods of immobilization also reduce tendon-bone junction strength.[19]

Early, limited, **protected motion** appears to provide greater tensile strength, less adhesion formation, and earlier organization, orientation, and remodeling of collagen, and it does not contribute significantly to gap formation.[12] The degree of motion (excursion within the tendon sheath) after injury and repair must be slight with protection from excessive stress, which would be detrimental to healing.

Clinical applications of rehabilitation techniques during tendon healing

Rehabilitation protocols during tendon healing reflect the extent of injury and indicate whether or not surgical repair and immobilization were used. Tendinitis is a common clinical pathologic process; generally, treatment focuses on pain management and reduction of swelling and involves RICE and nonsteroidal anti-inflammatory medications and physical therapy. Gradually a course of gentle stretching with resistive exercise emphasizing eccentric muscle contractions is used.[6] Some type of limited protection may be needed to avoid excessive, unwanted motion, and factors that exacerbate the pain are removed. For example, with patellar tendinitis (jumper's knee) it may be necessary to limit running and jumping activities; with bicipital tendinitis, it may be necessary to avoid overhead motions; and with tennis elbow (lateral epicondylitis), it may be wise to avoid using hand tools, playing tennis, or generally engaging in excessive wrist flexion, extension, pronation, and supination. Surgery and subsequent immobilization are quite rare as treatment. Naturally, modifications in activities are needed to reduce pain, but total cessation of activity is not usually needed. Many activi-

ties that cause pain can be removed and supplemented with other activities that do not cause pain. Specific tendon pathologies and comprehensive rehabilitation programs are covered in detail in later chapters.

More severe tendon injuries requiring surgical repair (although ruptured Achilles tendons may be casted instead of surgical repair in some cases) and subsequent periods of limited immobilization require judicious application of stress, exercise, weight bearing, and pain and swelling management. If stress (stretching and exercise) is added too soon or too vigorously after surgical repair or long periods of immobilization, stretching out of the repair and possible reinjury could occur.

REFERENCES

1. Akeson WH: An experimental study of joint stiffness, *J Bone Joint Surg* 43A:1022-1034, 1961.
2. Behm D: Debilitation to adaptation, *J Strength Cond Res* 7(2):65-75, 1993.
3. Booth FW, Seider MJ: Recovery of skeletal muscle after three months of hindlimb immobilization in rats, *J Appl Physiol* 47:435-439, 1979.
4. Caplan A et al: Skeletal muscle. In Woo SL-Y, Buckwalter JA, editors: *Injury and repair of the musculoskeletal soft tissues,* Rosemont, Ill., 1988, American Academy of Orthopaedic Surgeons.
5. Chavapil M: Physiology of connective tissue, Newton, Mass., 1967, Butterworth.
6. Curwin S, Stanish WD: *Tendinitis: it's etiology and treatment,* Lexington, Mass., 1984, Collamore Press, DC Heath.
7. Engles M: Tissue response. In Donatelli R, Wooden MJ, editors: *Orthopaedic physical therapy,* New York, 1989, Churchill Livingstone.
8. Eriksson E, Haggmark T: Comparison of isometric muscle training and electrical stimulation supplementing isometric muscle training in the recovery after major knee ligament surgery, *Am J Sports Med* 7(3):169-171, 1979.
9. Fitts RH, Brimmer CJ: Recovery in skeletal muscle contractile function after prolonged hind limb immobilization, *J Appl Physiol* 59:916-923, 1985.
10. Garrett W, Tidball J: Myotendinous junction: structure function, and failure. In Woo SL-Y, Buckwalter JA, editors: *Injury and repair of the musculoskeletal soft tissues,* Rosemont, Ill., 1988, American Academy of Orthopaedic Surgeons.
11. Garrett WE et al: Recovery of skeletal muscle after laceration and repair, *J Hand Surg* 9A:683-692, 1984.
12. Gelbermann R et al: Tendon. In Woo SL-Y, Buckwalter JA, editors: *Injury and repair of the musculoskeletal soft tissues,* Rosemont, Ill., 1988, American Academy of Orthopaedic Surgeons.

13. Goldspink DF: The influence of immobilization and stretch on protein turnover of rat skeletal muscle, *J Physiol* 264:267-282, 1977.

14. Gould N et al: Transcutaneous muscle stimulation to retard disuse atrophy after open meniscectomy, *Clin Orthop* 178:190-197, 1983.

15. Gould N et al: Transcutaneous muscle stimulation as a method to retard disuse atrophy, *Clin Ortho Rel Res* 164:215-220, 1982.

16. Halkjaer-Kristensen J, Ingemann-Hansen T: Wasting of the human quadriceps muscle after knee ligament injuries: II muscle fibre morphology, *Scand J Rehab Med* 13:12-20, 1985.

17. Järvinen M: Healing of a crush injury in rat striated muscle, *Acta Pathol Microbiol Scand* 142:47-56, 1976.

18. Johanson MA, Donatelli R, Greenfield BH: Rehabilitation of microtrauma injuries. In *Rehabilitation of the knee: a problem-solving approach,* Philadelphia, 1993, FA Davis.

19. Miller MD: *Review of orthopaedics,* Philadelphia, 1991, WB Saunders.

20. Nikolaou PK et al: Biomechanical and histological evaluation of muscle after controlled strain injury, *Am J Sports Med* 15:9-14, 1987.

21. Rozier CK, Elder JD, Brown M: Prevention of atrophy by isometric exercise of a casted Leg, *J Sports Med Phys Fitness* 19:191-194, 1979.

22. Tabary JC et al: Physiological and structural changes in the cat's soleus muscle due to immobilization at different lengths by plaster casts, *J Physiol* 224:231-244, 1972.

23. Tomanck RJ, Lund DD: Degeneration of different types of skeletal muscle fibers: II. Immobilization, *J Anat* 118:531-541, 1974.

24. Woo SL-Y et al: Mechanical properties of tendons and ligaments: II. The relationships of immobilization and exercise on tissue remodeling, *Biorheology* 19:397-408, 1982.

Gait and Joint Mobilization

In this section, the physical therapist assistant will be introduced to rudimentary concepts and compulsory scientific principles related to gait mechanics and peripheral joint mobilization techniques.

A basic, yet essential, component of orthopedic physical therapy management is the instruction and application of proper gait techniques following injury or disease of the musculoskeletal system. In order to safely and properly instruct patients in the use of assistive devices and to effectively apply fundamental gait techniques, the PTA must understand the components of the gait cycle and be able to instruct patients in appropriate gait patterns and identify deviations in gait. Therefore this section will clarify and describe the gait cycle, and introduce basic terms, definitions, and concepts. In addition, the PTA will be introduced to proper gait-pattern instruction, weight-bearing status, and the identification of gait abnormalities.

It is clinically relevant to clearly state that the delegation of selected mobilization techniques is entirely at the discretion of the physical therapist, and the application of peripheral joint mobilization is not universally accepted as a routine domain of clinical practice for the PTA. Therefore the information concerning peripheral joint mobilization is provided as a means of stimulating the PTA's awareness of the rationale for improving motion and for the reduction of pain as identified and prescribed by the physical therapist.

Fundamentals of Gait

KEY TERMS

Gait
Base of support
Center of gravity
Step length
Cadence
Stride length
Stance phase
Swing phase
Double support
Single support
Pelvic "list"
Heel strike
Foot flat
Midstance
Heel off
Toe off
Acceleration
Midswing
Deceleration
Antalgic gait
Steppage gait
Trendelenburg gait
Abductor "lurch"
Calcaneal gait
Four-point gait pattern
Three-point gait pattern
Two-point gait pattern
Nonweight-bearing
   (NWB)
Partial weight-bearing
   (PWB)
Touch down
   weight-bearing
   (TDWB)
Toe touch
   weight-bearing
   (TTWB)
Weight bearing as
   tolerated (WBAT)
Full weight-bearing
   (FWB)

Instructing patients concerning the appropriate use of assistive devices after orthopedic trauma requires an understanding of normal human locomotion as well as the ability to identify subtle deviations and abnormalities in gait. The physical therapist assistant is frequently assigned tasks related to instruction, supervision, and progression of various factors related to gait. To safely and effectively instruct patients in gait mechanics and to readily identify variations and deviations in gait, critical analysis of the individual components of the entire gait cycle, as well as the application of gait mechanics as they relate to function, is required. The physical therapist assistant must be able to accurately identify changes in a patient's gait pattern and articulate these changes to the physical therapist.

BASIC GAIT TERMS, DEFINITIONS, AND CONCEPTS

Normal, human locomotion requires a cyclic, coordinated pattern of motion focused on minimizing energy expenditure.[3] Certain factors are required for a normal, synchronous walking pattern. These factors include an adequate base of support, appropriate foot clearance during swing, adequate step length, and conservation of energy.[3] Although these factors are common components of walking, unique differences are seen in everyone's walking pattern or style.

Gait describes various styles of walking.[2] For example, some people have short, quick steps with very little trunk motion, while others may demonstrate long, slow strides with excessive arm swing and trunk motion.

A person's **base of support** provides both balance and stability to maintain an erect posture.[1] The base of support is the distance between a person's feet while standing and during ambulation. A wide base of support provides greater stability than a narrow base of support.

A person's **center of gravity** is approximately 5 cm anterior to the second sacral vertebra.[1] The center of gravity changes both vertically and horizontally during gait. The center of gravity during gait also contributes to balance and stability. A lower center of gravity (such as that while squatting) provides greater stability than a higher center of gravity (such as that while standing on the toes).

When describing a *gait cycle* (Fig. 10-1) (defined as the mechanical activity that occurs when foot contact is made with the ground and when the same foot contacts the ground again),[2] it is important to view each component separately. **Step length** describes the linear distance between the right and left foot during gait. Generally, this distance is measured from heel-to-toe contact with the ground of one foot to heel or toe contact with the ground of the opposite foot. **Cadence** refers to the total number of steps per minute. Normal cadence is between 70 and 120 steps or 90 and 130 steps per minute.[1,2]

Stride length is synonymous with the gait cycle. Leg length obviously influences the magnitude of stride length. Individuals with longer legs demonstrate longer stride lengths. Persons with shorter legs have a smaller stride length. Average values for stride length range from 70 to 82 cm.[1]

The **stance phase** of gait represents approximately 60% of the entire gait cycle (Fig. 10-1). Stance phase begins when foot contact is made with the ground and lasts until the same foot leaves the ground.[1,2,5]

The **swing phase** of gait occupies approximately 40% of the gait cycle (Fig. 10-1). During this phase, one limb is entirely nonweight-bearing; it applies throughout the gait cycle.

Double support represents the time within the gait cycle in which both feet are in contact with the ground and weight transfer occurs from one foot to the other.[1] **Single support** is defined as that time during the stance phase when only one foot is in contact with the ground.[1,2]

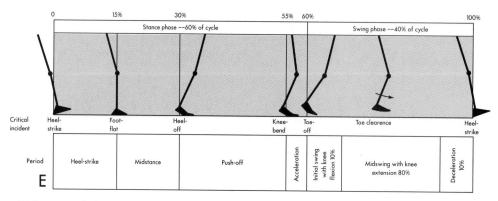

FIG. 10-1 Gait cycle. (From Tachdjian MO: *Pediatric orthopaedics,* ed 2, Philadelphia, 1990, WB Saunders).

Additional elements

In addition to the obvious contribution of the lower limbs to gait, other body parts also play a role in gait mechanics. During normal gait, the pelvis rotates approximately 8 degrees within the transverse plane of the body. This 8-degree rotation is broken down as 4 degrees of rotation to the right and 4 degrees of rotation to the left.[1] Pelvic rotation lengthens the femur during the swing phase through initial foot contact and helps to minimize vertical trunk displacement during gait to conserve energy.

The pelvis also rotates within the frontal plane of the body during gait, which is termed **pelvic "list."** This creates a downward motion of the pelvis of approximately 5 degrees on the nonweight-bearing limb during stance. The "listing" of the pelvis creates adduction of the weight-bearing limb and abduction of the nonweight-bearing limb, thereby improving the efficiency of the hip-abductor mechanism (Fig. 10-2).

The trunk, arms, and shoulders also rotate to ensure balance and stability during gait. Knee flexion in

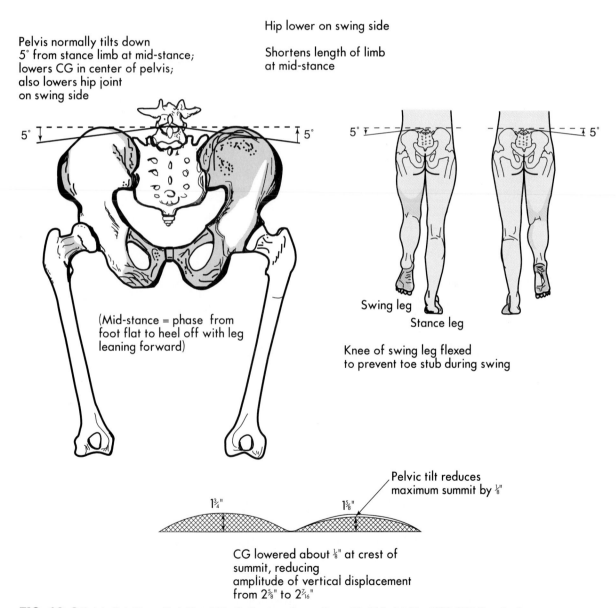

Pelvis normally tilts down 5° from stance limb at mid-stance; lowers CG in center of pelvis; also lowers hip joint on swing side

Hip lower on swing side

Shortens length of limb at mid-stance

(Mid-stance = phase from foot flat to heel off with leg leaning forward)

Swing leg

Stance leg

Knee of swing leg flexed to prevent toe stub during swing

Pelvic tilt reduces maximum summit by ⅛"

CG lowered about ⅛" at crest of summit, reducing amplitude of vertical displacement from 2⅜" to 2⁷⁄₁₆"

FIG. 10-2 Pelvic list. (From Tachdjian MO: *Pediatric orthopaedics,* ed 2, Philadelphia, 1990, WB Saunders).

KNEE FLEXION

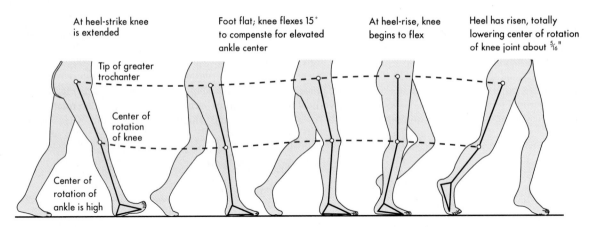

At heel-strike knee is extended

Foot flat; knee flexes 15° to compenste for elevated ankle center

At heel-rise, knee begins to flex

Heel has risen, totally lowering center of rotation of knee joint about $\frac{5}{16}$"

Tip of greater trochanter

Center of rotation of knee

Center of rotation of ankle is high

FIG. 10-3 Knee flexion during stance. (From Tachdjian MO: *Pediatric orthopaedics,* ed 2, Philadelphia, 1990, WB Saunders).

ANKLE ROTATION

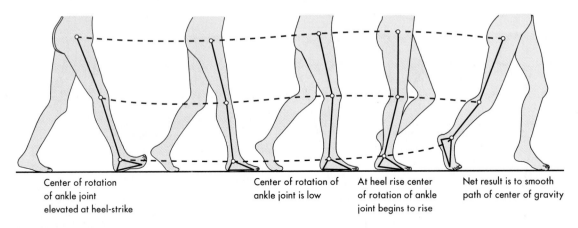

Center of rotation of ankle joint elevated at heel-strike

Center of rotation of ankle joint is low

At heel rise center of rotation of ankle joint begins to rise

Net result is to smooth path of center of gravity

FIG. 10-4 Foot and ankle motion. (From Tachdjian MO: *Pediatric orthopaedics,* ed 2, Philadelphia, 1990, WB Saunders).

stance also contributes to normal mechanics and energy conservation during gait. During stance, the weight-bearing knee must flex approximately 15 degrees to decrease impact (Fig. 10-3). Foot and ankle motion produces sequential dorsiflexion and plantar flexion during gait. The dorsiflexors contract eccentrically from initial heel contact with the ground, to keep the foot from "slapping" to the floor. The foot acts as a shock absorber by pronating during the stance phase. During "toe off," the foot serves as a rigid lever (Fig. 10-4).[3]

THE TWO PHASES OF GAIT

The swing phase and stance phase of gait are subdivided into 8 distinct periods (Table 10-1). The stance phase has five components:

TABLE 10-1

Phase	Period	Action	% Cycle
Stance			60
	Heel strike	Foot on ground	—
	Foot flat	Shock absorption	15
	Midstance	Roll over foot	15
	Heel off	Roll beyond foot	25
	Toe off	Knee flexes	5
Swing			40
	Acceleration	Limb begins to advance	5
	Midswing	Limb advances further	30
	Deceleration	Limb deceleration/ extension	5

From Miller MD: *Review of orthopaedics,* ed 2, Philadelphia, 1992, WB Saunders.

TABLE 10-2

Muscle	Action	Function
Gluteus medius	Eccentric	Controls pelvic tilt at midstance
Gluteus maximus	Concentric	Powers hip extension
Iliopsoas	Concentric	Powers hip flexion
Hip adductors	Eccentric	Controls lateral sway (late stance)
Hip abductors	Eccentric	Controls pelvic tilt (midstance)
Quadriceps	Eccentric	Stabilizes knee at heel strike
Hamstrings	Eccentric	Controls rate of knee extension (stance)
Tibialis anterior	Concentric	Dorsiflexes ankle at swing
	Eccentric*	Slows plantar flexion rate (heel strike)
Gastrocnemius/ soleus	Eccentric	Slows dorsiflexion rate (stance)

*predominate role
From Miller MD: *Review of orthopaedics,* ed 2, Philadelphia, 1992, WB Saunders.

- **Heel strike** or initial contact: The instant foot contact is made with the ground. Ideally, the heel initiates contact, but the midfoot or toe will be the point of initial contact in some pathologic gaits.
- **Foot flat** or loading response: The time the entire foot is in contact with the floor. Shock absorption is a primary action during this period.
- **Midstance** or single-leg support: When the body is directly over the weight-bearing leg. This action serves to roll the foot over into single-limb support during stance.
- **Heel off** or terminal stance: When the heel of the weight-bearing limb initially rises from the floor, weight is unloaded from the weight-bearing limb and shifted or transferred to the opposite limb.
- **Toe off** or preswing: When the knee of the weight-bearing limb flexes and prepares for the swing phase.

The swing phase has three components:

- **Acceleration,** initial swing, or preswing
- **Midswing:** When the nonweight-bearing limb is advanced to where the limb passes directly beneath the body
- **Deceleration** or terminal swing: The limb decelerates and is in a position of extension preparing for heel strike

It is important to recognize that most muscle action during the gait cycle is eccentric. When the hip flexors act concentrically to advance the limb during acceleration and midswing, the hamstrings contract eccentrically to control the rate of knee extension. The gluteus maximus and tibialis anterior also contribute concentric contractions during the gait cycle (Table 10-2).

GAIT DEVIATIONS

Gait abnormalities result from injury, muscle weakness, pain, or immobilization. The physical therapist assistant must be able to accurately identify both obvious and subtle gait deviations and to describe these pathologic characteristics to the physical therapist.

An exceedingly common gait deviation is the **antalgic gait.** It usually occurs in the presence of pain. This gait is characterized by a rapid swing phase of the uninvolved limb, with a reduction of the stance phase of the involved limb. There is an obvious, observable decrease in weight shifting over the stance leg to minimize weight bearing on the painful limb. Cadence is also reduced by the shortened step created by the decreased swing phase.

A **steppage gait** involves muscular weakness of the ankle dorsiflexors (tibialis anterior) and is characterized by extreme hip flexion and knee flexion during swing through to keep from dragging the toes on the floor. This gait is also characterized by the foot "slapping" the

TABLE 10-3

Gait Abnormalities Caused by Muscle Weakness

Muscle	Phase	Direction	Type of Gait	Treatment
Gluteus medius	Stance	Lateral	Abductor lurch	Cane
Gluteus maximus	Stance	Backward	Lurch (hip hyperextension)	
Quadriceps	Stance	Forward	Lurch/back knee gait	AFO
	Swing	Forward	Abnormal hip rotation	
Gastrocnemius/soleus	Stance	Forward	Flat foot (calcaneal) gait	± AFO
	Swing	Forward	Delayed heel rise	
Tibialis anterior	Stance	Forward	Foot drop/slap	AFO
	Swing	Forward	Steppage gait	

From Miller MD: *Review of orthopaedics,* ed 2, Philadelphia, 1992, WB Saunders.

ground because the weak dorsiflexors cannot adequately decelerate the foot during contact.

Muscular weakness is responsible for many identifiable gait abnormalities. To appreciate the specific gait deviations, it is best to review each muscle separately.

Weakness of the *gluteus medius* produces a **Trendelenburg gait** pattern, which is characterized by the pelvis dropping toward the unaffected limb during the single-limb support period of the stance phase. The pelvis drops because the gluteus medius cannot produce enough force of contraction (secondary to muscle weakness) from its attachment on the femur to keep the pelvis level during stance. With a weak gluteus medius, a patient may also demonstrate a gluteus medius or **abductor "lurch."** The patient laterally flexes the trunk over the involved limb to keep the center of gravity over the base of support.[1]

Weakness of the *hip flexors* (psoas muscles) produces difficulty in initiating swing-through.[1] To compensate for this specific muscular weakness, the patient externally or laterally rotates the leg and uses the hip adductors for swing-through. This circumduction of the hip exaggerates energy expenditure and produces extreme trunk and pelvis motion.

Gluteus maximus weakness results in rapid hip hyperextension during initial foot contact with the ground.[3] To compensate, the patient quickly extends the trunk during initial foot contact to maintain hip extension of the stance leg.[4]

Weakness of the *quadriceps muscle group* results in knee hyperextension during the stance phase of the gait cycle. Normally the quadriceps contract eccentrically to control the knee at heel strike or initial contact. When the quadriceps are weak, the knee quickly hyperextends at heel strike.

A **calcaneal gait** pattern occurs with weakness of the *gastrocnemius-soleus muscle group.* Because of weakness in the plantar flexion muscles, reduced foot propul-

sion occurs during the toe-off period of the stance phase. This weakness also creates a delayed rise of the heel at the initiation of swing phase.[3] Table 10-3 outlines the various muscles and resultant gait abnormalities caused by muscular weakness.

GAIT PATTERN INSTRUCTION

Instructing patients in the proper use of assistive devices, and identifying appropriate gait patterns are relevant clinical tasks for the physical therapist assistant. Several patterns are outlined here.

A **four-point gait pattern** is described as advancing the crutch opposite the uninvolved limb first, followed by the involved limb, then advancing the crutch toward the uninvolved limb, then finally advancing the uninvolved limb (Fig. 10-5). If the injured limb is the left leg, the four-point gait pattern looks like this:

Right crutch → Left foot → Left crutch → Right foot

The four-point gait pattern attempts to duplicate the normal reciprocal motion that occurs between the upper extremities and the lower limbs during normal gait.

A **three-point gait pattern** is commonly taught using bilateral axillary crutches (Fig. 10-6). The sequence of events begins by advancing both crutches and the involved limb. The noninvolved limb is then advanced forward and the sequence repeated.

A **two-point gait pattern** is described as advancing the left crutch and right lower extremity at the same time, then advancing the right crutch and left lower extremity together. (Fig. 10-7) This gait pattern is similar to the four-point gait pattern in which normal reciprocal motion and walking rhythm is encouraged.

For bilateral nonfunctioning limbs, a tripod gait pattern is used. Crutches are advanced, then the lower body is advanced. With a tripod gait, the body can be

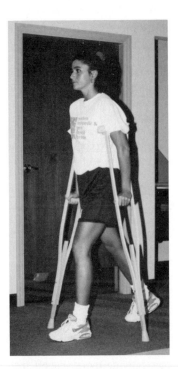

FIG. 10-5 Four-point gait pattern (see text for description).

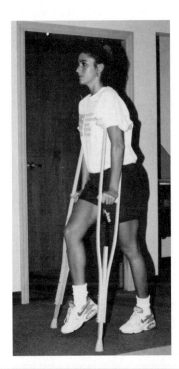

FIG. 10-6 Three-point gait pattern (see text for description).

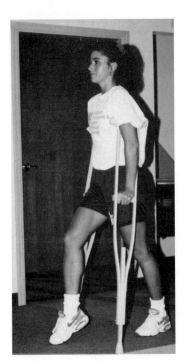

FIG. 10-7 Two-point gait pattern (see text for description).

lifted and advanced to the crutch or swung through and beyond the crutches.

WEIGHT-BEARING STATUS

Depending on the healing constraints of injured tissues (bone, ligaments, tendon, cartilage, muscle), certain weight bearing restrictions are imposed to protect the injured tissues from excessive stresses and loads, as well as to promote normal physiologic healing. If an injured limb is unable to support any weight, **nonweight-bearing (NWB)** status is assigned until sufficient healing has taken place to allow the limb to safely accept some degree of weight. **Partial weight-bearing (PWB)** is frequently graded in a percentage of the patient's weight (20%, 40%, 50%, and so on) or in pounds of pressure applied to the floor from the involved limb. When teaching PWB with orders to apply a certain amount of weight (such as 20 pounds or 50 pounds,), a bathroom scale can acquaint the patient with exactly how much weight is required to bear on the injured limb. The terms **touch down weight-bearing (TDWB)** and **toe touch weight-bearing (TTWB)** can be used synonymously to describe minimal contact of the involved limb with the ground. Generally, TDWB is used for balance purposes initially. As healing and pain allow, progressive weight-bearing can be instituted. **Weight bearing as tolerated (WBAT)** is assigned to patients in whom pain tolerance is the predominant limiting factor. Then the patient is allowed to bear as much weight on the injured limb as is comfortable. When a patient no longer requires an assistive device to accommodate pain or healing of injured tissues, **full weight-bearing (FWB)** status is generally allowed.

Weight-bearing status is a progressive process that involves constant assessment and reassessment of pain, joint stability, tissue healing constraints, and function. A patient with severe injuries will progress through each designation of weight-bearing as follows:

NWB → TDWB → PWB → WBAT → FWB

Less severe injuries may begin anywhere along the continuum and progress from there.

NEGOTIATING STAIRS WITH ASSISTIVE DEVICES

Ascending and descending stairs, steps, or curbs requires prudent instruction and careful supervision with necessary tactile and verbal cueing. The safety of the patient is the principal concern. Perhaps no other gait training technique elicits as much anxiety as negotiating stairs. Therefore the physical therapist assistant must accept the responsibility for clearly articulating the fundamentals of climbing and descending the stairs while both validating the patient's fears and providing confidence, encouragement, and a safe environment for instruction.

When instructing patients to ascend stairs using bilateral axillary crutches, the first step is to encourage the use of a handrail, if one is available. As the patient uses the handrail, both crutches are placed in the hand opposite the handrail. If at all possible, the patient should be instructed to use the handrail on the side of the injured limb. This may provide an added sense of stability and support. Ascending a step requires the noninvolved leg to step up first. Then the involved limb and crutches are advanced up to the same step.

When descending steps, the same instructions regarding the use of the handrail next to the injured limb should be repeated. The first step when descending stairs is to advance the crutches or cane to the step. The injured limb is then advanced down to the step, followed by the uninjured limb. It may help patients to remember, "Up with the good, down with the bad," when cueing them as to which limb to advance up or down the stairs. When providing support for the patient during stair climbing, the physical therapist assistant should stand behind the patient while giving appropriate verbal cues

and physical support at the waist. As a safety precaution, an interlocking gait belt should be applied and used during all phases of gait training. When instructing patients during stair descent, it is best to stand in front of the patient. However, enough space must be allowed between the therapist and patient to permit a technically correct and safe descent.

When no handrail is available, the patient should follow the same steps, except that both crutches are used as with normal walking with crutches.

SELECTION OF ASSISTIVE DEVICES

The initial selection of assistive gait devices depends largely on the age and activity level of the patient, the severity of the injury, and the weight-bearing status. Walkers can be prescribed for an elderly person because they are inherently stable and easy to use. Children may find using a pediatric walker easier and safer than axillary crutches.

Axillary crutches provide less stability than a walker, but compensate with greater mobility. Canes provide the least support of all assistive devices. However, some types of canes provide more support than others. For example, a wide-based quad cane (four points) allows more stability than a narrow-based quad cane or a single-point cane. A hemi-walker provides a wider, more stable base of support than a wide-based quad cane. Hemi-walkers and quad canes are frequently used by patients who have had a CVA with resultant hemiparesis.

As with weight-bearing status, patients may progress from one form of assistive device to another. As pain, healing, and function allow, a patient may move from using axillary crutches to a cane or from a walker to axillary crutches. Constant reassessment of a patient's balance, coordination, strength, endurance, weight-bearing status, and function will guide the physical therapist assistant in consulting with the physical therapist concerning appropriate gait devices.

REFERENCES

1. Epler M: Gait. In Richardson JK, Iglarsh ZA, editors: *Clinical orthopaedic physical therapy,* Philadelphia, 1994, WB Saunders.
2. Lippert L: Normal gait. In *Clinical kinesiology for physical therapist assistants,* ed 2, Philadelphia, 1994, FA Davis.
3. Miller MD: *Review of orthopaedics,* Philadelphia, 1992, WB Saunders.
4. Rothstein JM, Roy SH, Wolf SL: Gait. In *The rehabilitation specialists handbook,* Philadelphia, 1991, FA Davis.
5. Tachdjian MO: *Pediatric orthopaedics,* ed 2, Philadelphia, 1990, WB Saunders.

Concepts of Joint Mobilization

Providing comprehensive musculoskeletal rehabilitation requires that the physical therapist assistant understand the basic concepts related to joint mobilization. He or she must be able to accurately and skillfully apply the mobilization techniques as delegated by the physical therapist. This chapter focuses primarily on concepts, definitions, and general rationales for peripheral joint mobilization, including mobilization theory and compulsory scientific principles.

FUNDAMENTAL PRINCIPLES OF MOBILIZATION

The term **mobilization** refers to an attempt to restore joint motion, or mobility, and/or decrease pain associated with joint structures using manual, passive accessory-joint movement.[1,7]

The use of passive range of motion involves physiologic movements of a joint, which are motions that occur within the active or passive joint range of motion. These motions can be visualized and measured by goniometric assessment. Conversely, accessory movements involve motions specific to articulating joint surfaces.[1,7] These joint motions are referred to as **glide, spin, slide**, or **roll**.[1,4] Accessory and **physiologic joint motions** occur together during active range of motion. However, **accessory joint motion** cannot be selectively recruited, meaning that a patient cannot selectively perform joint roll, glide, or spin.[1] The application of accessory joint motion is defined as **"joint play"** or "motion that occurs within the joint as a response to an outside force but not as a result of voluntary movement."[1]

The concept of **joint congruency** and the terms **close-packed** and **loose-packed**, referring to joint position, are pertinent to the discussion of various grades of mobilization. *Congruence* refers to articular position with regard to concave and convex joint surfaces. A joint is congruent when both articulating surfaces are in contact throughout the total surface area of the joint.[1,4]

However, the study of arthrokinematics (joint movement) states that joints are rarely in total congruence. As joints move, the accessory motions of roll, spin, and glide alter total joint congruence.

MacConaill[4] has described close-packed positions as the most congruent positions of a joint,[1,4] where the joint surfaces are aligned and the capsule and ligaments are taut (Fig. 11-1). Generally, a close-packed position is used for testing the integrity and stability of ligaments and capsular structures. However, the close-packed position described by MacConaill[4] is not used for mobilization techniques. When the elbow and knee are fully extended, the ligaments and joint capsule are taut, allowing no freedom of movement. Therefore the knee and elbow in extension serve as two excellent examples of the close-packed position.

Any joint position, other than the close-packed position, is a loose-packed position. When the knee joint is flexed to 30 degrees, the intracapsular space is increased and supporting ligaments become more relaxed. The loose-packed position is ideal for applying joint mobilization techniques, but painful, stiff, and dysfunctional joints are rarely in "ideal resting positions" for the application of joint mobilization.

CONVEX-CONCAVE RULE

Anatomically, all articular surfaces are either convex or concave,[1,4] although the surfaces of some joints are not overtly of either shape. In these cases, fibrocartilage enhances and modifies the contour of the joint surfaces. On the convex joint surface, more cartilage is found at the center of the surface; on a concave joint surface, more cartilage is found at the periphery.[1]

The **convex-concave rule** specifically states, "When the concave surface is stationary and the convex surface is moving, the gliding movement in the joint occurs in a direction *opposite* to the bone movement."[1] Conversely, if the convex surface is fixed while the concave surface is mobile, the gliding motion occurs in the *same* direc-

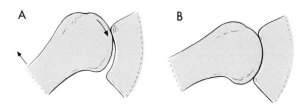

FIG. 11-1 The congruence of articular surfaces: **A**, Loose-packed position; **B**, Close-packed position. (From Gould: *Orthopaedic and sports physical therapy*, ed 2, St. Louis, 1990, Mosby).

tion as the bone movement.[1] This occurs because the convex bone surface always maintains an axis of rotation during joint motion (Fig. 11-2). The concept of accessory joint motions (spin, roll, slide, or glide), as they apply to joint congruency and the convex-concave rule, is clearly illustrated by MacConaill's classification of accessory movements (Fig. 11-3).

MOBILIZATION GRADES

Maitland[6] describes five grades of physiologic and accessory joint motions used in mobilization (Fig. 11-4). The terms **velocity, oscillation**, and **amplitude of movement** describe the degree of force and rate of motion used during any of the grades of mobilization, as follows:

Grade I mobilization: A small oscillation or small amplitude joint motion that occurs only at the beginning of the available range of motion.

Grade II mobilization: A larger amplitude motion occurring from the beginning of the range of motion to near midrange.

Grade III mobilization: A large amplitude motion that occurs from midrange of motion to the end of the available range.

Grade IV mobilization: A small oscillation or amplitude of motion that occurs at the very end range of the available joint motion.

Grade V mobilization: "A high velocity thrust of small amplitude at the end of the available range of motion."[1] This grade is not applied to mobilization techniques used by physical therapist assistants and will not be addressed in this text.

In general terms, a grade I or II small amplitude oscillation is used to treat pain or when joint motion produces pain.[1,7] Mobilization in grades III and IV, therefore, are used to treat joint restrictions.[1,7]

Traction is also used as a manual therapy technique either by itself or along with various mobilization techniques (Fig. 11-5). Traction can be classified in grades[3] or stages.[6] Generally, grade I or stage I traction is used for relief of pain and to minimize compressive joint forces during mobilization. The term **piccolo traction** describes a stage I traction technique. The force used to deliver grade I traction is not enough to actually separate the joint surfaces, but rather only neutralizes joint pressure.[1]

The term *slack* refers to the amount of normal looseness found in nonpathologic joint capsules and describes various degrees of joint tightness with stage II

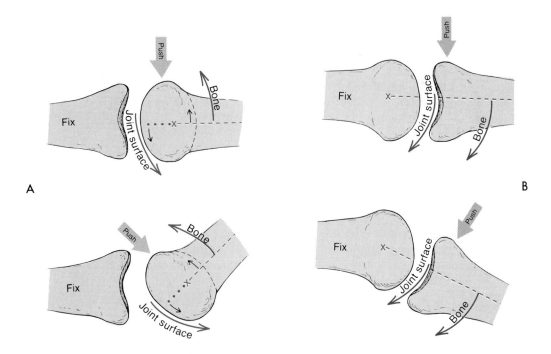

FIG. 11-2 A, Convex surface moving on concave surface. **B,** Concave surface moving on convex surface with a combination of roll, spin, and glide occurring in both simultaneously. (From Gould: *Orthopaedic and sports physical therapy,* ed 2, St. Louis, 1990, Mosby).

A

Convex on concave
Spin

B

Roll

C

Slide

Concave on convex
Spin

Roll

Slide

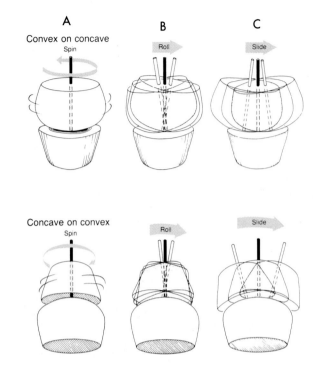

FIG. 11-3 MacConaill's classification of accessory movements: **A**, Spin; **B**, Roll; **C**, Glide. (From Gould: *Orthopaedic and sports physical therapy,* ed 2, St. Louis, 1990, Mosby).

and III traction. Stage II traction is defined as being able to "take up the slack" in the capsule of the joint being stretched; it is commonly used to treat pain. Stage III traction is more substantial, actually involving stretching of the soft tissues. These techniques are performed to stretch out joint tightness.

JOINT END-FEEL

There are various qualities of joint tightness or "play" during the application of passive range of motion. In normal, nonpathologic joints, three types of "end-feel" have been defined.[2,5] **Bone to bone** end-feel refers to a sudden, hard, nonyielding sensation felt at the end range of motion. Generally, the end-feel is not painful. Terminal elbow extension provides an example of a sudden bone to bone end-feel.

Another normal end-feel is **soft-tissue approximation**. This type of joint end-feel is characterized by a "yielding compression," as is typically encountered with knee flexion or elbow flexion.[5] The end-feel that occurs with soft tissue approximation results from muscular tissue compression during joint flexion. The ham-

string and calf muscles buttress and compress against each other during knee flexion, delivering a soft tissue approximation end-feel.

The third normal joint end-feel is described as a **hard or springy-tissue stretch**. The characteristic feature of this end-feel is "elastic resistance" or "rising tension."[5] This type of end-feel is the most common normal feel at the end range of joints. Terminal knee extension and wrist flexion provide a "springy" stretch that defines tissue stretch.

The physical therapist assistant must experience normal joint end-feel and be able to accurately identify distinguishing characteristics between bone-to-bone end-feel, soft tissue approximation, and tissue stretch.[2] The physical therapist assistant performing mobilization encounters abnormal joint end-feel and its precise identification requires considerable didactic and hands-on experience.[2]

The first type of abnormal end-feel is **muscle spasm**. The major component is pain accompanied by a sudden halt of movement that prevents full range of motion.[1,2,5]

In **springy block**, full motion is limited by a soft or "springy" sensation occasionally accompanied by pain.

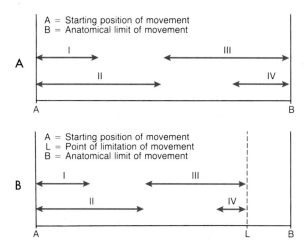

FIG. 11-4 A, Grades of oscillations used in manual therapy. **B,** Grades of oscillations used in manual therapy in relation to a joint with limited motion. (From Gould: *Orthopaedic and sports physical therapy,* ed 2, St. Louis, 1990, Mosby).

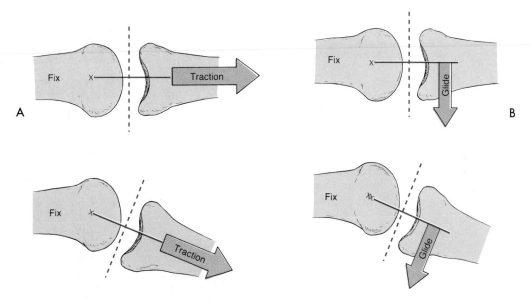

FIG. 11-5 A, Traction; **B,** Glide. (From Gould: *Orthopaedic and sports physical therapy,* ed 2, St. Louis, 1990, Mosby).

If a meniscus is torn in a knee, frequently the cartilage becomes caught in the joint, preventing terminal knee extension and its characteristic normal tissue stretch and feel.

In an **empty end-feel**, motion is very limited by significant pain without muscle spasm. Clinically, this end-feel is not characterized by any mechanical block, or restriction.

Another abnormal end-feel is described as **loose end-feel.**[1] Its primary feature is joint hypermobility, with no resistance typically felt at the end range of motion that signifies extraordinary joint looseness.

A **capsular end-feel**[5] is analogous to a normal tissue stretch, but the "elastic resistance" is encountered before the normal range of motion. This end-feel is related to a capsular restriction.[5]

CAPSULAR AND NONCAPSULAR PATTERNS

The physical therapist assistant must be aware that certain limitations of motion can be caused by lesions specific to the capsule and/or synovial tissues of a joint. All joints controlled by muscle activity possess a characteristic "pattern of proportional limitation."[5] For example, in the shoulder joint, the **capsular pattern** "involves external rotation as the most limited movement, abduction as less limited, internal rotation still less limited, and flexion as the least limited movement."[1,2] Any "characteristic pattern of limitation" is called a capsular pattern.

If a lesion causes a restriction of movement that does not correspond to a characteristic, predetermined capsular pattern, it is called a **noncapsular pattern**.[1,5] Cyriax[2] has identified three possible causes of noncapsular pattern restrictions:

1. *Ligamentous adhesions:* Frequently causes pain and limitation of motion. A noncapsular pattern would exist when injury to the capsule or accessory ligaments causes a restriction in one direction while other motions remain unaffected and pain free.

2. *Internal derangements:* A displaced or loose fragment within the joint. If the medial meniscus becomes wedged in the joint, knee extension will be affected while flexion remains normal.

3. *Extra-articular lesions:* Adhesions resulting from injury outside the joint. Muscular adhesions or acutely inflamed structures are examples.

INDICATIONS AND CONTRAINDICATIONS FOR MOBILIZATION

In the early stages after trauma, surgery, or immobilization, extreme caution must be employed before applying mobilization techniques. Although pain is an indication for the use of mobilization, care must be taken to avoid retarding or impairing the sequence of tissue healing during the acute inflammatory phase.

Pain and joint restrictions are rarely separated completely. In many instances of severe joint limitations, there may be only mild complaints of pain. Conversely, there may be little or no joint restriction but significant pain. Naturally, there are varying degrees of pain and joint limitations occurring as either major or minor components. Therefore pain is a *relative* indication for joint mobilization, depending on which stage of tissue healing is present. If an injury is acute or a patient is recovering immediately after a surgical procedure, mobilization may not be indicated because it is best not to disturb the immature scar. Healing that proceeds in an organized fashion encourages mature collagen formation. When injured tissues have progressed from the acute, intense inflammatory phase to fibroplasia and scar maturation, mobilization is then warranted to stress and remodel the scar.[7]

There are a few relative and absolute contraindications to the application of joint mobilization. Extreme caution is needed when considering mobilization in cases of osteoporosis, rheumatoid arthritis, joint hypermobility, and the presence of neurologic symptoms, all are therefore considered relative contraindications.[1,7] In cases of spinal mobilization, pregnancy and spondylolisthesis are relative contraindications. Absolute contraindications include bone diseases of the area treated, malignancy of the area treated, acute inflammatory and infectious arthritis, and central nervous system disorders.[1,7]

CLINICAL APPLICATION OF JOINT MOBILIZATION

Safe and effective joint mobilization requires the patient to be placed in a very comfortable position and the specific joint to be mobilized to be placed in a maximal resting or loose-packed position.[4] Before applying mobilization, patient compliance and relaxation can be facilitated by the judicious use of moist heat, ultrasound, transcutaneous electrical nerve stimulation (TENS), electrical muscle stimulation, ice, exercise, and the timely use of any physician-prescribed analgesics or muscle relaxant medications. If pain is the predominant feature of the joint to be mobilized, then grade I and II mobilization can be employed safely.

When using grade I and II mobilization, oscillations help modulate or minimize pain. Manually applied joint oscillations occur at a rate of 2 per second, or 120 per minute.[1] Typically, a mobilization grade technique is applied for 20 to 60 seconds only four or five times. This is recommended for the treatment of painful conditions on a daily basis or until pain is reduced.

For the treatment of joint restrictions, a program of mobilization is carried out two to three times per week.[1] Piccolo or stage I traction can be used simultaneously with grade I or II mobilization or by itself to reduce pain and "neutralize" joint pressure. When the limitation of joint motion is greater than the complaints of pain, grade III and IV mobilization can be used to help stretch the capsule and soft tissues around the joint.

Before applying any mobilization technique, the pathologic condition of the joint to be mobilized must be thoroughly understood. For example, it would be critical to avoid stressing the anterior capsule of the shoulder after an anterior dislocation, although mobilization to improve shoulder abduction may be warranted.[7]

In every case of joint mobilization, the physical therapist assistant must constantly observe and document the patient's tolerance, pain response, and swelling to determine whether to halt the procedure, reduce the grade of motion, or consult with the physical therapist regarding advancing the grade of mobilization.

As clearly stated in the beginning of this discussion, the physical therapist is responsible for delegating selected peripheral joint mobilization techniques to the physical therapist assistant. Although peripheral joint mobilization is an area of treatment not usually delegated to the PTA, beyond active and passive range of motion, understanding peripheral joint mobilization techniques and having an awareness of rudimentary concepts and principles of mobilization will provide the PTA with a broad understanding of the rationale for the application of certain techniques.

REFERENCES

1. Barak T, Rosen ER, Sofer R: Basic concepts of orthopaedic manual therapy. In Gould JA, editor: *Orthopaedic and sports physical therapy*, ed 2, St. Louis, 1990, Mosby.
2. Cyriax J: *Textbook of orthopaedic medicine, Vol 1, diagnosis of soft tissue lesions*, ed 8, London, 1982, Baillière Tindall.
3. Kaltenborn F: *Mobilization of the extremity joints: examination and basic treatment techniques*, Oslo, Norway, 1980, Olaf Norlis Bokhandel.
4. MacConaill MA, Basmajian JV: *Muscles and movements: a basis for human kinesiology*, Baltimore, 1969, Williams & Wilkins.
5. Magee DJ: *Orthopaedic physical assessment*, ed 2, Philadelphia, 1992, WB Saunders.
6. Maitland G: *Peripheral Manipulation*, ed 2, Newton, Mass., 1978, Butterworth-Heinemann.
7. Wooden MJ: Mobilization of the upper extremity. In Donatelli R, Wooden MJ, editors: *Orthopaedic physical therapy*, New York, 1989, Churchill Livingstone.

Management of Orthopedic Conditions

This section will introduce the physical therapist assistant to many of the diseases and injuries occurring in the musculoskeletal system. Each region of the body will be surveyed separately, and common and uncommon soft tissue injuries, fractures, and diseases will be outlined. This introduction defines specific orthopedic injuries and identifies criterion-based rehabilitation programs with an emphasis on practical applications.

Clinically, many orthopedic injuries are managed using a traditional protocol approach. This is based on a timetable, which is a written document that outlines and prescribes a progression for therapeutic interventions within the rehabilitation plan. Generally, a protocol lays out a systematic progression based on tissue healing constraints that should fall within certain time frames.

A more progressive way to manage rehabilitation is the criterion-based program, or critical mapping. This method, which is also known as critical treatment pathways, is "a description of the elements of care to be rendered . . . for a particular diagnosis. The pathway often takes the form of a chart or care path/care map that can be followed" by the clinician and patient.* Instead of using a timetable for progression, a set of criteria is developed that the patient must meet before progressing to the next phase of rehabilitation. These are based on tissue healing constraints as well as the patient's individual tolerance to the program. Therefore a criterion-based progression fosters close scrutiny of all objective and subjective data concerning the individual's performance.

The components required for effective management of orthopedic injuries by the physical therapist assistant are knowledge of musculoskeletal tissue healing principles, familiarity with various rehabilitation programs, skillful application of rehabilitation techniques, and a fundamental understanding of common and uncommon soft tissue injuries, fractures, and diseases of muscles, bones, and joints. Knowledge of specific indications and contraindications for certain therapeutic interventions is also helpful.

Orthopedic anatomy is not reviewed substantially in this section. Instead, chapters focus on mechanisms of injury, fracture classifications, clinical features of the injury, specific surgical procedures, and rehabilitation programs. Therefore the student clinician is strongly encouraged to review comprehensive musculoskeletal anatomy texts along with the study of each body part and disorder.

---

*APTA Guidelines for Physical Therapists Facing Changing Organizational Structures, APTA BoD, APP 3, 1995

Orthopedic Management of the Ankle, Foot, and Toes

This chapter will introduce the physical therapist assistant to injuries affecting the ankle, foot, and toes. Included are fractures as well as specific injuries to structures that influence ankle and foot mechanics.

LIGAMENT INJURIES OF THE ANKLE

Injuries to the lateral ligament complex (the anterior talofibular ligament, the fibulocalcaneal ligament, and the posterior talofibular ligament) account for approximately 25% of all sports-related injuries,[22] making **inversion ankle sprains** the most common sports injury and one of the more common orthopedic injuries seen in the emergency room.[34] Studies report that approximately 95% of all ankle sprains occur to the lateral ligament complex.[35] Therefore only about 5% of all ankle sprains involve the medial structures.

Lateral Ligament Injuries (Inversion Ankle Sprains)

Mechanisms of injury. Ligament sprains of the lateral aspect of the ankle are usually caused by plantar flexion, inversion, and adduction of the foot and ankle (Fig. 12-1). Large forces are not needed to produce an ankle sprain. Stepping off a curb, stepping into a small hole, or stepping on a rock can produce sudden plantar flexion and inversion motions. During athletic competition, stepping on an opponent's foot is a common occurrence leading to lateral ligament sprains of the ankle.

Classification of sprains. Classifying inversion ankle sprains can be difficult and quite confusing. The standard classification of ligament injuries (i.e., first, second, and third-degree sprains) requires elaboration when applied to inversion ankle sprains, specifically addressing grades, degrees, and descriptive severity of the injury (mild, moderate, or severe). A classification model described by Leach[24] is contrasted with the common standard classification of ankle sprains as a means of comparison and to illustrate the potential for confusion regarding classification of inversion ankle sprains:

- *First-degree sprain:* Single ligament rupture. The anterior talofibular ligament is completely torn. In the standard classification of ligament sprains a complete tear or rupture of a ligament is called a *grade III,* or *third-degree sprain* (Fig. 12-2).
- *Second-degree sprain:* Double ligament rupture. Both the anterior talofibular ligaments and the fibulocalcaneal ligaments are completely torn. The standard classification describes a partially torn single ligament as a grade II sprain (Fig. 12-3).

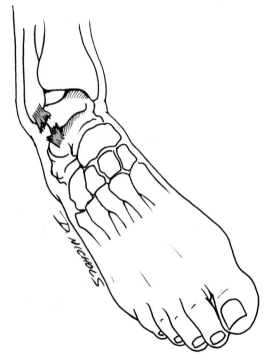

FIG. 12-1 Mechanism of injury to the lateral ligament complex of the ankle. Note the motion of plantar flexion, inversion, and adduction of the foot and ankle.

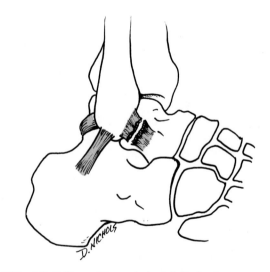

FIG. 12-2 Tear of the anterior talofibular ligament.

- *Third-degree sprain:* All three lateral ankle ligaments (anterior talofibular, posterior talofibular, fibulocalcaneal) are completely torn. In the standard classification a single ligament that is completely torn is defined as a grade III ligament sprain (Fig. 12-4).

Therefore it is essential that the system of classification used to describe the severity or complexity of injury be accepted and understood and not confused with another system or model of classification.

Clinical Examination

The physical therapist assistant must be aware of the organization and administration of examination procedures used to inspect inversion ankle sprains. Throughout rehabilitation, the assistant must communicate changes in the patient's status relative to initial evaluation data and make safe and appropriate modifications to the existing program, based on consultation with the supervising therapist.

Testing. Ankle stability tests are used by the physical therapist to identify and quantify the integrity of the lateral ligament complex. Injury to the anterior talofibular ligament can be clinically assessed by performing the anterior drawer test (Fig. 12-5). The patient must be in a relaxed seated or semirecumbent position with the involved leg flexed 90 degrees at the knee and the involved ankle slightly plantar-flexed. Stabilize the distal tibia and support it with one hand, while using the other hand to gently but firmly grasp the calcaneous and attempt to translate or pull the ankle forward. If the ligament is intact, no excessive motion is seen or felt. However, if the anterior talofibular ligament is torn, the ankle demonstrates excessive forward or anterior motion.

The talar tilt test examines the ankle ligament's resistance to maximal inversion stress (Fig. 12-6). While the patient is in the same position as the anterior drawer test, gradually stress the ankle by exerting constant pressure over the lateral aspect of the foot and ankle while applying counter pressure over the inner aspect of the lower leg until maximal inversion is reached.[3] Grade the severity of ligament injury according to the classification system used by the supervising physical therapist.

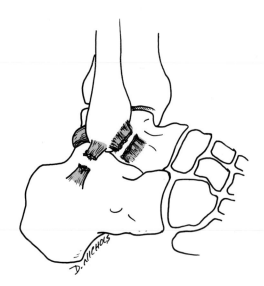

FIG. 12-3 Tears of the anterior talofibular ligament and fibulocalcaneal ligament.

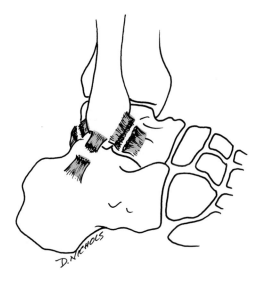

FIG. 12-4 Tears of the anterior talofibular ligament, fibulocalcaneal ligament and posterior talofibular ligament.

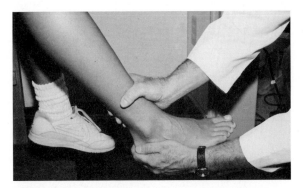

FIG. 12-5 Anterior drawer test of the ankle. With the affected foot slightly plantar-flexed, the distal tibia is stabilized with one hand while the other hand grasps the calcaneus and directs an anterior force in order to manually displace the calcaneus to test the integrity of the ATFL (anterior talofibular ligament).

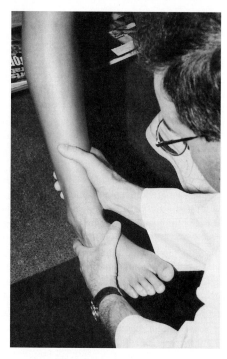

FIG. 12-6 Talar tilt test. The distal tibia is stabilized while the other hand "tilts" the talus to test the integrity of the lateral ligament complex.

Order of procedures. Box 12-1 outlines the procedure for evaluation of inversion ankle sprains. The mechanism of injury that produces an inversion ankle sprain may also cause other conditions that must be differentiated by the physician[34] and physical therapist, such as fracture of the base of the fifth metatarsal, malleolar fractures, osteochondral fractures, osteochondritis dissecans, midfoot ligament sprains, and **subluxing peroneal tendons.**

Rehabilitation

The specific rehabilitation program used to treat inversion sprains will depend on the severity of sprain (first, second, or third degree). Generally, first-degree and second-degree sprains can be effectively managed nonoperatively according to a closely supervised rehabilitation program.

Initial management of acute inversion ankle sprains calls for rest, ice, compression, and elevation (RICE). *Rest* is a relative term used to define avoidance of unwanted stress; it does not necessarily require complete avoidance of *all stress*. The application of ice, compression, and elevation is directed at minimizing and reducing intense inflammatory response, hemorrhage, swelling, pain, and "cellular metabolism" to provide the most conducive environment for tissue healing.[34]

Clinically, the most effective means to reduce swelling are elevation and compression. Elastic compression bandages (Ace wraps) are applied while elevating the injured limb above the heart. A three-phase (phase I—maximum protection; phase II—moderate protection;

BOX 12-1 Physical Therapist Initial Evaluation Outline for the Clinical Assessment of Inversion Ankle Sprains

History

1. How did the injury happen?
2. Where is the pain located?
3. Did you hear or feel a "pop" or "snap"?
4. Have you had a similar injury previously? If yes, explain.

Observation

1. Note any obvious deformity suggesting a fracture or dislocation.
2. Note the area and degree of swelling.
3. Evaluate complaints of pain.
4. Note any discoloration.
5. Perform a bilateral visual comparison of symmetry.

Palpation—Always begin palpation by explaining the procedure, then initially performing the procedure on the uninvolved side.

1. Distal tibia-fibula
2. Lateral ligament complex
3. Medial ligaments—deltoid ligament
4. Base of the fifth metatarsal
5. Peroneal tendons
6. Achilles tendon

Range of motion

1. Active and passive
2. Dorsiflexion
3. Plantar flexion
4. Inversion
5. Eversion

Strength

1. Manual muscle testing
   a. Dorsiflexion
   b. Plantar flexion
   c. Inversion
   d. Eversion

Clinical stability tests

1. Anterior drawer test
2. Talar tilt

phase III—minimum protection), criteria-based rehabilitation program is effective for the management of inversion ankle sprains. The maximum-protection phase calls for the RICE program to be used 3 to 5 times daily. Application of ice should be encouraged for 15 to 20 minutes, with a 1 to 2 hour rest period between applications. Protecting the torn ligaments from unwanted stress is the cornerstone of this phase. Joint protection and immobilization can be achieved through an array of commercial appliances, tape, casting, and braces; selection is left to the physician or physical therapist. Some physicians choose to use a short-leg walking cast or posterior plaster splint. More commonly, a plastic shell brace with an inflatable air bladder or a leather semirigid ankle support is used. Tape can be used for both compression and ligament support, but it must be applied skillfully and reapplied daily to be effective. The ankle must be positioned correctly during the application and use of all support devices. It should be neutral or slightly dorsiflexed as well as slightly everted to closely approximate the torn ligaments. Weight-bearing status and ambulation with assistive devices are individualized. A patient's pain tolerance guides the physical therapist assistant in the appropriate use of crutches and weight-bearing. Even during the maximum-protection phase, weight-bearing as tolerated should be encouraged.

An active range of motion (ROM) program must be used cautiously during the maximum-protection phase. It is imperative to *avoid* plantar flexion and inversion when instructing patients to perform ROM exercises.

Motion exercises are extremely important to help reduce pain and swelling as well as to help increase function of the joint. However, if certain motions (i.e., plantar flexion or inversion) are employed too early in the rehabilitation period, these "unwanted stresses" can disrupt the normal healing process. Electrical galvanic stimulation can also help reduce pain and swelling (see Chapter 2, properties of connective tissue).

Isometric strengthening exercises are initiated as soon as the patient's pain tolerance allows. Isometric dorsiflexion and eversion exercises are performed for two or three sets of 10 repetitions, holding each contraction for 10 seconds. Leg-strengthening exercises (leg extension, hamstring curls, hip abduction and adduction, and hip extension exercises) and general full body conditioning should be encouraged throughout the course of rehabilitation. Clinically, it is vital to view inversion ankle sprains as injuries that affect the whole person, rather than just the injured extremity. Maintaining aerobic fitness and strength during recovery is

particularly important in a population involved in sports.

Once the patient can bear weight on the injured limb without crutches, can perform all ROM and isometric exercises without undue complaints of pain, and can control the swelling, the moderate-protection phase can begin. This phase encourages the use of the RICE principle, full weight-bearing, and continued ligament support with the use of braces or tape. More progressive exercises are initiated, including concentric and eccentric contractions (Fig. 12-7) (with ankle

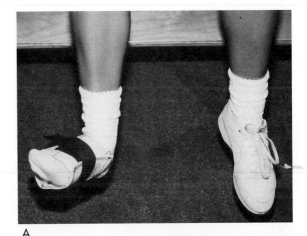

A

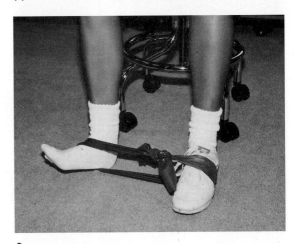

B

FIG. 12-7 A, Concentric and eccentric exercise with ankle weights. As the weight is slowly elevated to a position of dorsiflexion and eversion, encourage the patient to emphasize the eccentric or lowering phase of the exercise. **B,** Thera-band elastic band resistance for eversion and dorsiflexion.

weights or latex bands), heel cord stretching (Fig. 12-8) (towel stretch, wall stretch, or prostretch), and standing toe and heel raises.

Gradually and cautiously, plantar-flexion motions are added as pain allows. Stationary bicycling can be initiated with the seat height lowered slightly to encourage a more neutral ankle position instead of a plantar flexion position.

Proprioception exercises are generally initiated during the moderate-protection phase. Protection of the ligament must be encouraged during these challenging exercises. Balancing on the injured limb on a flat surface is progressed to use of a balance board, and then to a mini-trampoline—all excellent exercises that stimulate balance, coordination, and muscular endurance (Fig. 12-9).

Once the patient can perform all resistive exercises (ankle weight, Thera-band, and manual resistance), can ambulate without complaints of pain and without a limp, and can reduce swelling, the minimum-protection phase can begin.

From 4 to 8 weeks after injury, new collagen formation allows almost-normal stresses to be applied (see Chapter, 2 stretching of soft tissue contractures).[34] At this point, more functional activities are allowed, includ-

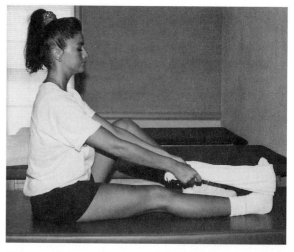

FIG. 12-8 Long-seated towel stretch.

ing straight-line jogging, large figure-of-eight running, jumping drills, and cutting activities.

The minimum-protection phase does not imply removal of all supportive devices. Maturation of the injured ligaments can take as long as 6 to 12 months.[34]

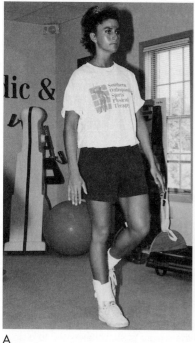
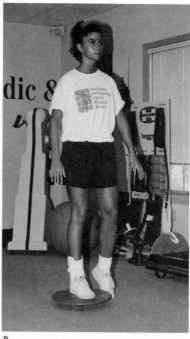
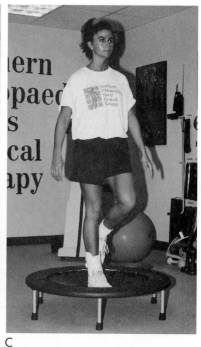

A   B   C

FIG. 12-9 A, Single-leg standing proprioception and balancing. Note the continued use of external support during the late stage of recovery. **B,** Single-leg standing proprioception and balancing using a wobble board or BAPS (biomechanical ankle platform system) board. **C,** Single-leg standing proprioception and balancing on a mini-trampoline. The highly unstable surface provides a challenging balance activity.

Therefore it is critical to encourage patient compliance with the use of either tape or a semirigid brace during all running activities.

Box 12-2 outlines a general three-phase rehabilitation program for an inversion ankle sprain. In all instances, if pain, swelling, or irritation persists, the patient is not taken to the next phase until he or she is pain free in the present phase. The ankle must be securely taped or braced when running, jumping, or otherwise performing aggressive, ballistic motions.

The treatment of grade III ankle sprains (using the standard classification) is somewhat controversial.[34] Some authors[3,5,38] report that surgery is needed because "surgical exploration often reveals that the torn ends of the fibulocalcaneal ligament are so widely separated that simple immobilization alone is not sufficient to allow the ligament to heal in a stable position."[3] However, other authors have found that "early controlled mobili-

zation (functional treatment) was the method of choice and provided the quickest recovery in ankle mobility and the earliest return to work and physical activity without compromising the late mechanical stability of the ankle."[34] Therefore depending on the physician's choice of treatment, a grade III sprain can be treated either surgically or with immobilization and supervised physical therapy.

Immobilization and joint protection last longer with grade III ankle sprains, than with grade I and II sprains. When these injuries are treated surgically, immobilization produces deleterious effects on muscle, bone, cartilage, tendons, and ligaments.

Deltoid Ligament Sprains (Medial Ligament)

Acute isolated sprains of the deep and superficial layers of the **deltoid ligament** are quite rare,[34] occurring in only 3% to 5% of all ankle sprains.[34,35] It is clinically important to recognize that "complete deltoid ligament ruptures occur in combination with ankle fractures."[34]

Rehabilitation. Partial tears are managed nonoperatively with physical therapy. Because complete ruptures occur with fractures, many authorities[7,10] advocate surgical repair and fixation of the fracture fragments. However, some authors[16] recommend casting, non–weight-bearing for 6 weeks, then progressive weight-bearing and physical therapy. In either case, rehabilitation focuses primarily on joint protection and the use of a semirigid orthosis.

The use of ice, compression, and elevation assists with pain and swelling. Progressive strengthening follows a three-phase plan of maximum, moderate, and minimum protection. Isometric exercises, latex rubber band strengthening exercises, active ROM (being careful to avoid unwanted stresses), and progressive weight-bearing are added as tolerated. Generally, a total body fitness program can be initiated during cast immobilization and non–weight-bearing.

CHRONIC ANKLE LIGAMENT INSTABILITIES

The physical therapist assistant, as an integral part of the rehabilitation team, must be aware of certain short-term and long-term complications that may arise from acute or chronic ligament injuries of the ankle. Complications after surgical repair or conservative treatment of ankle sprains are common. Renstrom and Kannus[34] report that between 10% and 30% of patients may have chronic symptoms of weakness, swelling, pain, and joint instability after inversion sprains. There are two types of

---

BOX 12-2   General Three Phase Rehabilitation Program for Inversion Ankle Sprains

Phase I—Maximum-protection phase

1. RICE
2. Electrical galvanic stimulation (EGS)
3. Weight bearing as tolerated (WBAT)
4. Joint protection (plastic, hinged orthosis, tape, air-cast, semirigid braces)
5. Active range of motion (dorsiflexion and eversion)
6. Isometric exercises
7. General fitness exercises

Phase II—Moderate-protection phase

1. RICE
2. Full weight bearing
3. Concentric and eccentric contractors (latex rubber band, ankle weights)
4. Continued joint protection
5. Heel cord stretching
6. Stationary cycling
7. Proprioception exercises
8. General fitness exercises
9. Avoidance of unwanted stresses (inversion and plantar flexion)

Phase III—Minimum-protection phase

1. Joint protection during activities
2. Running
3. Jumping
4. Plyometrics
5. Proprioception exercises
6. General fitness exercises
7. Isotonic exercises
8. Isokinetic exercises

instabilities associated with chronic ankle sprains: mechanical and functional.

Mechanical Instabilities

Mechanical instability is defined as laxity of the ankle ligaments. With mechanical instabilities, surgery may be required to stabilize the ankle joint. The Watson-Jones,[40] Evans,[15] Chrisman-Snook,[8] and Elmslie[8] procedures are common reconstructive surgical procedures used to help stabilize the lateral ligament complex of the ankle. In general, the peroneus brevis muscle is rerouted through a surgically constructed tunnel in the distal fibula (Fig. 12-10). The rerouting of the peroneus brevis dynami-

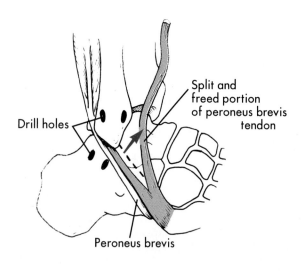

Drill holes

Split and freed portion of peroneus brevis tendon

Peroneus brevis

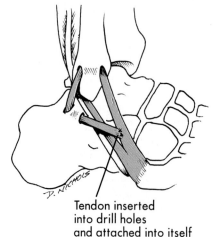

Tendon inserted into drill holes and attached into itself

FIG. 12-10 Chrisman-Snook procedure used for mechanical ankle instability.

cally stabilizes the lateral aspect of the ankle. Another method used to help stabilize chronic ligament laxity is a delayed anatomic repair of the ligaments. With this method, the ligaments are surgically cut, shortened, and reattached to the bone (Fig. 12-11).

Rehabilitation. The postoperative course of treatment after surgical correction of chronic ankle instability involves strict, rigid immobilization in a below-the-knee cast for approximately 2 weeks. After the cast is removed, the patient's involved limb is placed in a hinged rigid orthosis that allows adjustable limited ROM for 5 or 6 weeks. After immobilization has ended, passive dorsiflexion and plantar-flexion exercises are begun. Active motion is not permitted initially to allow the rerouted peroneus brevis muscle to scar down and heal properly. When tolerated, active ROM exercises begin with careful avoidance of excessive plantar flexion and inversion motions. Throughout the period of immobilization, a general body fitness program is encouraged. The use of aerobic exercises (stationary bicycle), leg strengthening exercises (leg extensions, hamstring curls), and proprioception exercises is vital throughout rehabilitation.

Dynamic muscular support is the foundation of various surgical procedures to correct chronic ankle instabilities. Therefore careful and thorough consideration is given to isometric stabilization exercises, Thera-band resistive exercises in all directions, manual resistance, isotonic resistance (with ankle weights), and isokinetic strengthening during the minimal-protective phase. In all cases, full ROM exercises with an emphasis on the eccentric contraction phase of each repetition should be encouraged.

In primary delayed repair or anatomic reconstruction, the ligament is surgically shortened and reinserted (imbricated). The healing time for ligaments is slightly longer and more tenuous than that for muscle and tendon reconstructions (tenodesis), so the period of immobilization may be prolonged. The progression of rehabilitation is the same as with a tenodesis. Active and passive ROM, control of swelling and pain, isometric and manual resistive exercises (being careful to avoid unwanted excessive plantar flexion and inversion motions), Thera-band and isotonic exercises, and isokinetics are used.

Generally, proprioceptive exercises are used extensively. Single-leg standing exercises, balance board activities, mini-trampoline exercises, and heel walking exercises are part of the moderate-protection and minimum-protection phases of rehabilitation. In all cases, joint protection with tape, braces, or a hinged orthosis is a rudimentary but critical principle throughout rehabilitation.

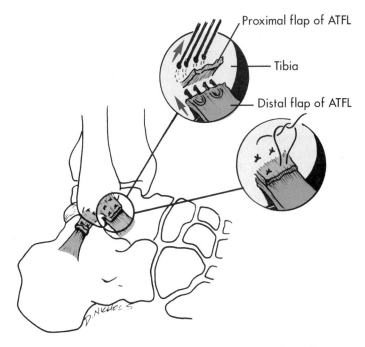

FIG. 12-11 Direct delayed-primary anatomic repair of torn ligaments.

Functional Instabilities

Functional instability refers to a subjective feeling of giving way without affecting ligament laxity. Unlike mechanical instability, functional instability involves a host of factors, including strength, proprioception, and ligament stability.

   Rehabilitation. The primary components of rehabilitation for chronic functional instabilities are closed-chain resistance exercises, proprioception maneuvers, dynamic muscular exercises (concentric and eccentric loads), and bracing for support. Single-leg support proprioception exercises with external resistance (Fig. 12-12) provide dynamic support and balance training. Balance board activities, heel-toe walking, and mini-trampoline activities are the cornerstone of proprioception exercises for the ankle throughout all phases of rehabilitation for functional ankle instabilities.

SUBLUXING PERONEAL TENDONS

The physical therapist assistant must recognize that certain anatomic variations as well as acute injuries can result in instability of the peroneal tendons and ultimate disability. This injury is classified as acute or chronic. The mechanism of injury involves passive dorsiflexion with the foot slightly everted.[14,27] Acute subluxation of the peroneal tendons can be misdiagnosed as a lateral

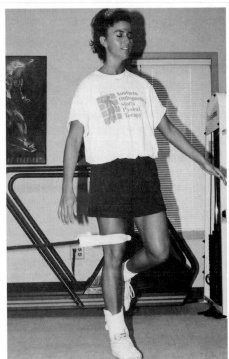

FIG. 12-12 Single-leg standing balance and proprioception exercise with the use of elastic cord to stimulate and encourage strength in a weight-bearing closed-chain functional position.

ankle sprain because of the close anatomic proximity of the tendons to the lateral ligament complex (Fig. 12-13).

Some patients who suffer dislocation of the peroneal tendons have a loose retinaculum (which supports the tendon within the peroneal groove) and may also have a very shallow peroneal groove. Acute injuries result in sprains (grades I, II, and III, using the traditional classification of sprains) to the peroneal retinaculum that cause anterior dislocation of the peroneal tendon over the lateral malleolus with ankle dorsiflexion.[14,27]

Management

Acute injuries are usually treated initially with conservative measures,[39] including rigid-cast immobilization and non–weight-bearing gait for approximately 6 weeks.[39] However, in some cases,[21,39] the patients ultimately require a surgical repair to correct the disability.[39] Many authorities still recommend cast immobilization and non-weight-bearing for 6 weeks for acute injuries,[21] but operative care is the treatment of choice for cases involving recurrent or chronic subluxing peroneal tendons. Keene[21] reports the five basic types of surgical repair procedures for correction of chronic subluxing peroneal tendons, as follows:
- Bone block procedures
- Rerouting procedures
- Periosteal flaps
- Groove deepening procedures
- Tendon slings

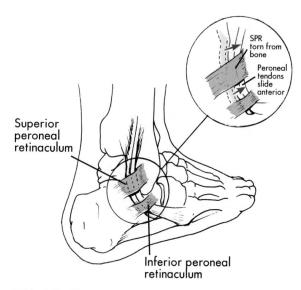

FIG. 12-13 Subluxing peroneal tendons. Note anatomic position of the peroneal tendons in relation to the lateral ligament complex of the ankle.

Rehabilitation

The postoperative care of subluxing peroneal tendons requires excellent communication between the physical therapist assistant, physical therapist, and surgeon. The exact procedure performed should be explained to the physical therapist, who should articulate the key points of the surgery to the physical therapist assistant and outline the indications and contraindications for rehabilitation. Usually postoperative care involves the use of immobilization for a few weeks and instruction in weight-bearing as tolerated. Keene[21] recommends plantar flexion and dorsiflexion exercises 3 weeks after surgery.

All immobilization is terminated 6 weeks after surgery. While immobilized, the patient progresses through a general body-conditioning program of aerobic exercise and strengthening. After immobilization, active ROM and isometric strengthening exercises are begun. As pain allows, manual resistive and Thera-band strengthening exercises can be added. Care must be taken with extreme dorsiflexion and eversion maneuvers after surgery. Depending on which procedure was used, soft tissue healing and bone healing constraints must be carefully observed to avoid placing excessive stress on the surgically repaired tissues.

Initially, limited ROM dorsiflexion strengthening exercises should be used. As pain, swelling, and strength improve, greater degrees of dorsiflexion motion can be added. Proprioception exercises on a flat surface can be initiated soon after immobilization ends. Progression to balance board activities and mini-trampoline exercises depends on the patient's tolerance. Keene[21] recommends that when ROM has been achieved and the involved limb reaches 80% of the strength of the noninvolved limb, a running program can begin.

At first, slow straight-line jogging is attempted. If there is no pain, swelling, or complaints of instability, longer distances are tried. As symptoms allow, sprints can be attempted with careful observation of symptoms.

Plyometric exercises and rapid cutting maneuvers can be included for the athletic patient. For example, jumping in place, side-to-side hops and quick figure-of-eight sprints are progressive functional activities that involve rapid change of direction and ballistic concentric and eccentric open and closed-chain loading. In most cases, full return to activity can be achieved about 16 weeks after surgery.

ACHILLES TENDINITIS

Achilles **tendinitis** is an overuse injury resulting from repetitive microtrauma and accumulative overloading of the tendon[21] (Fig. 12-14). The primary feature of Achilles tendinitis is localized pain at the midportion, distal third, and insertion on the calcaneus.

Many intrinsic and extrinsic factors can lead to Achilles tendinitis. Intrinsic factors are "decreased vascularity, aging and degeneration of the tendon, anatomic deviations such as heel-leg or heel-forefoot malalignment and poor gastroc-soleus flexibility."[21] Extrinsic factors include variations in training, running-surface changes, and poor or inappropriate footwear.

The general features of Achilles tendinitis include soft tissue swelling, pain, and crepitus.

Rehabilitation

Most cases of Achilles tendinitis are managed conservatively with various physical agents, oral medications, relative rest, and progressive exercises. Initial management includes the use of ice massage or ice packs for 15 to 20 minutes, three to five times daily. The treating physician may prescribe a nonsteroidal anti-inflammatory drug to help reduce swelling and pain. All aggravating motions must be stopped. For example, an athletic patient who runs must stop running temporarily until symptoms subside. A program of aerobic exercise using a stationary bicycle or a swimming program can take the place of the running program. Sometimes a small felt heel-lift can be placed in everyday shoes to help

reduce the stress on the tendon. As symptoms are reduced, the heel wedge is gradually diminished. It is not advisable to suddenly remove the heel-lift support when symptoms improve because occasionally pain and swelling return.

Ultrasound can also be used to help reduce pain and assist with collagen synthesis.[19] Generally, ultrasound can be used immediately before an exercise program to improve circulation, enhance relaxation of the soft tissues, and reduce pain. Occasionally, phonophoresis (ultrasound used with a topical hydrocortisone cream) is used in cases of severe pain.

Flexibility exercises are used to increase dorsiflexion motion and reduce the effects of scarring in prolonged cases of Achilles tendinitis. Researchers have pointed out that a lack of dorsiflexion is a common denominator for patients suffering from Achilles tendinitis.[23]

Initially, active dorsiflexion exercises are used. Towel stretches are added gradually as pain allows. In many cases, it may be helpful to apply ice packs or ice massage to the tendon before stretching and strengthening exercises. Standing heel cord stretches can be added to the flexibility program as soon as towel stretches do not cause pain or swelling. In all cases of stretching, it is advisable to avoid any ballistic motions, to stretch gently and firmly, and to hold each stretch for 10 to 30 seconds.

Standing heel cord stretches can be performed on a small block or with a commercial appliance to produce greater dorsiflexion motion. A soleus stretch is also used for Achilles tendinitis. The patient faces a wall with his or her knees touching the wall while keeping the heels on the floor (Fig. 12-15).

Strengthening exercises often prove very beneficial for patients with Achilles tendinitis. However, most full ROM strengthening and stretching exercises also cause complaints of pain. A safe and effective exercise program focuses initially on limited ROM and submaximal exercises. When the patient can perform all exercises without pain, the next phase of more vigorous exercise can begin.

Initially, Thera-band plantar-flexion exercises can be used. Use of the Thera-band for plantar flexion motion should emphasize the eccentric phase of the exercise.[12] Curwin and Stanish[12] advocate eccentric exercises for treatment of many types of tendinitis. For example, when strengthening the gastroc-soleus muscle group using standing heel raises, the patient is instructed to rise up on the balls of the feet using the noninvolved limb. Before the descent phase, the body weight is transferred to the involved limb and then the body is slowly lowered. As symptoms improve, more concentric

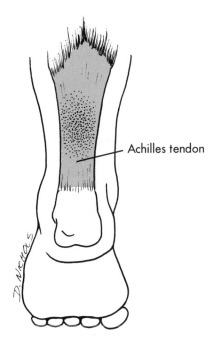

— Achilles tendon

FIG. 12-14 Achilles tendinitis.

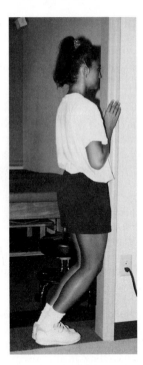

FIG. 12-15 Standing soleus stretch. Flexing the knees will enhance the stretch to the gastroc-soleus complex.

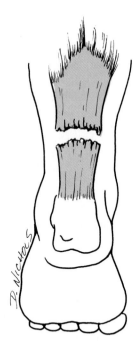

FIG. 12-16 Complete rupture of the Achilles tendon.

lifting is allowed gradually, with greater dorsiflexion motion.

In some severe cases of Achilles tendinitis, physicians may prescribe rigid cast immobilization of the ankle for 10 days.[23] The entire program of rehabilitation after cast immobilization progresses at a slightly slower rate because of the limited ROM and strength loss associated with immobilization. In all cases of Achilles tendinitis, the patient is instructed in a general body fitness program. Aerobic exercise can be achieved with either an upper body ergometer (UBE), a seated bicycle ergometer with the seat height corrected to prevent plantar flexion, or with a swimming program. Upper-body and lower-body stretching and strengthening exercises are encouraged as long as the tendon suffers no undue stress or pain.

RUPTURES OF THE ACHILLES TENDON

Complete ruptures of the Achilles tendon can occur with excessive sudden plantar flexion (Fig. 12-16). These ruptures usually involve the area "3 to 4 cm proximal to its insertion on the calcaneus, within the area of decreased vascularity" and occur mostly to men 20 to 50 years old.[21] In acute Achilles tendon rupture, palpation reveals a defect or gap in the continuity of the distal third of the tendon. The Thompson test, a very sensitive test, clinically assesses the integrity of the Achilles tendon. To perform this simple test, the patient lies prone on an examining table with the feet extending off the end. Expose the entire lower leg, from knee to toes. Grasp the belly of the calf of the noninvolved limb and squeeze so that the foot will plantar flex. If the tendon is ruptured on the involved limb, when the calf is squeezed, no plantar flexion motion results (Fig. 12-17).

Management and Rehabilitation

A ruptured Achilles tendon can be treated surgically or with cast immobilization. Nonoperative treatment of Achilles tendon ruptures requires the patient to be immobilized for as long as 8 weeks.[21] However, with nonoperative treatment, researchers[2,15,20] have documented rerupture rates from 8% to 39%. In addition, there is a greater loss of strength, power, and endurance compared to surgically repaired tendons.[2,17,20,21] Surgically repaired Achilles tendons have a much lower rate of rerupture (0% to 5%), and there is a significant increase in the ultimate recovery of muscular strength, power, and endurance. However, Nistor[33] reports only minor differences between surgical and nonsurgical management. Some surgeons[33] prefer nonoperative management because there are fewer complications re-

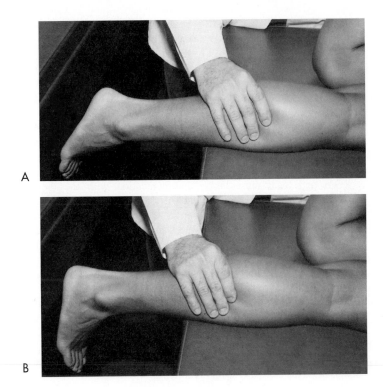

FIG. 12-17 Thompson test to confirm or deny the presence of a ruptured Achilles tendon. **A,** A negative Thompson test is demonstrated by observation of plantar flexion of the foot when squeezing the calf. **B,** A positive Thompson test reveals no plantar flexion of the foot when the calf is squeezed.

lated to surgery, reduced complaints, no hospitalization, and no significant differences in function compared to surgically treated patients. Keene[21] reports various techniques used to repair acute Achilles tendon ruptures, including end-to-end primary repair and direct repair and augmentation with tendon grafts or synthetic grafts.[21]

The rehabilitation program used after nonoperative immobilization of an Achilles tendon rupture requires the physical therapist assistant to appreciate the time-dependent nature of tendon healing as well as plastic and elastic deformation principles (see stretching of soft tissue contractures, Chapter 2). Throughout the course of immobilization, the patient should be instructed in a general body conditioning program that does not stress the involved tissues. The muscles of the noninvolved limb (quadriceps, hamstrings, gastroc-soleus, and so on) should be vigorously strengthened along with the thigh and hamstring muscles of the involved limb. Aerobic exercise is also encouraged. Stationary bike ergometers using only the noninvolved limb (a toe clip is necessary for single-limb cycling) and UBEs are appropriate and safe cardiovascular fitness tools. When the cast is re-

moved and after the initial evaluation by the physical therapist, the physical therapist assistant will proceed with thermal agents as indicated. Moist heat followed by ultrasound can be used before ROM and flexibility exercises. If pain and swelling are present, a cold whirlpool or ice packs with compression can be applied.

Regaining full dorsiflexion and plantar flexion motion is an exceedingly slow process after cast removal. Gentle active dorsiflexion and plantar-flexion exercises are initiated immediately. Typically a small heel-lift is used in everyday shoes to minimize stress on the healing tendon. Because the tendon was not surgically repaired, the process of regaining tensile strength and collagen alignment must be approached cautiously (see stretching of soft tissue contractures, Chapter 2). Progressive active motion is an essential component for full return to function. However, if the tendon is stressed too soon or too vigorously, the tendon may rerupture. The heel-lift is worn for 3 to 4 weeks and is gradually reduced in size to prevent sudden excessive stress on the tendon.[21]

Progressive plantar-flexion and dorsiflexion exercises using a latex band are encouraged as pain and motion allow. Proprioception exercises can be employed early, depending on the patient's tolerance. Generally, proprioception exercises begin with the patient in a seated position (Fig. 12-18) and progress as tolerated. If rerupture occurs, it is usually within 4 weeks after immobilization.[21] During this maximum-protection phase, the patient is encouraged to avoid sudden forceful plantar flexion or dorsiflexion motions.

As motion increases gradually, closed-chain resistive exercises can be initiated, based on the patient's ROM, pain tolerance, swelling, and the length of time after cast removal. Seated stationary cycling can be used for aerobic fitness as well as ROM and local muscular endurance. The seat must be adjusted to avoid excessive plantar flexion or dorsiflexion, however. Step-ups can be used (with heel-lift) to encourage weight-bearing eccentric loading.

Weight-bearing plantar flexion can begin gradually once the patient has successfully completed the prescribed program of ROM and strengthening exercises without complications. Standing plantar flexion is initiated without a block to stand on. The patient is instructed to gradually rise up on the toes using primarily the noninvolved limb, then lowers himself or herself down using both feet. As strength improves, the patient gradually uses more of the involved limb to rise up on the balls of the feet. Adding a small block of wood on which to rise up adds greater dorsiflexion stress and motion. Seated calf-raises can be performed by modifying a leg extension machine (Fig. 12-19). The seated position may be more comfortable for some patients initially.

The physical therapist assistant reassesses the patient's ROM, strength, pain, and swelling on a daily basis. Modifications are necessary if the patient is having undue pain with any phase of the program. Daily communication with the therapist allows continuous restructuring of the rehabilitation plan based on the patient's needs as assessed by the physical therapist assistant. Isokinetic testing for plantar flexion, dorsiflexion, ROM, strength, power, and local muscular endurance is generally reserved for the minimal-protection phase. However, isokinetic strengthening exercises can be employed early if done at higher speeds and performed submaximally under limited ROM conditions.

Postoperative rehabilitation follows a similar criteria-based rehabilitation program. Keene[21] reports that isokinetic strengthening exercises are begun 2 to 4 weeks after immobilization (which usually lasts 6 weeks).

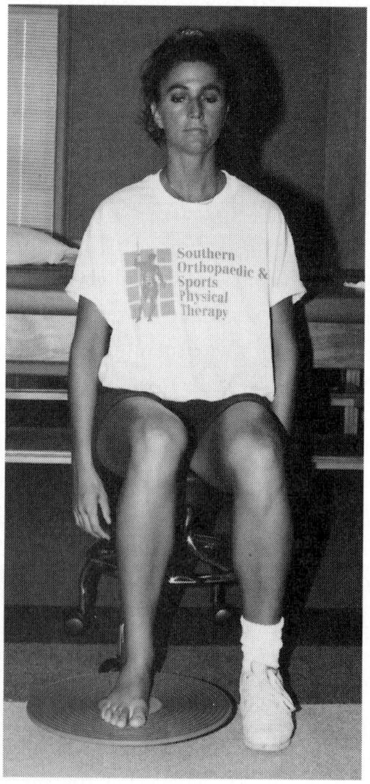

FIG. 12-18 Initial proprioception activities can begin in a seated position using a wobble board.

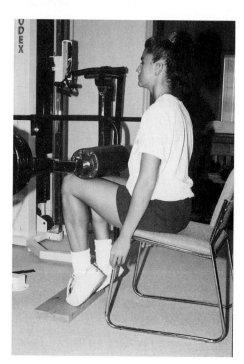

FIG. 12-19 Seated heel or calf raises are performed by modifying and adjusting a knee-extension machine with a range-limiting device.

When strength values are at least 70% of the noninvolved limb, a gradual, progressive jogging program can begin.[21] Recovery from a surgically repaired Achilles tendon rupture varies from patient to patient, but generally good results are seen in 6 months.

COMPARTMENT SYNDROMES

Compartment syndromes of the lower leg are defined as either acute or chronic elevated tissue pressure within a closed fascial space, resulting in occlusion of vessels and compromised neuromuscular function.[1,36]

Acute compartment syndromes of the leg are most commonly associated with tibial fractures, direct trauma to the area, muscle rupture, muscle hypertrophy and circumferential burns.[22,34] **Acute elevated intracompartmental pressure within the lower leg is considered a medical emergency.**

Chronic compartment syndromes are also referred to as exertional compartment syndrome or exercise-induced compartment syndrome. Muscular contractions and exertion have been shown to cause increases in muscle size, leading to increased intracompartmental pressure.[22,34] This results in ischemia and reduced neuromuscular function. In order to understand this series of events, it is necessary to review pertinent anatomy of the lower leg.

There are four well-defined compartments of the leg, divided by nonyielding fascia.[1,36] The *anterior compartment* of the lower leg contains the tibialis anterior, anterior tibial artery and vein, and foot and toe extensor muscles. The *lateral compartment* contains the superficial peroneal nerve, and short and long peroneal muscles. The *superficial posterior compartment* contains the soleus muscle and plantaris and gastrocnemius tendons. The *deep posterior compartment* contains the posterior tibial muscle, the peroneal artery and vein, tibial nerve, and posterior tibial artery and vein. If swelling occurs in one or more of these compartments, reduced capillary blood perfusion results in neurovascular and muscular dysfunction.

Clinical symptoms of acute compartment syndrome include pain, palpable swelling or tenseness, and paresthesias.[1,36] The skin may be warm, shiny, and tense. Passive stretching of the muscles of the lower leg may produce severe pain.

Symptoms of chronic or exertional compartment syndromes include a dull aching pain within the muscle during and after long-term exercise. Paresthesias may also develop as the syndrome progresses. The compartments most commonly affected with chronic exercise-induced compartment syndromes are the anterior and deep posterior compartments of the lower leg.

Management and Rehabilitation

Acute compartment syndrome is treated with a surgical procedure called a fasciotomy.[1,36] When nerve and muscle ischemia last longer than 12 hours, severe and irreversible damage occurs.[1] If, however, the ischemia can be reduced in less than 4 hours, usually no permanent damage occurs.[1]

A surgical fasciotomy is designed to relieve intracompartmental pressure by opening or releasing the fascial compartment, thereby allowing the pressure to be reduced. It is interesting to note that the surgical incision is left open and is managed with sterile dressings.[1] Immediately following surgery, ice packs and leg elevation are necessary to reduce swelling. Walking as tolerated and active and passive gentle ROM of the ankle and knee are begun two days following surgery. Treatment with ice and leg elevation are continued following exercise. A general conditioning program can begin with strethening exercises and aerobic exercises utilizing a single-leg ergometer or UBE. Once the patient shows improved motion, reduced pain, and reduced swelling, light resistance exercises can begin for the involved leg. However, very light resistance should be encouraged since heavy and intense exercise, which leads to muscular hypertrophy, is contraindicated following fasciotomy for acute compartment syndromes.

The management of chronic exercise-induced compartment syndromes is similar to that of acute compartment syndromes. However, chronic compartment syndromes do not represent a surgical emergency. Therefore subcutaneous fasciotomy need only be used when pain and symptoms affect function. The postoperative management of fasciotomy following chronic compartment syndromes parallels the rehabilitation program outlined for acute compartment syndromes.

ANKLE FRACTURES

The most widely accepted classification of ankle fractures is described by **Lauge-Hansen**.[29] The organization and classification of ankle fractures frequently involve the direction of force, which results in specific patterns of injury (Fig. 12-20). For example, a Lauge-Hansen pronation-abduction or pronation-lateral rotation injury may result in a malleolar or bimalleolar fracture of the ankle (Fig. 12-21).

Ankle fractures include lateral malleolar fractures, medial malleolar fractures, bimalleolar fractures (combined medial and lateral malleolar fractures), and trimalleolar

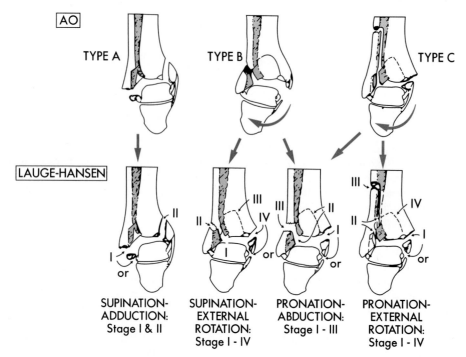

FIG. 12-20 AO and Lauge-Hansen classification of ankle fractures. (From Sangeorzan BJ, Hansen ST: Ankle and foot: trauma. In Poss R, editor: *Orthopaedic knowledge update* III, Park Ridge, Ill., 1990, American Academy of Orthopaedic Surgeons).

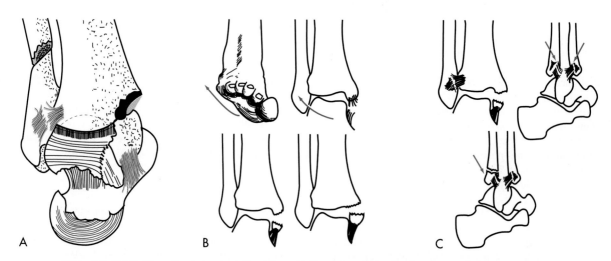

FIG. 12-21 A, Pronation-lateral rotation injury; **B,** Pronation abduction injuries; **C,** Pronation abduction injury. (From McRae R: *Practical fracture treatment,* ed 3, New York, 1994, Churchill Livingstone).

fractures (bimalleolar fractures plus the posterior margin of the tibia). Most fractures are managed with an open reduction with internal fixation (ORIF) procedure. Typically, these fractures are fixed with various screws and plates to hold the fragments in place (Fig. 12-22).

In many cases of ankle fractures repaired with an ORIF procedure, the patient will be in a semirigid postoperative removable splint for 2 weeks. This splint can be removed to allow for active dorsiflexion and plantar flexion ROM exercises. Because of the mecha-

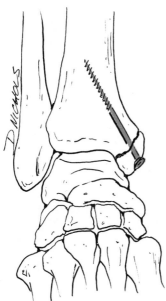

FIG. 12-22 ORIF screw fixation for medial malleolar fracture.

nism of injury that caused the malleolar fracture as well as the position of the internal fixation devices, no inversion or eversion exercises are performed.

Once the patient achieves full plantar flexion and dorsiflexion ROM, a walking cast is applied. Before casting, the surgical wound must be fully closed, sutures removed, infection absent, and no drainage present. A general full-body conditioning program is prescribed throughout immobilization. Both aerobic fitness and strengthening exercises are also advocated.

Once the cast is removed, ROM exercises, isometric strengthening, stationary cycling, and weight-bearing exercises are begun. Progressive exercises employ latex rubber tubing, manual resistive exercises, proprioception exercises, and isokinetic strengthening. The physical therapist assistant must be acutely aware of the signs and symptoms of possible hardware loosening (increased pain, swelling, crepitus, motion) so as to swiftly inform the therapist and make all necessary modifications in the present program. If, for example, after cast removal following an ORIF procedure for a medial malleolar fracture, the physical therapist assistant recognized increased swelling and complaints of crepitus when strengthening exercises were increased, stressing inversion of the ankle, the assistant should halt those particular exercises and inform the physical therapist.

DISTAL TIBIA COMPRESSION FRACTURES (PILON FRACTURES)

Distal tibia compression fractures (pilon fractures) occur as a result of vertical or axial loads that "drive" or compress the tibia into the talus. The initial management of these injuries usually involves an ORIF procedure, external fixation, or skeletal traction with a calcaneal pin.[29] Because of the nature of these fractures, weight-bearing activities are usually deferred for as long as 12 or more weeks. Weight-bearing creates vertical compression and compromises the natural course of healing needed for a stable outcome. Secondary osteoarthritis is a common complication with severe multifragmented compression fractures.[29] Typically, throughout immobilization a general conditioning program is allowed as long as no weight-bearing occurs.

After immobilization, active motion and general ankle strengthening exercises are performed to the patient's tolerance. Care is taken to protect the articular surface of the distal tibia and talus. Initially, non–weight-bearing strengthening exercises and ROM maneuvers are allowed. Progressive loading (compression) can proceed cautiously using latex surgical tubing for long sitting plantar flexion strengthening. Partial weight-bearing repetitive motion activities such as a stationary bicycle ergometer can be used to enhance ankle motion and endurance. Weight-bearing activities are generally painful until satisfactory healing has occurred. However, toe-touch weight-bearing progressing to partial weight-bearing is well tolerated, helps restore proprioception, and assists with healing.

CALCANEAL FRACTURES

Calcaneal fractures are intraarticular depression fractures usually caused by falls from a height and resulting in compression of the calcaneus from the talus (Fig. 12-23). McRae[29] describes seven common patterns of calcaneal fractures:

1. Vertical fractures of the calcaneal tuberosity
2. Horizontal fractures
3. Fractures of the sustentaculum tali
4. Anterior calcaneal fractures
5. Fracture of the body of the calcaneus without involvement of the subtalar joint
6. Calcaneal fractures with lateral displacement and involvement of the subtalar joint
7. Central calcaneus crushing fractures

Depending on the type of fracture pattern, the patient can be treated conservatively with casting or with an ORIF procedure.[29] Physical therapy management begins when the patient is casted (with or without ORIF) and as

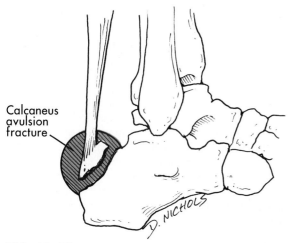

FIG. 12-23 Fractured calcaneus type II with avulsion.

pain allows. Active and active assisted plantar flexion with inversion and dorsiflexion with eversion are usually allowed. Supportive measures to control pain and swelling are used as required. The cornerstone in recovering from a calcaneal fracture lies in regaining motion and strengthening the plantar flexors. Multiangle isometric plantar flexion can be initiated and progressed to full ROM manual resistance dorsiflexion and plantar flexion. The use of latex rubber tubing for plantar flexion in a long seated position is an appropriate and challenging calf strengthening exercise during the moderate protection phase of rehabilitation. Strengthening of the soleus can be achieved by having the patient lie prone with the affected leg flexed 90 degrees at the knee and placing ankle weights around the foot of the affected leg (Fig. 12-24).

FRACTURES OF THE TALUS

The talus can be fractured by falling from a height and landing on the foot in a crouched position.[29] This produces an axial compression load between the talus and the calcaneus. There are four classifications of **talar fractures**:[29]

Type I: Talar neck fracture without displacement

Type II: Talar fracture with subtalar subluxation (the incidence of avascular necrosis is as high as 50%)[29]

Type III: Talar fracture with further subtalar subluxation (the incidence of avascular necrosis is as high as 85%)[29]

Type IV: The talar head dislocates from the navicular in association with a type III injury

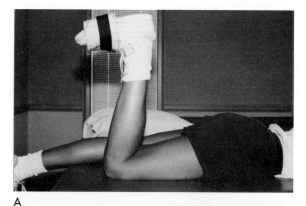

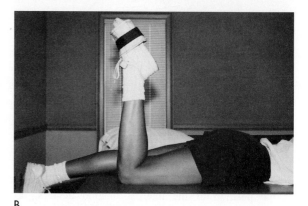

FIG. 12-24 Prone gastroc-soleus strengthening. **A,** Starting position with the knee of the affected limb flexed to 90 degrees. **B,** The patient actively plantar-flexes the foot against gravity and the applied resistance.

These fractures can be treated with closed reduction and cast immobilization or with an ORIF procedure. To allow for proper healing, these fractures require 3 months of non–weight-bearing. The rehabilitation program can proceed during this immobilization period with single-leg stationary cycling, aerobic training, or a UBE. Strengthening exercises include knee extension and hamstring curl maneuvers as well as non–weight-bearing hip abduction, adduction, flexion, and extension. Usually, the patient is immobilized in a posterior splint that can be removed for exercise periods. Range-of-motion exercises and supportive measures for pain and swelling control can be used during the maximum-protection phase of the rehabilitation program.

Because of the duration of immobilization and non–weight-bearing status, osteoarthritis is a common long-term complication with talar fractures.

STRESS FRACTURES OF THE FOOT AND ANKLE

A stress fracture is a partial or complete fracture of bone caused by unrelenting stress and force that do not allow for osteoblastic repair of bone and in turn cause accelerated bone resorption. Common sites for stress fractures in the foot and ankle are the metatarsals, lateral malleolus, OS calcis, navicular, and sesamoid.

Clinically, pain is the predominant feature of a stress fracture. The pain usually increases with activity and subsides with rest. The incidence of stress fractures in the foot and ankle is related in part to participation in demanding physical activity. If stress and forces are applied to bone and are not removed in order to allow the bone to repair, osteoclast activity overtakes the rate of osteoblast activity and stress fractures occur.

The development of stress fractures can be viewed in part as resulting from a linear progression or continuum of excessive external forces that lead to intrinsic reactions of muscle, bone, and periosteum. For example, with increased muscular forces resulting from continued and excessive use (marathon running, recreational jogging, aerobic dance, occupations that require standing or walking all day) there is an associated increased rate of bone remodeling around the area of increased stress.[37] If the stress is not removed, this increase in bone remodeling is followed by a greater rate of bone resorption. If the stress continues, the bone eventually will respond by developing microfractures, periosteal inflammation, and resultant stress fractures.[37] If stressed further, and the bone and soft tissues are not allowed to recover fully and heal properly, the development of linear fractures and ultimately displaced fractures can occur.[37]

There are certain stress fractures that pose a greater risk of delayed union, nonunion, and displacement than others.[28] The base or proximal diaphysis of the fifth metatarsal is described as "no man's land" and is "at risk" for delayed union or nonunion following a stress fracture.[28,34] Usually, complete rigid-cast immobilization is indicated for a period of 6 to 8 weeks when conservative, relative rest has failed to arrest symptoms of pain.[28,34,35] Other stress fractures termed *at risk*[22] are tarsal navicular fracture, sesamoid fractures, and all intraarticular fractures.

The management of "not at risk"[28] stress fractures of the foot and ankle can be effectively rehabilitated with activity modification, relative rest, therapeutic agents to relieve pain and swelling, as well as specific leg, ankle, and foot stretching and strengthening exercises. For example, the therapist may suggest arch strengthening exercises with the use of marbles, gastroc strengthening, dorsiflexion strengthening, ankle-eversion-and-inversion exercises, as well as closed kinetic chain proprioception exercises. A low-impact aerobic exercise is quite useful in athletic patients who run a great deal. For example, instead of running or jogging, have the patient use a stationary cycle ergometer, UBF, or stair stepper, or have the patient run in a non–weight-bearing manner under water.

For stress fractures of the foot and ankle that are "at risk"[28] (fifth metatarsal, navicular sesamoids, intraarticular fractures), more caution is required during the advancement of closed-chain activities to protect the healing bone from unwanted forces. With at-risk stress fractures, some form of external support can be used to brace the area. Usually some type of bracing, padding, casting, or orthosis is applied to control stress and forces to the healing bone.[28] The application of therapeutic exercises must be approached cautiously. Submaximal isometric exercises are encouraged initially. As pain allows, active ROM and light concentric and eccentric loads are added. Obviously, vertical compressive loads and shearing forces (jumping, running, cutting, and so on) are strictly prohibited in order to allow proper healing. Modifications in aerobic activity and general physical conditioning can allow the patient to continue to participate in strenuous physical conditioning, provided no stress is applied to the healing tissues. The initiation of closed-chain functional activities must be deferred until radiographic confirmation by the physician documents stable bone healing.

MEDIAL TIBIAL STRESS SYNDROME

Musculoskeletal overuse injuries of the lower leg involving the distal third of the posterior medial border of the tibia have historically been referred to as shin splints. This term has no place in orthopedic management and should be discarded as a nonspecific term used to describe any pain occurring in the lower leg.[1] A more precise and descriptive term is *medial tibial stress syndrome,* which describes pain over the distal and middle thirds of the tibia along the posterior medial border.[3] Differential assessment by the physician and physical therapist will include stress fractures of the tibia and fibula, ischemic disorders, and deep-compartment syndromes of the lower leg. Therefore medial tibial stress syndrome includes musculotendinous inflammation and periosteal inflammation of the muscle-tendon-bone interface at the posterior medial border of the tibia.

Specifically, the tissues most often responsible for the pain associated with medial tibial stress syndrome include the posterior tibialis muscle and the medial origin of the soleus muscle.[1,30] Investigators have shown through cadaver dissection, electromyographic studies, and bone scans that clinical findings of pain associated with medial tibial stress correlate with the medial origin of the soleus and not the posterior tibialis muscle.[30] However, excessive traction on the posterior tibialis muscle and tendon (which originates at posterior surfaces of the tibia, interosseous membrane, and fibula and inserts into the undersurfaces of the navicular, all three cuneiforms and the second, third, and fourth metatarsals) can occur from excessive foot pronation, thereby causing stress and strain on supporting soft tissue of the lower leg.[1]

Because pain is the predominant feature of medial tibial stress syndrome, it is quite helpful to classify and describe the severity of pain related to the patient's ability to perform activities.[18] Grade I describes pain that is experienced after activities. Grade II defines pain both during and after activities, but does not affect the actual performance of activities. Grade III pain is felt before, during, and after activities and affects the patient's ability to perform activities. Grade IV pain is so significant that no activities can even be attempted.

In general, grade I pain refers to muscle soreness and minor soft-tissue inflammation. Grade II pain is viewed as a mild or moderate soft tissue inflammation. Grade III pain involves significant soft tissue inflammation, and bone microfractures. Grade IV pain defines an actual stress fracture.

A patient experiencing minor pain (grade I) will typically describe transient muscle soreness and general tenderness following activities. Treatment generally consists of ice packs or ice massage, physician prescribed nonsteroidal antiinflammatory drugs (NSAIDs), rest and gradual stretching and strengthening exercises for the entire lower leg.

With grade II pain, the patient is able to localize the exact site of the pain and typically has had symptoms for a few weeks.[18] It is significant to note that along with treatments involving ice, medications, and exercise, the therapist will make a significant attempt to decrease the volume of activity and to modify activities that exacerbate the pain. A reduction of 10% to 25% of the total volume of activity usually is appropriate to allow for sufficient healing.[18]

With a major soft-tissue inflammation (grade III) the patient is able to clearly define an exact or focal area of pain (point tenderness). The patient may demonstrate other evidence of inflammation, including heat, erythema, swelling and crepitus. Because of the significance of pain and dysfunction associated with grade III

pain that is localized to the posterior medial border of the tibia, the physician may order a bone scan in addition to radiographs, in order to determine whether periostial inflammation and bone breakdown are present. Treatment of major soft tissue inflammation will focus on pain and swelling reduction. Therapeutic interventions will include ice packs or ice massage, oral analgesics, antiinflammatory medications (NSAIDs), complete rest from the aggravating activity, and specific stretching exercises for the gastroc-soleus complex, intrinsic foot musculature, and posterior tibialis. Upon resumption of activities, a 25% to 75% reduction in volume is warranted until full pain-free motion is achieved. This grade of pain can be considered a pre-stress fracture syndrome if not managed appropriately. If stress is not removed, the condition can worsen.

Grade IV pain is usually constant and activity is severely affected. In addition to the five cardinal signs of inflammation (redness, swelling, pain, heat, and dysfunction) the patient may also demonstrate reduced range of motion and muscular atrophy.[18] This level of pain signifies a breakdown of the periosteal-bone interface and a stress fracture. Complete rest, crutches, ice, medications, therapeutic agents, iontophoresis, and phonophoresis may be indicated to control swelling and pain.

In general terms, treatment of medial tibial stress syndrome is highly individualized and specifically related to the comprehensive evaluation performed by the physical therapist. If the physical therapist determines that the patient demonstrates excessive foot pronation, custom molded orthotics may be prescribed to relieve stress on the medial soleus and reduce traction on the tibialis posterior muscle and tendon. Cryokinetics (ice packs or ice massage in conjunction with stretching and strengthening exercises) are usually advocated as a means to control pain and swelling and to encourage motion and function. Relative rest is prescribed in most cases of medial tibial stress syndrome. That is, instead of complete rest and immobilization, the patient's activity level is modified to accomodate the patient's complaints of pain and dysfunction. For example, a patient who is an avid jogger may be encouraged to jog in a pool instead. If an upper body ergometer (UBE) is available, the patient can still actively perform aerobic conditioning activities without the associated stress on the lower leg. Overall, modifications in the patient's activity level (relative rest) and the judicious use of physician-prescribed NSAIDs and or analgesics, as well as a highly specific gastroc-soleus stretching program and lower-leg strengthening regimen, proves effective in the management of medial tibial stress syndrome.

PLANTAR FASCIITIS (HEEL SPUR SYNDROME)

Chronic inflammation of the plantar aponeurosis, with or without an associated calcaneal heel spur, is called **plantar fasciitis** (Fig. 12-25). Leach and coworkers[25] describe plantar fasciitis as repetitive microtrauma leading to injury, attempted repair, and chronic inflammation. Brody[6] describes plantar fasciitis as an "inflammatory reaction due to chronic traction on the plantar aponeurosis (fascia) at its insertion into the calcaneus."

Patients frequently complain of pain along the medial border of the calcaneus on the plantar surface. Many patients report that pain is worse in the morning when the foot contacts the floor in getting out of bed. Palpation of the plantar fascia usually reveals tenderness at the medial tuberosity of the os calcis or throughout the entire course of the fascia.[4] Palpation is performed with the toes flexed, which reduces tension on the fascia, or with the toes extended, which increases tension on the fascia.[4]

Management

Many patients respond well to conservative physical therapy procedures. All causative factors must first be eliminated or modified for healing to proceed. Ice massage or ice packs and physician prescribed nonsteroidal antiinflammatory medications along with a plastic heel cup are initial management procedures used to reduce pain and swelling. Specific stretching exercises are employed to help reduce tension on the plantar fascia. General calf-stretching exercises are initiated and progressed according to the patient's tolerance. Specific soleus stretching exercises are also used. Occasionally, ultrasound, phonophoresis, or iontophoresis is used to reduce pain and swelling. Additional stretching exercises should include toe-extension stretches with a towel. As pain and swelling improve, specific strengthening exercises can be used to strengthen the intrinsic and extrinsic foot muscles.

Toe curls are effective when used in conjunction with stretching, ice, and/or ultrasound (Fig. 12-26). The picking up of marbles with the toes or the repeated "gripping" with the toes of a towel placed on the floor strengthens the foot muscles.

Occasionally the physician may inject a local steroid to help decrease pain and swelling in more severe cases. Because many patients complain that the most severe pain is in the morning, some physicians and physical therapists prescribe night splints, which place the foot in a position that decreases stress on the plantar fascia. In

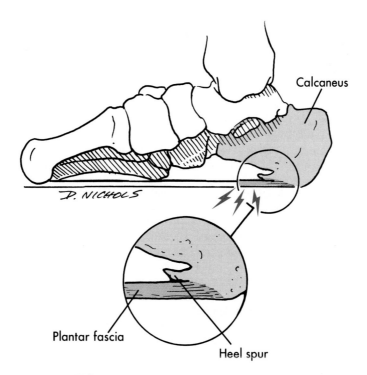

D. NICHOLS

Calcaneus

Plantar fascia

Heel spur

FIG. 12-25 Plantar fasciitis with heel spur.

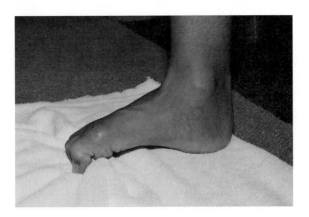

FIG. 12-26 Resistive toe curls are performed by gripping a towel.

an athletic population, plantar fasciitis occurs from running and competitive sports participation. During recovery from plantar fasciitis, it is imperative to maintain aerobic fitness and general body strength. Aerobic exercises can be performed without weight-bearing in a pool or with a UBE to decrease repetitive loading on the plantar fascia. Stationary cycling is an excellent alternative.

With some patients who do not respond to conservative therapy, the physician may decide to correct the problem surgically. Surgical options include plantar fascia release (fasciotomy) and excision of calcaneal exostosis (spur).

ARCH DEFORMITIES (PES PLANUS AND PES CAVUS)

Pes planus (flatfoot) is a congenital or acquired deformity of the foot where the medial longitudinal arch of the foot is reduced, causing the medial border of the foot to contact the ground when standing.[26] The usual cause of acquired pes planus is muscular weakness, laxity of ligaments that support the medial longitudinal arch, paralysis, or a pronated foot.[26] Pes planus deformity can be classified as mild, moderate, or severe.

During the initial evaluation, the physical therapist will measure the degree of hindfoot (tibiofibular joints; talocrural joint-articulation between the talus, medial malleolus of the tibia, and the lateral malleolus of the fibula; and the subtalar joint) and forefoot (tarsometatarsal joints, intermetatarsal joints, metatarsalphalangeal joints, interphalangeal joints) varus and valgus.[26] A 4-degree to 6-degree hindfoot valgus and a 4-degree to 6-degree forefoot varus is classified as a mild pes planus. A moderate pes planus is associated with a 6-degree to 10-degree hindfoot valgus and a 6-degree to

10-degree forefoot varus. Severe pes planus results from a 10-degree to 15-degree hindfoot valgus and an 8-degree to 10-degree forefoot varus. In addition, the therapist will assess the deformity in weight-bearing and non–weight-bearing positions.[35] With a rigid pes planus deformity, the foot appears to have an abnormally low arch in both weight-bearing and non–weight-bearing positions.[35] With a flexible pes planus deformity, the foot appears to have a normal arch in a non–weight-bearing position, but an abnormally low or flat arch in weight-bearing.

No specific therapeutic interventions are required if there is no associated pain or dysfunction. However, because the area is a terminal component of the closed kinetic chain during weight-bearing (the arch can affect the knee, hip and spine in a closed kinetic chain), treatment that is specific to the arch may be indicated if associated pain and dysfunction are experienced in other joints along the kinetic chain. For example, pes planus can affect the normal neutral-to-pronation sequence of the foot during the gait cycle. Because the foot is already pronated (with pes planus) the reduced normalized motion from neutral to pronation is affected during gait. Therefore the knee and other joints along the kinetic chain must compensate for this reduced motion. If pain and resultant dysfunction occur in one or more of these associated joints, then corrective action is needed to place the foot in a more neutral position to enhance the normal physiologic motion of the entire kinetic chain. Usually, the use of a custom fabricated orthotic is indicated to create a more normal mechanical arch. An orthosis or orthotic device is defined as an "apparatus or appliance that is used to correct or control a structural abnormality of a body part."[9] Materials used in orthotics include cork, leather, rubber, foam, felt, and plastic.[9] The rationale for the use of a custom molded orthotic to correct a symptomatic pes planus is supported by the work of D'Ambrosia,[13] who documented that 90% of patients with pes planovalgus reported effective relief of symptoms with the use of orthotics.

Pes cavus, on the other hand, describes an abnormally high arch.[26,35] Pes cavus usually is a result of neurogenic pathologic processes, muscle imbalances, and congenital abnormalities; both medial and lateral longitudinal arches are affected. Clinically, patients may complain of painful callouses beneath the metatarsal heads due to the mechanical friction and pressure that occurs with metatarsal heads. Osteoarthritic changes are not uncommon in the tarsal area because of the altered biomechanics of the foot.

Treatment for pes cavus is again focused on pain and dysfunction. No treatment is indicated if no symptoms exist, although the therapist may document this deformity during a lower-quarter evaluation. Felt pads can be used to control the pain of metatarsal head callousities. Unfortunately, D'Ambrosia[13] found little benefit (25%) from the use of orthotics with patients who had pes cavus.

MORTON'S NEUROMA (PLANTAR INTERDIGITAL NEUROMA)

Patients with a **neuroma** may complain of diffuse, occasionally radiating pain into the toes and proximally to the dorsal or plantar surface of the foot.[11] A neuroma usually occurs at the 3-4 interspace and less frequently at the 2-3 interspace[31] (Fig. 12-27). Morton's neuroma occurs bilaterally only 15% of the time with the patient complaining of a "burning," "cramping," or "catching" sensation.[31,11] A painful mass can be palpated in approximately one third of the cases.[31]

Treatment

Conservative care calls for the use of a metatarsal pad, change of footwear to a wider, softer shoe, and local corticosteroid injections. Surgical excision of the neuroma may be necessary when all attempts at conservative care fail to relieve pain.

Physical therapy care involves early active motion to limit postoperative stiffness and fibrosis. Postoperative care dictates that the patient be weight-bearing as tolerated and progressed to full weight-bearing as pain allows. Compression bandages are used with elastic tape to assist with swelling and pain management. Generally, physical therapy care begins 2 to 3 weeks after surgery, once the sutures are removed. Typically, however, patients are encouraged to perform active ankle, foot, and knee ROM exercises during the early healing phase before physical therapy.

Thermal agents used to reduce swelling and pain include whirlpool baths and cryotherapy. In addition, ultrasound can be used under water in conjunction with active motion exercises to improve circulation, reduce tissue congestion, and improve motion. Active ROM exercises include ankle motion in all directions, knee flexion and extension, and specific toe-extension exercises with toe curls and splaying of the toes as tolerated. Occasionally, passive mobilization of the metatarsals may be needed to avoid the development of movement limitations. As soon as the pain allows, strengthening exercises can be initiated.

All strengthening exercises for the ankle and knee are included with specific intrinsic foot strengthening exercises. Resistive toe curls can begin as an open kinetic chain exercise and progress to a closed kinetic chain exercise as strength and patient tolerance allow.

General body strengthening exercises and aerobic fitness are encouraged during all phases of recovery from surgical resection of a Morton's neuroma.

HALLUX VALGUS

Hallux valgus is a lateral or valgus deviation of the great toe with both soft tissue and bony deformity (Fig. 12-28). This condition is made worse by improper footwear (narrow toe box), and often the pain can be relieved by removing the shoes. Examination should include assessment of the deformity in a standing position, which often accentuates the deformity, [11,31] and measurement of the hallux valgus angle (normal is <15 degrees) to determine the degree of deformity and angle of deviation.

Management options include both conservative care and operative procedures. Initial care is supportive, with a change in footwear to include a wider toe box (this alone can significantly reduce symptoms), insoles, arch supports (orthotics), and pads to dissipate stress and relieve pain. Modifications in activity may profoundly

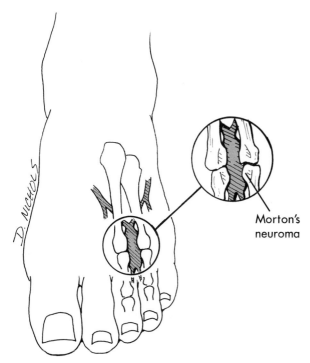

Morton's neuroma

FIG. 12-27 Morton's neuroma.

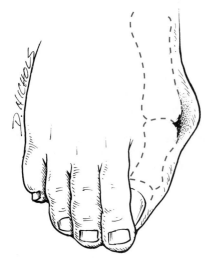

FIG. 12-28 Hallux valgus.

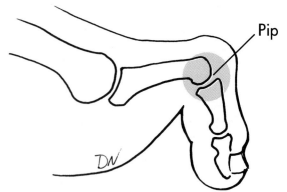

FIG. 12-29 Hammer toe.

reduce symptoms. In an athletic population, changing from running activities to swimming or bicycling can reduce pain caused by the repetitive pounding of running.

Many surgical options are available, depending on the severity of the deformity. General physical therapy management of postoperative bunionectomy is designed to reduce pain and swelling, improve ROM, and increase strength to enable a return to normal daily activities. Generally, the patient wears a wooden-soled shoe, progressing to an open-toed sandal. Gauze padding and toe spacers are used to maintain proper alignment after the surgical procedure. Once the sutures are removed and the wounds closed, whirlpool treatments can begin, with active ROM exercises for both flexion and extension of the great toe. Manual resistive toe-extension and the toe flexion exercises can begin as pain allows. Gait mechanics must be carefully reviewed and correct walking encouraged after bunionectomy. Usually weight-bearing patterns and restrictions of movement affect proper gait mechanics, especially the strength, power, and motion needed for toe-off. Restoration of joint motion and stability, as well as toe flexion and extension strength, forms the foundation of the rehabilitation program.

LESSER TOE DEFORMITIES (HAMMER TOES, MALLET TOES, AND CLAW TOES)

Three distinct types of lesser toe deformities are **hammer toes, mallet toes,** and **claw toes.** All three deformi-

ties are worsened by wearing improper shoes (narrow toe box).

Hammer toe (Fig. 12-29) is characterized by deformity of the metatarsophalangeal (MTP) joint, proximal interphalangeal (PIP) joint, and distal interphalangeal (DIP) joint. The MTP joint is either in neutral position or extension. The PIP joint is held in flexion, with the DIP in either flexion or extension.

Mallet toe (Fig. 12-30) is characterized by a neutral MTP joint, a neutral PIP joint, and a flexed DIP joint.

Claw toes (Fig. 12-31) are often associated with neuromuscular disease and are similar in appearance to hammer toes. Claw toes are distinguished by MTP hyperextension, PIP flexion, and DIP flexion. This deformity usually results from "simultaneous contraction of the extensors and flexors."[31]

The physician or physical therapist will determine if the lesser toe deformity is either rigid (fixed) or flexible. Flexible deformities are usually correctable with conservative, passive measures, whereas fixed deformities may require surgery.

Management and Rehabilitation

Nonoperative conservative care of lesser toe deformities focuses on modifying activities that exacerbate pain, changing footwear to a wider, softer toe box (to avoid pressure and the occurrence of soft or hard callus formation over bony prominences), padding areas subjected to blistering and corn formation, and using supportive measures to reduce pain and swelling (such as custom fabricated orthotics or "off the shelf" orthotics). Whirlpool baths, ultrasound, stretching exercises for the toes, and foot and ankle strengthening exercises may help reduce pain and swelling.

Surgical repair is reserved for fixed or rigid deformities, although some flexible deformities also require

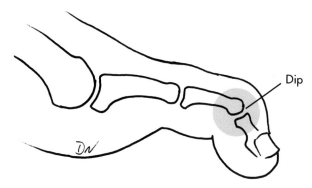

FIG. 12-30 Mallet toe.

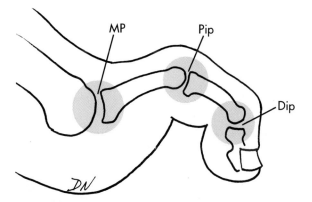

FIG. 12-31 Claw toe.

operation. Typically, sutures and pins are removed about 3 weeks after surgery.[11] The patient will be weight-bearing as tolerated initially, with a progression to full weight-bearing as pain allows. The affected extremity is held in a rigid-solid open-toe postsurgical boot to protect the repair from unwanted excessive flexion and extension of the toes.

For about 6 weeks after surgery, taping, padding, and protecting the repair are emphasized before progressing to weight-bearing toe-off proper gait mechanics. This time is needed to protect the surgical repair and to allow for the healing of bone and tendons (tenotomies are done for flexible lesser toe deformities). Throughout the rehabilitation program, from the immediate postoperative period until discharge, it is important to maintain strength, flexibility, and aerobic fitness. The affected extremity may be strengthened with open-chain resistive exercises (knee extension and leg curls), and aerobic fitness can be achieved with a stationary bike ergometer with the seat height lowered to maintain a neutral ankle position at the bottom of the pedal stroke. If the patient

cannot operate the bike in this fashion, the opposite, noninvolved extremity can be used alone (single-leg pedaling) using toe clips. A UBE can also be an effective aerobic conditioning tool during rehabilitation.

Once the pins and sutures are removed at 3 weeks, physical therapy management can begin. Whirlpool baths, ultrasound, active ROM, and gentle stretching and strengthening exercises (open-chain progressing to closed-chain toe curls with a towel or marbles) can be employed. The toes must be protected from unwanted stress throughout the maximum-protection phase (6 to 8 weeks after surgery) of rehabilitation. Coughlin[11] recommends avoiding all running activities for 9 to 12 weeks after surgery to allow for proper healing.

COMMON MOBILIZATION TECHNIQUES FOR THE ANKLE, FOOT, AND TOES

Limitations of movement resulting from fibrosis after trauma, surgery, or disease of the foot, ankle, or toes frequently require specific mobilization procedures to regain normal joint function. Mobilization techniques are typically used in conjunction with thermal modalities to control pain and swelling and aid in relaxation; these modalities include hot packs, ultrasound, whirlpool baths, and ice packs. Active and passive exercises, specific stretching exercises, strengthening exercises (open progressing to closed chain), and proprioception tasks help the patient regain balance, coordination, and function. The choice of mobilization technique, direction of application, grades, amplitude of force, velocity, oscillations, and distractions is made by the physical therapist based on the specific pathologic condition involved, tissue-healing constraints, and overall appropriateness with regard to the short-term and long-term goals of the rehabilitation program.

The following techniques are general procedures used for a wide variety of specific joint limitations. These techniques can be modified by the therapist depending on the specific nature of the limitations involved. This list is not intended to be a comprehensive review of all techniques for each joint of the ankle, foot, and toe. These methods are commonly used, easily practiced, effective procedures for treating a host of joint limitations. It is clinically relevant to restate that the delegation of selected mobilization techniques to be used by the PTA is entirely at the discretion of the physical therapist and peripheral joint mobilization is not universally accepted as a routine domain of practice of the PTA. Information concerning peripheral joint mobilization has been provided as a means to stimulate the PTA's awareness of the rationale for improving motion and for the reduction of pain as identified and prescribed by the physical therapist.

Ankle Mobilization

Anterior and posterior glides are best performed with the patient in a supine or "long-sitting" position with the lower leg firmly and comfortably supported. For anterior glide of the calcaneus, the hand position, stabilization, and direction of force are similar to those for the anterior drawer test for ligament stability testing of the anterior talofibular ligament. Place one hand firmly on the distal anterior surface of the tibia and fibula. Use the application hand to firmly "cup" the calcaneus and provide an anterior-directed force (Fig. 12-32).

The posterior glide technique is performed with the patient in the same position as the anterior glide. Stabilize the distal tibia and fibula with the palm of one hand. Place the application hand on the dorsal surface of the talus to provide a posterior-directed force (Fig. 12-33).

Traction is achieved through long-axis distraction of the talus caudally from the tibia and fibula. The patient can be either supine or prone with the lower leg firmly and comfortably supported. Firmly grasp the dorsal surface of the talus with the open palm of one hand, while using the other hand to firmly grasp and cup the calcaneus. Apply the force simultaneously with both hands along the long axis of the tibia and fibula (Fig. 12-34), effectively distracting the talus from the mortise.

Metatarsal Mobilization

Distal metatarsal glides are performed while the patient is supine with the lower leg supported. Use the hand, thumb, and fingers of one hand to stabilize the ray of the second metatarsal while the hand, thumb, and fingers of the application hand firmly grasp the first ray at the metatarsal head. Apply force in a plantar and dorsal direction (Fig. 12-35).

PIP Joint Mobilization

Long-axis distraction of the PIP joint is achieved by stabilizing the affected metatarsal ray with one hand while using the application hand to firmly grasp the affected phalanx. The thumb and fingers apply long-axis traction (distraction) (Fig. 12-36).

Plantar and dorsal PIP glides are performed with the patient supine and the lower leg supported. Use one hand to firmly grasp the first metatarsal ray at the

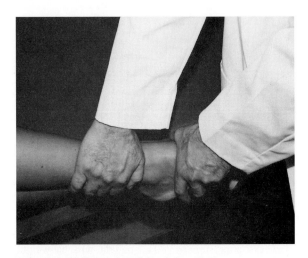

FIG. 12-33 Posterior glide of the talus.

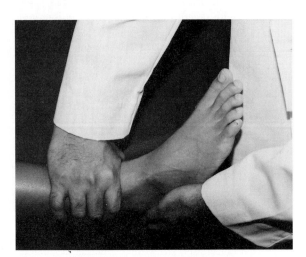

FIG. 12-32 Anterior glide of the calcaneus.

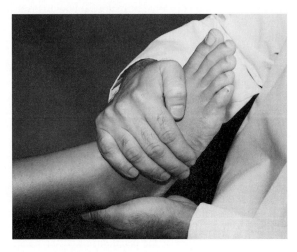

FIG. 12-34 Long-axis distraction of the talus.

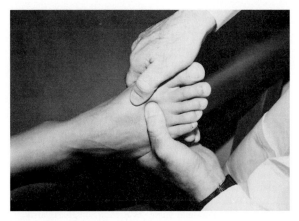

FIG. 12-35 Distal metatarsal anterior-posterior glides.

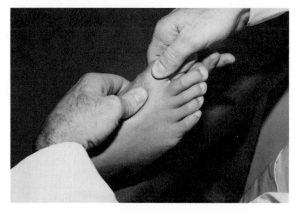

FIG. 12-37 Proximal interphalangeal (PIP) plantar and dorsal glides.

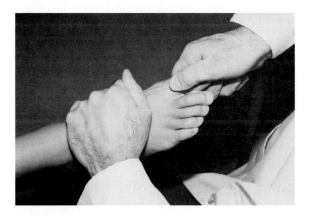

FIG. 12-36 Long-axis proximal interphalangeal (PIP) distraction.

metatarsal head. The thumb of the stabilizing hand must be placed on the dorsal surface of the metatarsal head. Use the application hand to grasp the proximal phalanx and apply a plantar and dorsal force while stabilizing the metatarsal head (Fig. 12-37).

REFERENCES

1. Andrish JT: The Leg. In DeLee JD, Drez D editors: *Orthopaedic sports medicine, principles and practice,* vol. 2, Philadelphia, 1994, WB Saunders.
2. Beskin JL et al: Surgical repair of Achilles tendon ruptures, *AM J Sports Med* 15:1-8, 1987.
3. Black HM, Brand RL: Injuries of the foot and ankle. In Scott NW, Nisonson B, Nicholas J, editors: *Principles of sports medicine,* Baltimore, 1984, Williams & Wilkins.
4. Bordelon RL: Heel pain. In DeLee JD, Drez D, editors: *Orthopaedic sports medicine: principles and practice,* vol 2, Philadelphia, 1994, W. B. Saunders.
5. Brand RL, Collins MDF, Templeton T: Surgical repair of ruptured lateral ankle ligaments, *Am J Sports Med* 9:40-44, 1981.
6. Brody DM: Running injuries: prevention and management, *Clinical Symposia* 39(3):28, Ciba-Geigy, 1987.
7. Canale ST: Ankle injuries. In Crenshaw AH, editor: *Campbell's operative orthopaedics,* vol 3, ed 7, St. Louis, 1987, Mosby.
8. Chrisman OD, Snook G: Reconstruction of lateral ligament tears of the ankle: an experimental study and clinical evaluation of seven patients treated by a new modification of the Elmslie procedure, *J Bone Joint Surg* 51A:904-912, 1969.
9. Clanton TO: Sport shoes, insoles and orthoses. In DeLee JD, Drez D, editors: *Orthopaedic sports medicine, principles and practice,* vol 2, Philadelphia, 1994, WB Saunders.
10. Conrad JJ, Tannin AH: Trauma to the ankle. In Jahss MH, editor: *Disorders of the foot,* Philadelphia, 1982, WB Saunders.
11. Coughlin MJ: Conditions of the forefoot. In DeLee JD, Drez D, editors: *Orthopaedic sports medicine: Principles and practice,* vol 2, Philadelphia, 1994, WB Saunders.
12. Curwin S, Stanish W: *Tendinitis: it's etiology and treatment,* Lexington, Mass., 1984, The Callamore Press.
13. D'Ambrosia RD: Orthotic devices in running injuries, *Clin Sports Med* 4:611-618, 1985.
14. Eckert WR, David EA: Acute rupture of the peroneal retinaculum, *J Bone Joint Surg* 58A:670-673, 1976.
15. Evans DL: Recurrent instability of the ankle: a method of surgical treatment, *Proc R Soc Med* 46:343-344, 1953.
16. Harper MC: The deltoid ligament: an evaluation of need for surgical repair, *Clin Orthop* 226:156-168, 1988.
17. Inglis AE, Sculco TP: Surgical repair of ruptures of the tendo Achilles, *Clin Orthop* 156:160-168, 1981.
18. Jackson DW: Shin-splints: an update: *The Physic and Sports Med* 6(10):51-61, 1978.
19. Jackson BA, Schwane JA, Starcher BC: Effect of ultrasound therapy on the repair of Achilles tendon

injuries in rats, *Med Sci Sports Exer 23(2):*171-176, 1991.

20. Jacobs D et al: Comparison of conservative and operative treatment of Achilles tendon rupture, *Am J Sport Med* 6:107-111, 1978.

21. Keene JS: Tendon injuries of the foot and ankle. In DeLee JD, Drez D, editors: *Orthopaedic sports medicine, principals and practice,* vol 2, Philadelphia, 1994, WB Saunders.

22. Lassiter TE, Malone TR, Garrett W: Injury to the lateral ligaments of the ankle, *Orthop Clin North Am* 20:629-640, 1989.

23. Leach RE, James S, Wasilewski S: Achilles tendinitis, *AM J Sports Med* 9(2):93-98, 1981.

24. Leach R: Acute ankle sprains: vigorous treatment for best results, *J Musculoskel Med* 1:68-76, 1983.

25. Leach RE, Seavey MS, Salter DK: Results of surgery in athletes with plantar fasciitis, *Foot Ankle* 7(3):156-161, 1986.

26. Magee DJ: Lower leg, ankle and foot. In: *Orthopaedic physical assessment,* ed 2, Philadelphia, 1992, WB Saunders.

27. Marti R: Dislocation of the peroneal tendons, *AM J Sports Med 5* (1):19-22, 1977.

28. McBryde A: Stress fractures of the foot and ankle In DeLee JD, Drez D editors: *Orthopaedic sports medicine, principles and practice,* vol 2, Philadelphia, 1994, WB Saunders.

29. McRae R: *Practical fracture treatment,* New York, 1994, Churchill Livingstone.

30. Michael RH, Holder LE: *The soleus syndrome:* a cause of medial tibial stress (shin splints), *Am J Sports Med* 13(2):87-94, 1985.

31. Miller M: *Review of orthopaedics,* Philadelphia, 1992, WB Saunders.

32. Myerson MS: Injuries to the forefoot and toes. In Jahss MH editor: *Disorders of the foot and ankle: medical and surgical management,* vol 2, ed 2, Philadelphia, 1991, WB Saunders.

33. Nistor L: Surgical and nonsurgical treatment of Achilles tendon rupture, *J Bone Joint Surg* 63A:394-399, 1981.

34. Renstrom P, AFH, Kannus P: Injuries of the foot and ankle. In DeLee JD, Drez D, editors: *Orthopaedic Sports medicine, principles and practice,* vol II, Philadelphia, 1994, WB Saunders.

35. Riddle DL: Foot and ankle. In Richardson JK, Iglarsh ZA, editors: *Clinical orthopaedic physical therapy,* Philadelphia, 1994, WB Saunders.

36. Riehl R: Rehabilitation of lower leg injuries. In Prentice WE, editor: *Rehabilitation techniques in sports medicine,* ed 2, St. Louis, 1994, Mosby.

37. Stanitski CL et al: On the nature of stress fractures, *Am J Sports Med,* 6:391-396, 1978.

38. Staples OS: Ruptures of the fibular collateral ligaments of the ankle: results study of immediate surgical treatment, *J Bone Joint Surg* 57A:101-107, 1975.

39. Stover CN, Bryan D: Traumatic dislocation of peroneal tendons, *AM J Surg* 103:180-186, 1962.

40. Watson-Jones R: Recurrent forward dislocation of the ankle joint, *J Bone Joint Surg* 34B:519, 1952.

Orthopedic Management of the Knee

KEY TERMS

As a vital team member, the physical therapist assistant is frequently challenged to safely and effectively manage acute, chronic, and postsurgical orthopedic conditions of the knee. This chapter presents common pathologic conditions of the ligaments, meniscus lesions, patellofemoral diseases, extensor mechanism disorders, and fractures of the knee as well as rehabilitation procedures related to total knee joint replacement. This chapter gives the physical therapist assistant an appreciation of various knee ailments, mechanisms of injury, and specific tissue healing constraints, and provides an introduction to the rationale behind criterion-based rehabilitation programs for the knee.

The knee is an extraordinarily complex joint. Therefore the physical therapist assistant is strongly encouraged to review pertinent knee joint anatomy and functional mechanics before and throughout this study.

LIGAMENT INJURIES

Ligament injuries of the knee refer to various degrees of sprains that may lead to frank ruptures of the ligament, manifested by loss of joint function. Knee ligament sprains and joint instability are complex and sophisticated problems involving various degrees of straight-plane and/or combined rotatory instability. Knee ligament sprains may be defined as follows:

- *Mild: Grade I, first-degree ligament sprain:* An incomplete stretching of collagen ligament fibers resulting in minimal pain, minimal or no swelling, no loss of joint function, and no clinical or functional instability.
- *Moderate: Grade II, second-degree ligament sprain:* A partial loss of ligament fiber continuity. A few collagen ligament fibers may be completely torn; however, most of the ligament remains intact. This degree of sprain is characterized by moderate (more intense than first-degree) pain, moderate swelling, some loss of joint function, and some loss of joint stability.
- *Severe: Grade III, third degree sprain (rupture):* The entire collagen ligament fiber bundles are completely torn. There is no continuity within the body of the ligament. This is usually characterized by profound pain, intense swelling, loss of joint function, and instability.

Anterior Cruciate Ligament (ACL) Injuries
Pertinent history and physical examination. The natural history of an **anterior cruciate ligament (ACL)** sprain usually involves combined forces of external rotation, valgus stress, and internal tibial rotation alone or combined with knee hyperextension while the affected foot is planted (Fig. 13-1).[43] In contrast to many other knee injuries, the typical ACL sprain involves a noncontact, deceleration, closed kinetic chain (CKC) mechanism of injury, rather than external forces affecting the ligament. The resultant sprain can rapidly develop a tense hemarthrosis (blood within the joint) requiring arthrocentesis (aspiration of fluid from within a joint). Removal of blood can signal a ligament tear, whereas blood with fat droplets may reveal a fracture or ligament sprain. Removal of synovial fluid without blood may indicate a chronic meniscus lesion or synovitis.[40]

The physical therapist assistant must recognize that the cruciate ligaments are intracapsular structures, which, when injured, can produce a joint effusion. This anatomic relationship is contrasted with the medial and lateral collateral ligaments, which are extracapsular structures. When the medial collateral ligament (MCL) is sprained, there is generally less swelling and no intraarticular effusion because the resultant bleeding from the injured tissues can evacuate the area and the fluid is therefore not restrained within the joint capsule.

Ligament stability tests. The physical therapist assistant must be aware of various clinical ligament stability tests to accurately and effectively communicate changes in a patient's stability to the supervising physical therapist and physician. Although ligament stability tests are part of the initial evaluation procedures used by

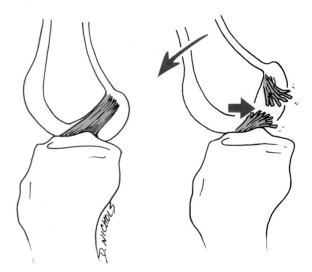

FIG. 13-1 Mechanism of injury to the anterior cruciate ligament (ACL). Typically, the ACL is injured in a noncontact deceleration mechanism of combined forces of external tibial rotation, valgus stress, internal tibial rotation, and knee hyperextension.

the physician and physical therapist, the physical therapist assistant can better understand the static and dynamic restraints of the knee and develop a more comprehensive view of rehabilitation when exposed to the rudimentary concepts of ligament stability testing.

Degrees of instability are graded similarly to degrees of ligament sprains. Hughston[26] has divided ligament instabilities into three degrees, as follows:

Mild instability: Graded 1+; characterized by 5 mm or less of joint surface separation

Moderate instability: Graded 2+; joint surface separation of 4 to 10 mm

Severe instability: Graded 3+; joint surface separation of 10 mm or more

Perhaps the most common, clinically useful, and easily taught and performed ligament stability test for the ACL is the Lachman examination (Fig. 13-2).[26] The patient is supine on an examining table with the affected knee flexed to approximately 25 to 30 degrees. Use one hand to stabilize the distal femur, and with the other hand grasp the proximal tibia. Gently direct an anterior and posterior force to the proximal tibia. Observe the integrity (stability) of the ACL, noting the degree of joint motion (5 mm to 10 mm) present.

The anterior drawer test (Fig. 13-3) is another clinical examination used to approximate the degree of anterior tibial translation relative to the fixed femur. This examination is used less frequently than the Lachman test and is a less sensitive test to challenge the stability of the ACL. Hughston[26] describes the validity of the anterior drawer test in flexion this way:

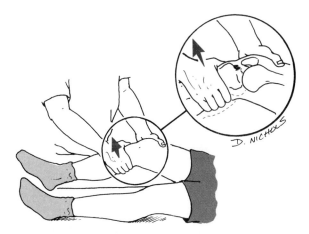

FIG.13-2 The Lachman exam. This examination tests the stability of the ACL with the knee flexed 25 degrees to 30 degrees. If the tibia can be displaced anteriorly in reference to the stabilized distal femur, then an injured ACL should be considered.

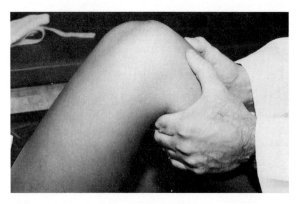

FIG. 13-3 The anterior drawer test. With the injured knee flexed to 90 degrees, the clinician grasps the proximal tibia and provides an anteriorly-directed force. If the tibia displaces anteriorly in reference to the stabilized distal femur, then the ACL may be considered injured.

The anterior drawer test in flexion has long been incorrectly perceived to test for a tear of the anterior cruciate ligament, but this ligament is relatively relaxed at 80 to 90 degrees of knee flexion. Instead, the anterior drawer test in flexion assesses the meniscotibial ligaments and the mobility of the menisci on the tibia.

The examination is performed with the patient supine and the affected knee flexed to approximately 90 degrees. Stabilize the affected limb by sitting on the foot of the affected limb. Use both hands to grasp the proximal posterior tibia, with the thumbs of both hands on the anterior joint line of the knee. Exert an anterior and posterior force to the proximal tibia and observe the amount of joint separation of the tibia relative to the femur.

Other relevant tests for the stability of the ACL incorporate multidirectional rotation examinations to acknowledge the presence of anteromedial rotatory instability (AMRI), posteromedial rotatory instability (PMRI), and posterolateral rotatory instability (PLRI). Anterolateral rotatory instability (ALRI) is the more common multiplanar instability encountered.[43,26] The Hughston jerk test and pivot shift test are commonly used examinations to sublux and reduce the tibia relative to the femur.[26]

Mechanical ligament stability tests. Various instrumented ligament stability devices help quantify degrees of instability (Box 13-1).The most common devices used with the greatest reliability[10] are the KT1000 and KT2000 knee ligament arthrometers.[10] The patient is supine with both knees flexed approximately 20 degrees to 25 degrees over a plastic bolster. The device is attached to the tibia with Velcro straps while the patella is stabilized (seated) with the patella reference pad. A handle is used to direct an anterior and posterior force to the proximal tibia. Audible tones are encountered when various pounds of force are applied to the tibia. The needle on a small dial on the surface of the device deflects in a positive or negative direction, quantifying the degree of tibial translation relative to the stable femur in millimeters of displacement.

Throughout the performance of this examination, complete muscle relaxation of the hamstrings, quadriceps, and gastroc-soleus muscle group must be maintained. Swelling, intraarticular effusion, and muscle spasm falsely stabilize the knee,[29] rendering the examination meaningless.

Operative management. The physical therapist assistant must recognize the various surgical procedures used to correct functional instabilities related to injuries of the ACL and be aware of the short-term and long-term ramifications of ligament healing to more effectively deliver sound rehabilitation programs and to better appreciate the complex nature of surgical repair and rehabilitation. Therefore this section provides a rudimentary description of the most common ACL surgical procedures as they relate to the scope and practice of the physical therapist assistant.

Central one-third bone-patellar tendon-bone autograft. An **autograft** uses tissue from the body of the patient. Various tissues are used for grafts, including the gracilis tendon, fascia lata, semitendinosus tendon, and quadriceps muscle tendon. The bone-patellar

tendon-bone autograft is the strongest one used for ACL reconstructions.[14]

An **allograft** refers to biologic tissue taken from another human body.[14] The major risks of using allograft involve disease transmission (risk of human immunodeficiency virus infection) and problems with effective sterilization procedures.[14]

Artificial ligaments include synthetic devices (Gore-Tex), tissue-scaffold devices, and **ligament-augmentation devices (LAD).** The major disadvantage of using prosthetic ligaments is that this material tends to deteriorate over time and cannot repair itself.[14]

The arthroscopic central one-third bone-patellar tendon-bone autograft procedure involves harvesting the graft from the involved knee (Fig. 13-4) and surgically routing this structure through tunnels placed in the femur and tibia in a way that duplicates normal ACL anatomy, then securing (fixing) the graft to the bone to allow for stable healing (Fig. 13-5). A small stab wound is made in the knee, and a small diameter drainage tube is inserted to help evacuate the joint of residual bleeding, which, if allowed to accumulate, increases arthrofibrosis. This small drain is usually removed after a few days when the bleeding is controlled. Even with the placement of the drain, postoperative arthrofibrosis is a clinically significant problem that occurs frequently.

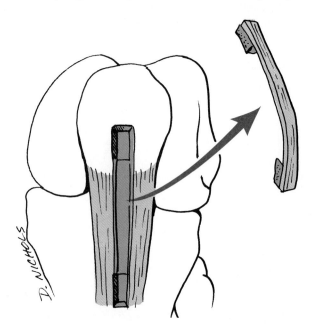

FIG. 13-4 Bone-patellar-tendon-bone harvest. A pedicle of bone from the tibial tubercle and the patella is removed along with a full-thickness graft of the patellar tendon to be used to anatomically reconstruct the ACL.

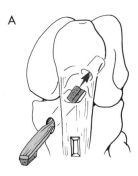

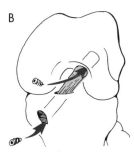

FIG. 13-5 The central one-third arthroscopically-aided bone-patellar-tendon-bone autograft procedure. **A,** The placement of the graft within the knee joint, through tunnels drilled in the tibia and femur. **B,** The graft tissue and bone pedicles being secured with anchor screws.

Sterile bandages are placed over the incisions, and the patient's leg is placed in a brace or knee immobilizer locked in 0 degrees of flexion.

Healing of the graft after surgery. Ligament healing processes and revascularization of graft material are vital concerns in the prescribed rehabilitation program designed by the supervising physical therapist. The appropriate progression of the rehabilitation program depends on the physical therapist assistant's awareness of the various stages of healing after an autograft procedure.

Once the graft is harvested and surgically routed within the knee, it begins a gradual process of avascular necrosis over the first 6 to 8 weeks.[14] The graft gradually loses strength and is quite fragile during the first 2 months after surgery, so excessive loads and forces that would compromise the healing of the graft must be avoided during this phase. The graft slowly revascularizes, and at approximately 3 months the tensile strength of the graft is less than 50% of its original strength.[14,38] Graft strength may take as long as a year to mature and it will never reach preoperative levels.

Rehabilitation after ACL reconstruction. The rehabilitation program after ACL reconstruction is designed to protect the graft; reduce pain and swelling; increase joint motion while improving strength, endurance (local muscular endurance as well as aerobic fitness), flexibility, and proprioception; and ultimately return the knee to full function. This task is organized sequentially and is constantly modified, based on the patient's individual response to surgery and rehabilitation. By design, set "cookbook" type protocols for rehabilitation after ACL surgery are rapidly losing favor among rehabilitation specialists. The physical therapist and physical therapist assistant must work together to assess and adjust programs based on the individual's ability to recover and adapt. As stated by Einhorn et al,[14] "each patient reacts differently to the surgical intervention. Loss of strength, swelling, and range of motion (ROM) are unpredictable. Patient personality, attitude, and pain tolerance vary greatly with each case." Therefore the physical therapist and physical therapist assistant must design and implement a rehabilitation program based on goals and criteria the individual must achieve before advancing to a more challenging phase.

In general terms, ACL reconstruction rehabilitation can be organized into three broad, interconnecting phases:

- *Maximum-protection phase:* From the first day postoperatively to approximately 6 weeks after surgery.[43]
- *Moderate-protection phase:* From approximately the seventh to the twelfth weeks after surgery.[43]
- *Minimal-protection phase:* From the thirteenth week after surgery until return to activity.[43]

This section will review each phase separately and introduce the physical therapist assistant to the many variables and individual differences among patients. The importance of reassessment of initial evaluation data and the need for open communication and team work with the supervising physical therapist cannot be emphasized too strongly.

Maximum-protection phase. As the graft slowly loses its strength (6 to 8 weeks after surgery), excessive loads and forces that stress the ACL must be avoided. These forces are controlled primarily by joint protection with range-limiting hinge braces and avoidance of anterior tibial translation and shearing forces as well as rotatory motions.

Control of swelling is important throughout each phase of rehabilitation. Even with suction drains inserted at the time of surgery, postoperative swelling can have a profound negative effect on the progress of the patient. Swelling inhibits muscle contractions, contributes significantly to pain, limits joint motion, and can stimulate arthrofibrosis. The use of elastic compression wraps along with the application of ice packs and elevation of the limb help to minimize swelling. For convenience and ease of application for the patient to use at home, commercial cold and compression appliances are available.

The patient's ability to achieve early active range of motion (ROM) is an essential component of the maximum-protection phase. While the newly placed graft is struggling to revascularize, it must be protected from anterior translatory and rotatory forces by use of an adjustable range-limiting brace. However, regaining full knee extension and flexion must proceed.

Frequently, patellar motion (caudal, cephalic, medial, and lateral glide) must be an immediate goal for knee flexion and extension to improve. Scarring from the graft harvest site and suprapatellar pouch typically inhibits free patellar motion. Initially, the physical therapist assistant must provide gentle stretching of the patella (Fig. 13-6) and instruct the patient to perform these stretches two to three times daily. Generally, full knee extension is achieved soon after surgery; if not, passive prone or supine knee extension stretches can be used judiciously to gradually increase knee extension (Fig. 13-7). In addition to active and passive knee flexion and extension, some authors[14,39,43] advocate the use of a continuous passive motion (CPM) device for a limited time very early in this phase. The use of a CPM device is based on studies that show: "Instituting CPM immediately after surgery helps maintain a normal articular surface and prevent degenerative changes that

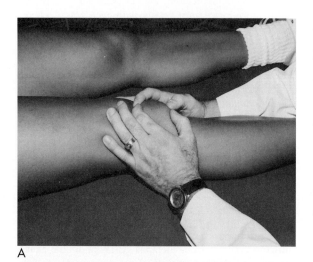

A

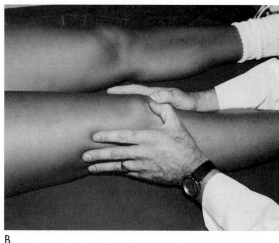

B

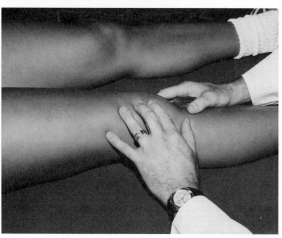

C

FIG. 13-6 Postoperative manual patellar stretching is used to enhance knee motion. If the patella becomes "adhered" to surrounding tissues, normal knee flexion and extension cannot occur. **A,** A caudal (inferior)-directed force applied to the patella. **B,** A cephalic (superior)-directed force. **C,** The patella being directed medially.

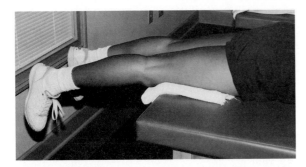

FIG. 13-7 Prone passive knee-extension stretch. Note the application of a folded towel under the thigh to elevate the leg and avoid compression of the patella and patellar tendon against the end of the table.

might occur as a result of ACL reconstruction."[43] Other investigators[14,39] have shown that CPM may help evacuate synovial joint hemarthrosis and aid in the prevention of knee joint contracture. The use of CPM is generally limited to the period immediately after hospitalization and is reserved for daytime use only.[14]

Ambulation and weight-bearing status are somewhat controversial in terms of when to allow full weight-bearing. In general, weight-bearing with crutches is allowed as tolerated as soon as possible after surgery. Daniel et al[11] advocate weight-bearing as tolerated for 5 to 6 weeks with crutches. Einhorn et al[14] recommend full weight-bearing by 2 to 4 weeks. Timm[43] encourages non–weight-bearing for the first week postoperatively, progressing to weight-bearing as tolerated.

Strengthening exercises during the maximum-protection phase focus on isometric cocontractions of the quadriceps and hamstrings. The physical therapist assistant must recognize that passive terminal knee extension is allowed but open-chain active knee extension with or without resistance causes an anterior tibial translation force relative to the femur that stresses the new graft. Cocontraction of the quadriceps and hamstring muscles within the hinged brace help to stabilize the joint and provide for muscular activity. Open kinetic-chain knee-extension exercises may be used during the maximum-protection phase if the resistance is placed proximal to the knee joint and the patient is not allowed to extend the knee in the final 40 degrees of extension "because of the high tensile forces on the ACL."[14] The primary focus of strengthening the postoperative ACL patient during the maximum-protection phase is to encourage quadriceps control (be able to demonstrate active quadriceps-hamstring setting) and hamstring strength. The hamstrings act as dynamic stabilizers to limit anterior tibial shearing forces,[14,38,39,43] and work on hamstring strength begins within the first week

postoperatively.[14] Both standing leg-curls and supine leg-curls can be initiated during this phase if a brace is used. New studies[5] offer the following exercise protocol that does not strain the ACL:[5]

- Isometric hamstring muscle contraction exercises at 15, 30, 60, and 90 degrees
- Isometric quadriceps contractions at 60 and 90 degrees
- Simultaneous contraction of the quadriceps and hamstring muscles at 30, 60, and 90 degrees of knee flexion
- Active flexion-extension motion of the knee from 35 degrees to full flexion
- Passive flexion-extension motion of the knee without muscle contraction

Four-way (flexion, extension, abduction, adduction) hip strengthening exercises as well as calf strengthening exercises are also encouraged during this phase. The criteria to be achieved by the patient before advancing to the moderate-protection phase include the following:

- ROM from 0 degrees extension to 120 degrees of flexion
- Full weight-bearing (encourage normal gait mechanics)
- Quadriceps control
- Hamstring control
- Controlled pain and swelling
- A minimum of 6 weeks from the day of surgery

Moderate-protection phase. As stated by Malone,[32] "Rehabilitation must degenerate into function!"; therefore the moderate-protection phase begins the process of functional recovery and focuses on CKC tasks and proprioceptive activities.

Progression from one phase to another is a slow, interrelated process with a strong carryover from one phase to the next. For example, at the beginning of the moderate-protection phase, the patient continues with all of the rudimentary exercises initiated in the maximum-protection phase. To advance to the next level at the beginning of the moderate-protection phase requires strong compliance from the patient in performing all stretching and strengthening exercises as well as demonstrated progress in weight-bearing status and proper gait mechanics. Generally, immobilization is discontinued around the fifth or sixth week postoperatively.[11] Control of pain and swelling continues as indicated.

CKC exercises and progressive proprioceptive tasks (to stimulate the afferent neural input system) are initiated and progressed throughout this phase. Studies[1,3] have demonstrated that "the ligaments of the knee have a rich sensory innervation that allows them to act as the first link in the 'kinetic chain .'"[3] Loss of the mechanoreceptor "stabilizing reflex"[3] may result in reduced afferent neural input system function, which may contribute to "progressive instability and disability."[3] Therefore gradual CKC progressive loads are essential to encourage functional muscle control and confidence in the use of the affected limb during weight-bearing (functional) activities. As previously mentioned (Chapter 3), CKC exercises are a system of interdependent articulated links in which motion at one joint produces motion at all other joints in the system in a predictable manner. The reasons for the early use of CKC activities are that these exercises are more functionally relevant, stimulate neuromuscular coordination, enhance joint approximation, and influence the joint mechanoreceptor system.

Initial instruction in CKC exercises begins with the patient braced to protect the healing graft. Standing and shifting of body weight from the nonaffected limb to the affected limb is a safe and appropriate introduction to CKC exercises. Once the patient can demonstrate confidence, muscle control, and stability, the brace is removed (with prior consultation and concurrence from the supervising physical therapist) and the patient is allowed to shift weight without braced support. The leg press is used as a CKC exercise in a short-arc motion

early in the moderate-protection phase while the patient is braced (Fig. 13-8). Progressive ROM exercises are allowed as the patient tolerates them. Standing wall slides are also introduced during the moderate protection phase if the affected limb is braced and the tibia is kept as vertical as possible to avoid an anterior tibial translation force (Fig. 13-9). The short-arc step-up is an

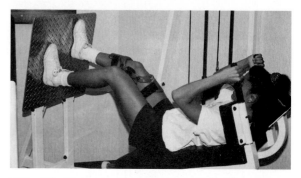

FIG. 13-8 Closed–kinetic-chain leg press with the knee braced. The noninvolved leg is used to support the weight and provide confidence during the application of the short-arc leg press.

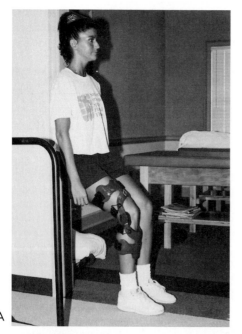
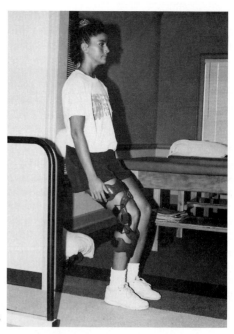

A   B

FIG. 13-9 Closed-chain short-arc wall slides. As the knee is braced in order to avoid unwanted anterior tibial translation, the patient is introduced to quadriceps strengthening (concentrically, eccentrically, and isometrically) in a vertical weight-bearing position. **A,** A partial wall slide with the patient holding an isometric position. **B,** Note the use of a small ball placed behind the patient to encourage greater balance and control.

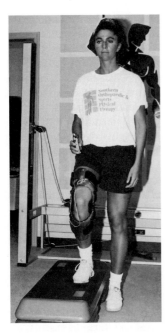

FIG. 13-10 The use of portable biofeedback or electrical muscle stimulation (EMS) can be used to enhance greater quadriceps control during short-arc step-ups.

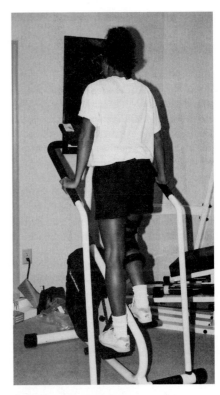

FIG. 13-11 Stair-steppers can be used as a closed-chain functional (stair climbing) exercise, provided the knee is braced and the intensity controlled to avoid excessive unwanted forces.

excellent exercise used to stimulate quadriceps control and strength. Often a biofeedback system is used in conjunction with step-ups to encourage appropriate quadriceps control (Fig. 13-10).

Stationary cycling is also encouraged throughout the moderate-protection phase of ACL rehabilitation. The height of the seat may require adjusting to accommodate the limited knee flexion ROM. The stationary cycle is used primarily to encourage range of motion, but during the middle and later stages of this phase, the cycle can be used as an aerobic conditioning tool if the patient has achieved the required ROM, strength, and stability to perform endurance activities. Stair-steppers can also be introduced during this phase if the ROM and intensity of the resistance on the apparatus are modified and controlled initially to allow for protected joint motion (Fig. 13-11).

To stimulate greater strength and local muscular endurance of the quadriceps, the patient can be instructed to perform the stair-stepper in a reverse manner. Throughout this phase the patient is encouraged to maintain patellar-stretching, hamstring-stretching, and quadriceps-stretching exercises, normal gait mechanics, a general fitness program of strength and endurance activities that do not stress the affected limb, ice application after exercises, and joint-protection principles.

Criteria that must be met by the patient before progressing to the next phase include the following:
- Full ROM (flexion, extension, patellar mobility)
- Normalized full weight-bearing gait and removal of brace as indicated
- Improved quadriceps strength
- Improved hamstring strength
- Continued control of pain and swelling
- A minimum of 12 to 13 weeks from the day of surgery

Minimal-protection phase. The minimal-protection phase signals the return to more normalized activities and the introduction of more challenging functional activities.

Isolated knee ligament stability tests, including manual clinical examinations (such as Lachman test, anterior drawer test, and pivot shift test) and instrumented stability examinations (KT1000 knee ligament arthrometer) are performed at the discretion of the physical therapist and physician, usually during the moderate-protection and minimal-protection phases of rehabilitation. Ongoing documentation of the stability of the affected limb is essential to justify progression to more challenging exercises and to quantify the clinical results of the surgery. The use of isokinetic testing of the involved limb is also left to the judgment of the physical therapist and physician. Generally, isokinetic examinations are reserved for the moderate-protection and minimal-protection phases. Because of the long-term nature of graft healing and the tibial translation forces produced with isokinetic testing and training, certain precautions must be taken to minimize these forces and protect the graft. Timm[43] states that isokinetic exercise "requires the use of an antishear device or a proximally positioned input pad to protect the reconstructed ACL against excessive anterior tibial translation forces."

As clinical testing demonstrates improved strength, neuromuscular control, and stability of the ligament, more progressive proprioceptive exercises can be initiated. The use of a balance board and mini-trampoline further challenges the mechanoreceptor system (Fig. 13-12). Standing knee extension with resistance provided by elastic tubing is an excellent CKC exercise that encourages quadriceps control in more functional positions (Fig. 13-13). Slide board activities are usually reserved for a more athletic population but can be modified for the general population to be less intense and less sports specific. Straight-line jogging progressing to faster running is initiated for patients inclined toward participation in sporting activities.

Progressive strengthening of the entire lower extremity includes isokinetic velocity spectrum training, isotonic eccentric quadriceps strengthening, leg presses, and squatting exercises. The physical therapist assistant must be constantly aware that rehabilitation after ACL reconstruction involves the entire body and not just the affected limb. Care must be taken to involve all muscle groups as well as the sensory input systems and aerobic system throughout each phase of rehabilitation. Returning the patient to functional activities is the primary focus of the rehabilitation team.

Frequently other structures are injured along with the ACL. The rehabilitation plan outlined does not account for possible injury to the **meniscus, posterior cruciate, medial or lateral collateral ligaments,** or joint capsule; associated fractures; or impaired neurovascular struc-

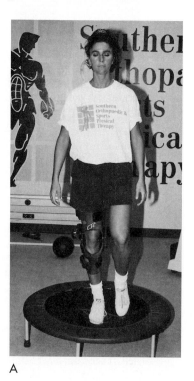
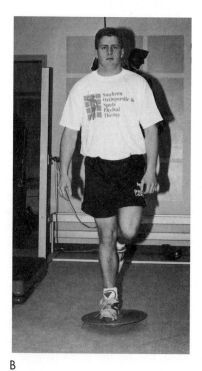

A　　　　　　　　　　　　　　B

FIG. 13-12 Closed–kinetic-chain balance and proprioception exercises. **A,** The use of the mini-trampoline is a challenging and effective balancing exercise. **B,** Single-leg standing on a wobble board.

tures. The complex nature and vast array of combined injuries dictates modifications at each level of rehabilitation and prolongs the healing process.

The physical therapist assistant must also be aware that isolated single or partial ACL injuries and various circumstances may dictate a nonsurgical course of treatment. The physician must decide if the patient is best suited for surgery or should be treated nonoperatively. If the patient is treated nonoperatively, the rehabilitation program progresses at a faster pace, although the injured ligament must still be protected and allowed to heal. Therefore absence of surgery does not mean the patient is allowed unprotected motion and nonrestricted activities. Daniel and Fritschy[11] suggest approximately 12 weeks for a return to running for patients treated nonoperatively for a single-ligament ACL injury.

Posterior Cruciate Ligament (PCL) Injuries

Isolated PCL injuries occur less often than ACL injuries.[3,9,12] Four specific injury mechanisms can produce a PCL injury, with the most common being a "posteriorly-directed force on the anterior aspect of the flexed knee."[12] Hughston[26] describes a second mechanism in which a patient falls on a flexed knee, making contact with the tibial tuberosity and forcing the tibia posteriorly (Fig. 13-14). A third mechanism of injury can occur from hyperflexion of the knee without a resultant force on the tibia.[12] A fourth mechanism usually results in both an ACL and PCL injury and involves knee hyperextension with the foot planted.

Clinical examination of the PCL can be confusing. While assisting the physical therapist with the initial evaluation data, the physical therapist assistant may observe two distinct tests used to define the presence and degree of a PCL injury. In the first examination—the anterior and posterior drawer test—the tibia "sags" or subluxes posteriorly relative to the femur if the PCL is torn (Fig. 13-15). The examiner may produce a "false positive" anterior drawer sign, wherein the posterior tibial sag is actually being reoriented to the neutral position rather than a true anterior translation occurring (Fig. 13-16).

A more sensitive test is the Godfrey posterior tibial sag test. The patient is supine with the hip and knee of

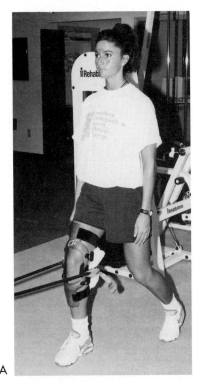
A

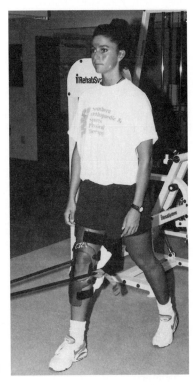
B

FIG. 13-13 Functional closed-chain resistive knee extension in the standing position. **A,** Starting position with affected knee flexed. **B,** End position with affected knee extended.

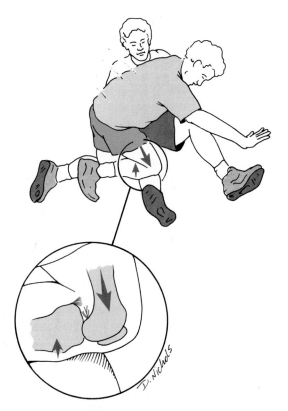

FIG. 13-14 Mechanism of posterior cruciate ligament injury (PCL). With the knee flexed, the proximal tibia is driven in a posterior direction.

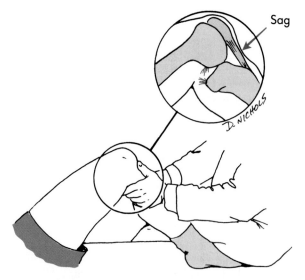

FIG. 13-15 Starting position of the anterior drawer test. If the PCL is torn, the proximal tibia will be in a posterior tibial sag initial reference position.

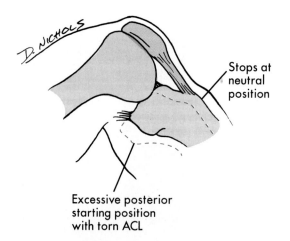

FIG. 13-16 A false positive anterior drawer test can be seen when the tibia translates forward during the drawer test. This is because the torn PCL places the tibia posterior to the femur, so when the clinician directs an anterior force the tibia appears to actually displace anterior to the femur.

the affected limb held at 90 degrees. Hold the heel of the affected limb and allow the tibia to translate, sublux, or sag posteriorly by gravity (Fig. 13-17).

Management and rehabilitation. Many straight-plane and combined rotatory instabilities exist with ligament injuries. Various circumstances, including acute trauma, chronic instability, isolated ligament injury, and complex combinations of injury to multiple structures, profoundly alter the course of rehabilitation. As stated by Hughston:[27] "It must be understood that there is no way the knee can be subjected to a force sufficient to tear the PCL without simultaneously tearing other ligamentous structures about the knee." Hughston[27] elaborates by saying the resultant accessory ligament instabilities are "no greater than mild." Therefore this discussion focuses on the care and rehabilitation of defined straight-plane isolated single-ligament PCL injury and does not delve into the complex nature of the many PCL injuries identified.

There is much disagreement about how best to manage a PCL injury. Some patients appear to respond well to surgical repair while others do very well without surgery.[12,15,27] One common denominator that exists in both groups is the high incidence of articular cartilage degeneration that results from various degrees of instability.[9,12,15,27]

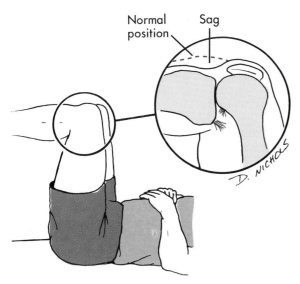

Normal position   Sag

FIG. 13-17 Godfrey tibial sag test. This is a clinically-sensitive test to view the reference of the proximal tibia in relation to the distal femur with the leg flexed to 90 degrees.

Nonoperative rehabilitation. The single most significant factor in the rehabilitation of PCL injuries treated nonsurgically is quadriceps strengthening.[15,37] Studies demonstrate[37] that satisfactory results can be achieved when the quadriceps strength of the affected limb exceeds the quadriceps strength of the uninvolved limb. Less than satisfactory results are seen when the strength of the quadriceps is less than 100% of the quadriceps strength of the uninvolved limb.[37]

In the acute phase a knee immobilizer or hinged knee brace is used for patient comfort. Rest, ice, compression, and limb elevation (RICE) are used to minimize swelling and control pain. The treating physician may prescribe a nonsteroidal anti-inflammatory medication in some cases. Full weight-bearing is allowed as soon as the patient is able. Isometric quadriceps sets and straight-leg raises can commence immediately. The immobilizer is removed to allow active and passive ROM exercises of the knee on a daily basis.

As swelling, pain, and quadriceps control improve, the brace is removed and the patient is instructed in CKC quadriceps-strengthening exercises. No open-chain resistive hamstring exercises are allowed during the early or maximum protection phase because of the posterior tibial translatory forces provided by the hamstrings, which stress the healing PCL.

Short-arc leg-press exercises, step-ups, and wall squats are initiated early to stimulate quadriceps strength

and balance, cocontraction of the quadriceps and hamstrings, and the joint mechanoreceptor system. Gradually, short-arc eccentric hamstring curls are added when ROM has improved and the patient can demonstrate good quadriceps strength and control during all open-chain and closed-chain exercises. Quadriceps strength is tested isokinetically to determine when to initiate more advanced functional exercises. An excellent CKC exercise is the stair stepper used in reverse fashion. Quadriceps strength and cocontraction of the hamstrings are enhanced. The stair-stepper used in the forward position allows the patient to push off on the balls of the feet, minimizing the work of the quadriceps. A reverse motion eliminates the plantar flexors and encourages greater quadriceps work. Standing knee extensions using rubber tubing placed behind the knee help encourage strong quadriceps control in a weight-bearing position.

After acute isolated PCL injuries treated nonoperatively, DeLee et al[12] suggest patients can return to full activity within 8 weeks.

Postoperative rehabilitation. Common graft choices used to surgically reconstruct the PCL include the medial gastrocnemius tendon,[27] central one-third bone-patellar tendon-bone autografts, and Achilles tendon allografts.[12,15] Depending on the surgeon and the procedure used, either an arthroscopically assisted or an open arthrotomy technique can be performed (Fig. 13-18).

A postoperative knee immobilizer or hinged range-limiting brace is applied and maintained until the patient demonstrates quadriceps control, full extension, and full weight-bearing. Some authors[15] recommend a conservative approach to weight-bearing after PCL reconstruction, advocating limited full weight-bearing for 4 to 6 weeks or longer in some cases. Other authorities[12] encourage full weight-bearing initially. While early range of motion is encouraged for the patellofemoral joint and knee extension, minimizing full knee flexion to 50 to 60 degrees is needed to protect the healing graft. Generally, full knee-flexion ROM can be achieved in 2 months after surgery.[12]

The maximum-protection phase of rehabilitation focuses on early isometric and progressive resistive exercises for the quadriceps. Goals throughout the early phases of rehabilitation include patellar-mobility exercises, early knee extension, controlled-limited knee flexion, weight-bearing as tolerated, and control of pain and swelling with RICE and thermal agents as prescribed.

Progressive exercises employ CKC activities to stimulate quadriceps control and cocontractions of the quadriceps and hamstring muscle groups. Engle et al[15] do not advocate isolated resisted hamstring exercises until 12 weeks after surgery. Others[12] suggest that

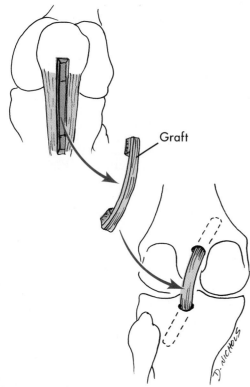

FIG. 13-18 Central one-third arthroscopically-aided bone-patellar-tendon-bone autograft for posterior cruciate ligament reconstruction. As with the ACL, the patellar tendon along with pedicles of bone from the patella and tibial tubercle is harvested and then surgically routed through tunnels drilled through the femur and tibia.

isometric hamstring exercises can be performed early if cocontractions of the quadriceps are performed. Hamstring exercises are progressed to limited-range (10 to 60 degrees) prone, eccentric resistance exercises (while braced during the early postoperative phase).[12]

The moderate-protection phase of rehabilitation defined by Timm[43] begins at the thirteenth week after surgery and progresses to the twenty-fourth week. This phase focuses on weight-bearing CKC exercises. Generally, stair-climbers, step-ups, leg presses, and partial squats are advanced throughout this phase. Progression within this phase is dictated by the patient's individual tolerance to exercises as well as clinically documented objective findings from the KT1000 knee ligament arthrometer, manual clinical stress tests (drawer sign, tibial sag), and isokinetic testing.

The physical therapist assistant must constantly be aware of the healing constraints of repaired or reconstructed tissues throughout each phase of rehabilitation.

The early or maximum-protection phase coincides with the fibroplasia stage of healing.[15] Timm[43] suggests this phase lasts approximately 6 weeks and is characterized by the following goals:

- Protect the articular cartilage of the healing knee
- Reduce the possibility of scar tissue adhesion formation
- Ensure adequate circulation to the surgery site and the remodeling tissues
- Reestablish normal tibiofemoral and patellofemoral arthrokinematics
- Attain voluntary control over joint forces through muscle reconditioning

The moderate-protection phase generally corresponds with the early maturation and late-fibroplasia stages of healing.[15] Similar goals during the early phase of the moderate-protection rehabilitation program include the following:

- Control forces while protecting the graft
- Stimulate collagen fiber maturation and remodeling
- Promote revascularization of the graft
- Obtain normal functional ROM and strength[43]

The minimal-protection phase is directed at returning the patient to the premorbid functional state. The late stage of healing is collagen maturation, which signals the initiation of more vigorous, functional activities that are the hallmark of the minimal-protection phase. Because controversy exists among physicians and therapists concerning when to initiate motion, weight-bearing, and various functional activities after PCL reconstructive surgery, the physical therapist assistant must recognize that the cornerstone of any prescribed rehabilitation program comprises tissue healing principles and the patient's ability to attain certain criteria before beginning more advanced activities.

Medial Collateral Ligament (MCL) Injuries

Injuries to the MCL are the most common ligament injuries seen in the knee.[17,30,47] The MCL can be injured by a direct external force or by a noncontact abduction or rotational stress. In contact sports, the MCL is often injured by a valgus-directed force to the lateral aspect of the knee causing injury to the medial structures (Fig. 13-19). Non–contact-related MCL sprains occur frequently as the lower leg is fixed, the tibia is rotated externally, and a valgus force is directed through the knee (Fig. 13-20).

Injury to other ligaments (ACL, PCL) and associated structures (medial meniscus and lateral meniscus) are often seen in more severe MCL injuries. Studies[16] show an increasing correspondence of associated ligament injuries (most frequently the ACL) with the more severe

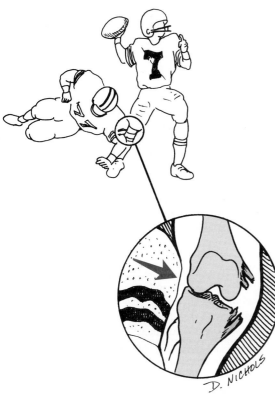

FIG. 13-19 Medial collateral ligament sprain (MCL) from an external force contacting the lateral aspect of the knee, causing the medial knee structures (MCL) to be torn.

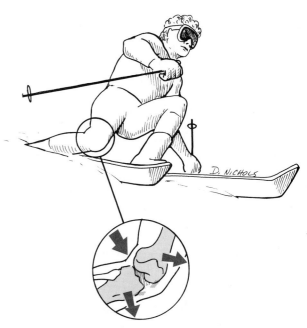

FIG. 13-20 The MCL can also be sprained from non-contact forces.

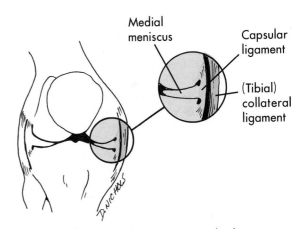

FIG. 13-21 The medial meniscus can also become injured in conjunction with the MCL because of its intimate anatomical relationship with the MCL.

grades of MCL injuries. Fetto and Marshall[16] demonstrate a 20% occurrence of associated ligament injuries with grade I MCL sprains, 52% in grade II sprains, and 78% with grade III sprains.

There is an intimate anatomic relationship between the MCL and the medial meniscus of the knee. O'Donoghue[36] is credited with describing the "unhappy triad" as combined injury to the MCL, ACL, and medial meniscus. Because the MCL and medial meniscus are strongly attached to one another (Fig. 13-21), it is clear that the meniscus may become injured along with more severe MCL injuries. However, the more common triad is the MCL, ACL, and lateral meniscus.[34]

Ligament stability tests. The severity of ligament injury can be classified as follows:[34]

Grade I: 0 to 5 mm of joint opening with no instability

Grade II: 5 to 10 mm of joint opening with some degree of instability

Grade III: 10 to 15 mm of joint opening with moderate instability

Grade IV: Greater than 15 mm of joint opening with gross ligament instability

Others report a slightly different classification model:[30]

Grade I: 1 to 4 mm

Grade II: 5 to 9 mm

Grade III: 10 to 15 mm

Specific end-feel classifications during MCL stress testing help clarify the significance of joint injury (see Chapter 11). For example, Linton and Indelicato[30] describe grades I and II as having a definite end-feel to the stress tests, while grade III tears have a soft or "loose" end-point. The end-point, or "feel," is what the physical therapist is looking for during the examination.

The most sensitive test to describe the severity of an MCL sprain is the valgus stress test. This test is performed with the patient supine on an examining table while the examiner stands to the side of the affected limb at the level of the distal tibia. Test the affected knee in 30 degrees of knee-flexion. Firmly grasp the medial aspect of the distal tibia with one hand, while using the other hand to apply a valgus-directed force to the lateral proximal joint line, in effect causing the medial joint line to gap or "open." Also perform this test with the knee in full extension. If the knee gaps open in terminal extension, this signifies a rather significant injury to the MCL, ACL, PCL, and posterior capsule. Even with a complete rupture of the MCL, however, if the PCL and posterior capsule of the knee are not injured, the knee may not demonstrate significant instability when tested in full extension.[30] This clearly shows the ultimate stabilizing effect of the PCL and capsule in terminal extension.

Rehabilitation. Although some authorities[36] advocate surgical repair of selected MCL tears, most physicians now treat isolated grade I, II, and even III MCL tears nonsurgically.[17,30,34,47] However, protection of the ligament during healing is paramount if full function and stability are to be achieved. Wilk[47] outlines four critical conditions that must be observed for MCL healing, as follows:

- Maintenance of the torn fibers in close continuity
- Intact and stable ACL and other supporting ligaments of the knee
- Immediate controlled motion and stresses to the healing ligament
- Protection of the MCL against deleterious stresses (valgus and external rotation stresses)

The concept of early protected motion is the foundation for rehabilitation of MCL sprains. Generally, a three-phase (maximum, moderate, and minimal protection) criteria-based program is used. A knee immobilizer or range-limiting hinged brace is used initially to control unwanted valgus and rotational stress. Ice, elastic compression wraps, and elevation are used to control pain and swelling. Isometric quadriceps sets, straight-leg raises, and ankle pumps are initiated as soon as the patient can tolerate execution of the exercises. Generally, weight-bearing with crutches as tolerated is pre-

scribed. The immobilizer is removed daily for active and passive knee flexion and extension exercises. Seated assisted knee flexion and supine wall slides are used to assist with painful knee flexion. Clearly, all valgus forces and rotational stresses must be avoided to protect the healing ligament. As pain lessens and quadriceps strength increases, the crutches are discarded. Wilk[47] suggests nonassisted ambulation by the eighth day after injury. When strengthening the nonoperated MCL, care must be taken to protect the medial structures from all valgus and rotational forces. By placing resistance above the joint line, hip adduction strengthening can be achieved if the knee is protected with a functional brace. Bracing for knee support is generally organized into three distinct categories,[13] as follows:

- Prophylactic
- Rehabilitative
- Functional

In some cases a prophylactic hinged brace can be used during the moderate-protection and minimal-protection phases of MCL injury rehabilitation because these braces allow for full flexion and extension and may limit valgus stresses to the knee.

CKC exercises are gradually added as pain allows. Stair steppers, leg presses, step-ups, and wall squats can be instituted as ROM and pain tolerance dictate. Patient compliance with home exercises and joint protection are significant factors that must be reinforced by the physical therapist assistant during each phase of rehabilitation.

Active knee flexion range should progress steadily without increased complaints of pain and swelling. If the patient does not regain knee flexion or has increased complaints of pain and swelling, the possibility of a torn meniscus must be examined. Daily communication with the therapist quickly identifies the necessary modifications in the rehabilitation program. In addition, through daily communication, the physical therapist assistant can establish a cycle of scheduling physical therapy reevaluations based on clinical observation.

As with all injuries, the whole patient, not just the injured body part, must be treated. A full body fitness program that does not produce unwanted valgus or rotation forces is encouraged beginning with the maximum-protection phase. In an athletic population of patients, adding lateral slide board activities and running drills during the minimum-protection phase is appropriate to allow a functional return to sporting activities.

A general set of criteria can be applied for a safe and effective progression from one phase of recovery to the next. Holden et al [24] believe that the requirements for advancing through the very early stages of recovery (2 to 3 weeks) should include the following:

- No significant effusion
- Decreasing tenderness
- Full ROM

Clinically significant warning signs during recovery through the second week are as follows:[24]

- Persistent effusion
- Continued pain
- Reduced ROM

Criteria for advancing through the third week, according to Holden et al,[24] include these points:

- No effusion
- No femoral condyle or tibial tenderness
- Full ROM
- No change in valgus stability test

Other signs to be aware of during the early (maximum-protection to moderate-protection phases) recovery period as outlined by Holden et al[24] include the following:

- Subjective complaint of knee giving out with increased stress
- Locking

MENISCUS INJURIES

The functions of the meniscus include:[8,22,23,25]

- Stability
- Shock absorption
- Load transmission
- Nutrition
- Lubrication
- Control of motion

The menisci are fibrocartilaginous tissues containing primarily (90%) type I collagen.[2] The medial and lateral menisci of the knee serve as "extensions of the tibia"[2] and provide for reception of the femoral condyles onto the surface of the tibia (Fig. 13-22).

Injury to the meniscus can result in many patterns of tears (Fig. 13-23). Five main types have been identified,[18] as follows:

- Horizontal tears
- Longitudinal tears
- Degenerative tears
- Flap tears
- Radial tears

In younger patients, longitudinal tears account for 50% to 90% of meniscus tear patterns, whereas horizontal tears are more common among the older population of patients.[18]

Mechanisms of Injury

The meniscus can be injured by sudden trauma or by gradual degeneration.[2,8,18,23] Traumatic meniscus injuries are most common in a younger, active population,

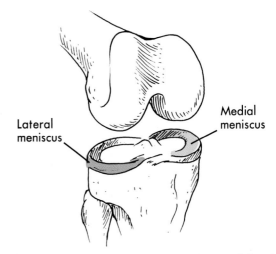

FIG. 13-22 Anatomical relationship of the medial and lateral meniscus to the tibia and femur.

while degenerative tears occur more frequently to individuals over age 40.[2] Noncontact, weight-bearing injuries to the meniscus usually involve combined forces of knee flexion, rotation, compression, and shear[2,8,18] (Fig. 13-24). Degenerative tears can be quite subtle and do not usually involve a history of sudden overt trauma. Generally, with degenerative tears, some type of insignificant activity (squatting, getting out of a car) precedes the symptoms of pain, swelling, and locking of the knee.

Clinical Examination

A history of some type of twisting injury followed by symptoms of pain, swelling, locking, or "catching" may indicate meniscal injury. While assisting the physical therapist during the initial clinical examination, the physical therapist assistant will observe various manually applied stress tests to identify if a meniscal lesion is present.

Apley's compression and distraction test[40a] is used to determine if the injury is ligamentous or meniscal. To perform this test, the patient is prone with the affected knee flexed to 90 degrees. Stabilize the distal femur with a strap or with a hand. Use the free hand to grasp the distal tibia and provide a distraction and internal-external rotation force to the tibia. Pain signifies the possibility of a ligament tear. The compression component of this examination is performed in the same manner, except that the free hand applies a compression and rotational force to the distal tibia. Pain with compression and combined internal and external rotation on the flexed knee signifies the presence of a meniscal lesion.

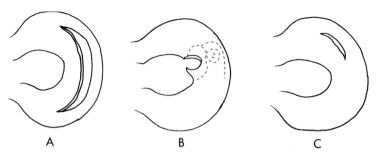

FIG. 13-23 Various patterns of tears can occur to the meniscus. **A,** Bucket-handle tear. **B,** Parrot-beak tear. **C,** Longitudinal tear.

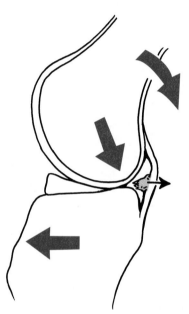

FIG. 13-24 Mechanism of injury to the meniscus. Combined forces of flexion, rotation, and compression can tear the meniscus.

The McMurray test[18,40a] is also used to reproduce symptoms of a torn meniscus. The patient is supine with the hip and knee of the affected limb fully flexed. To test for the presence of a medial meniscus lesion, apply a valgus force to the knee with one hand while applying an external rotation force and extending the knee by holding the distal tibia with the other hand. To test for a lateral meniscus tear, provide a varus force with internal tibial rotation. With either internal or external rotation of the knee, if a tear is present, the patient may experience pain and an audible or palpable snap or "pop."

The "bounce home" test[40a] is designed to determine if a torn meniscus is preventing knee extension. The patient is supine with the affected knee flexed and supported by the examiner's hand. Passively extend the knee to full extension. If the meniscus is torn, the knee may not fully extend because the torn tissue blocks extension and creates a rubbery, springy end-feel.[32]

Management

The rationale for treatment options is directly related to the location of the tear in the meniscus and the ability of the meniscus to repair itself. The vascular anatomy of the medial and lateral meniscus is reserved for the peripheral 10% to 30% of its width (Fig. 13-25).[2] The remaining portions are relatively avascular and aneural. Researchers and surgeons[2,22,23,40a] recognize a zone classification of injury related to the vascular supply of the meniscus. The injured meniscus may or may not heal or repair itself, depending on the location of the tear. A

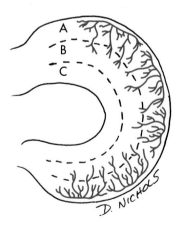

A-Red-on-red zone
B-Red-on-white zone
C-White-on-white zone

FIG. 13-25 The vascular anatomy of the meniscus. The vascular supply to the meniscus is reserved for the peripheral 10% to 30% of the meniscus.

zone I tear is recognized as "red-on-red" because the location of the tear is vascular on both sides (Fig. 13-26). Injuries in this area may heal better than those in other areas because of the blood supply. A zone II tear is located in the "red-on-white" area of the meniscus (Fig. 13-27). A tear in this area has a vascular supply on only one side. These tears may also heal because of the communication with a blood supply.

A zone III tear is located in the nonvascular central body of the meniscus called the "white-on-white" area (Fig. 13-28). An injury in this area does not heal because there is no blood supply to support the healing process.

The rationale for management is clearly supported by the severity and location of the tear in the meniscus. Surgical options include total meniscectomy (removal of the entire meniscus), subtotal or partial meniscectomy (removal of only the torn portion of the cartilage), and **meniscal repair** (suturing the torn meniscus together). If the tear is located in the "red-on-red" area, some surgeons elect a nonsurgical course of treatment. Fu and Baratz[18] identify a few variables to consider—"the age of the patient, the stability of the knee, the location of the tear, and the integrity of the meniscus"—when deciding on the course of treatment.

Degenerative arthritic changes, joint space narrowing, and osteophyte formation[2,18,40a] are common problems associated with total meniscectomy. These destructive changes also occur in a significant number of patients after **subtotal meniscectomy.**[18] The goal of surgical care for meniscal tears is to maintain as much viable tissue as possible by avoiding total meniscectomy and investigating the possibility of surgical repair.

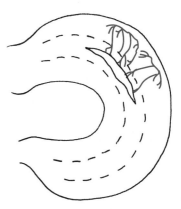

FIG. 13-27 Tear of the meniscus in the "red-on-white" zone. This zone II tear refers to the tear being vascular on only one side. This is also a reparable tear.

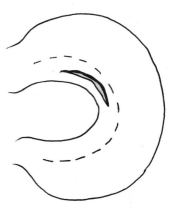

FIG. 13-28 Tear of the meniscus in the "white-on-white" zone. This zone III tear refers to the tear being avascular on both sides, therefore this tear is considered not reparable.

Rehabilitation After Subtotal Meniscectomy

Preservation of the load-bearing functions of the meniscus is the foundation for a partial meniscectomy. Rehabilitation after subtotal meniscectomy focuses initially on management of pain and swelling using RICE, TENS, thermal agents, and nonsteroidal antiinflammatory drugs (NSAIDs) as prescribed by the physician. ROM is progressed by using a number of techniques:

- Supine wall slides
- Stationary cycle for ROM
- Seated assisted knee flexion
- Standing wall squats
- Prone knee-extension hangs

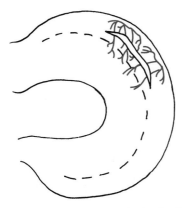

FIG. 13-26 Tear of the meniscus in the "red-on-red" zone of the meniscus. This zone I tear refers to the tear being vascular on both sides, therefore being reparable.

Early weight-bearing as tolerated is progressed to full weight-bearing as pain allows. Progressive strengthening exercises during the early phases of recovery focus on isometric quadriceps control, hamstring isometrics, straight-leg raises, hip abduction-adduction, and hip extension.

The physical therapist assistant must carefully oversee the advancement of CKC exercises and observe, document, and communicate any objective or subjective changes in pain or swelling, and report to the physical therapist regularly concerning each positive or negative change.

Many patients can tolerate a progressive program of early weight-bearing, ROM activities, and strengthening exercises and may develop a chronic effusion that necessitates a significant modification in the rehabilitation plan.

In general, these patients are allowed to advance through the maximum-protection phase rather quickly. An older, less active population of patients may require a slower progression, depending on whether there is **articular cartilage** degeneration. Some surgeons advocate the use of a knee immobilizer during the first week after surgery to assist with early weight-bearing and to provide support for the quadriceps.

During the moderate-protection phase, from the fourth to the eighth week,[43] the patient may begin with more functional CKC exercises. Step-ups, wall squats, leg presses, and stair steppers promote cocontraction of the quadriceps and hamstrings and stimulate the joint mechanoreceptor system to allow improved support. Proprioceptive exercises, including single-leg standing, balance board activities, and the mini-trampoline, can begin during this phase, as can isokinetic velocity spectrum training (sets of exercises at progressively faster speeds).

The minimum-protection phase begins at the ninth postoperative week and advances to the twentieth week.[43] The goal of this phase is to normalize gait, attain full range of motion, and enhance functional activities.

The fact that many meniscal injuries occur in conjunction with injuries to other structures (ACL, MCL, joint capsule) is significant and must be fully appreciated by the physical therapist assistant. The rehabilitation program for combined subtotal meniscectomy and the presence of other joint pathologic conditions must be modified to account for the healing of other structures.

The long-term consequences of subtotal meniscectomy must be clearly understood when addressing functional activities (ADLs) and a return to athletics. Early degenerative changes are seen with both total and partial meniscectomy[2,18] and include narrowing of the tibiofemoral joint space, formation of bone spurs (osteophytes), and degeneration of the femoral articular surface on the side of the surgery. Counseling and education of the patient focus on modifying ADLs related to stair-climbing and repetitive vertical compressive loading.

Rehabilitation After Meniscal Repair

The physical therapist assistant must understand the fundamental differences between complete and partial removal of the meniscus and meniscal repair. Because many meniscal injuries occur in conjunction with associated ligament injuries (ACL, PCL, MCL) as well as in isolated cases, the ultimate course of treatment for combined meniscal repairs and associated ligament injuries depends largely on the surgical procedure used to correct the ligament instability. In one study,[42] meniscal repairs done in conjunction with reconstruction of the ACL actually healed better (90%) than meniscal repairs done on stable knees (57%). Here discussion includes concepts involving isolated meniscal repair. Associated ACL reconstruction and meniscal repairs generally follow a more progressive program focusing on the principles of ACL rehabilitation as well as enhancing recovery from the meniscal repair. Combined surgical repairs for the ACL and meniscus require highly individualized rehabilitation programs in which the surgeon and physical therapist carefully consider many short-term and long-range issues for the patient, including the following:

- Age
- Level of activity
- Joint stability

The foundation and contrasting difference between meniscectomy and meniscal repair rehabilitation is allowing the surgically repaired (sutured) meniscus to heal by avoiding (limiting) loads and stresses (ROM) that compromise the repair site.

Initially, after the repair of isolated meniscal injury without ACL reconstruction, the patient is non–weight-bearing, gradually progressing to full weight-bearing in 4 to 6 weeks.[18,25,40a,42] This delay in weight-bearing status for meniscal repairs is necessary to avoid vertical compressive loads that may disrupt the suture site.[25] The patient may also be immobilized in a range-limiting brace for approximately 4 weeks.[18] Limiting knee flexion to approximately 90 to 100 degrees for 4 to 6 weeks is required to avoid excessive motion at the suture site. Throughout the maximum-protection phase,[43] pain and swelling management is essential. The use of ice, elastic compression bandages, elevation, and electrical stimulation may reduce symptoms related to the surgery.

Regaining quadriceps control and controlled ROM can be initiated immediately after surgery. Quadriceps sets, straight-leg raises, hamstring sets, short-arc knee extensions, hip abduction-adduction and extension, and calf pumps are initiated and progressed from the first day after surgery throughout the maximum-protection phase. ROM activities (prone knee flexion, supine wall slides) are progressed gradually and limited to approximately 100 degrees for the first 4 to 6 weeks. The initiation of isotonic exercises (knee extension and leg curls) can begin during the later stages of the maximum-protection phase (3 to 4 weeks) and throughout the moderate-protection phase (weeks 4 to 8).[43]

Stationary cycling to increase ROM begins during the later stages of the maximum-protection phase (3 weeks) and progresses as tolerated through the moderate phase. These patients cannot begin CKC exercises (such as leg presses, squats, step-ups, and stair-climbers) until at least 8 weeks after repair. As motion improves, swelling and pain are controlled and full weight-bearing without crutches is achieved at 6 weeks. Then a very gradual program of short-arc leg presses, treadmill walking, and step-ups can begin. Access to an underwater treadmill is advantageous because the buoyancy of the water allows for limited weight-bearing and normalized gait mechanics before full weight-bearing. To reduce injury to the repaired meniscus, weighted and full squats must be strictly avoided for up to 3 to 6 months after repair.[18] While the general concepts of regaining lost motion and improving strength and function are the same after subtotal meniscectomy and meniscal repairs, obvious delays in initiating weight-bearing, full ROM, and CKC exercises are required to enhance healing of the repaired meniscus.

As mentioned, meniscal repairs are also seen in conjunction with ACL reconstructions. The program of recovery for these patients may be different to address both ligament and cartilage healing. Tenuta and Arciero[42] compared protocols involving ACL rehabilitation with meniscal repairs and rehabilitation programs with cruciate-stable knees. Their study shows a "significant decrease in the completely healed meniscal repairs in patients who followed an aggressive rehabilitation program after ACL reconstruction that made little effort to protect the meniscal repair." To minimize postoperative problems associated with ACL reconstructions, the rehabilitation program calls for accelerated weight-bearing and motion. With this in mind, it is clear to see why some meniscal repairs may fail to heal completely if the principles of non–weight-bearing and controlled motion are not followed.

PATELLOFEMORAL PATHOLOGIC CONDITIONS

Injuries and diseases of the patellofemoral joint and the extensor mechanism (quadriceps, quadriceps tendon, patella, patellar tendon, patellofemoral articulation) are quite complex. The physical therapist assistant must understand the anatomic relationships and rudimentary mechanics of the patellofemoral articulation and the extensor mechanism to fully appreciate the rationale for rehabilitation of the many problems that can occur in this area. This requires careful review of the anatomy and kinesiology of the knee and extensor mechanism to gain a broad understanding of the relationships between mechanical deviations and resultant patellofemoral abnormalities.

This section outlines a few of the more commonly encountered problems affecting the patellofemoral joint, focusing mainly on fundamental rehabilitation concepts involving lateral patellar compression and patellar tracking disorders, retropatellar articular cartilage arthrosis, patellar subluxation, and rehabilitation programs related to proximal and distal surgical realignment procedures.

Lateral Patellar Compression and Patellar Tracking Disorders

Often the underlying cause of anterior knee pain[25] is mechanical deviations of patellar tracking during knee flexion and extension. The resolution of pain and dysfunction related to patellar tracking problems is centered on therapeutic exercises that strengthen the quadriceps, stretching exercises to gain flexibility in the hamstrings and lateral knee structures, supportive bracing and taping, NSAIDs, thermal modalities, and various surgical interventions.

Before discussing specific rehabilitation procedures, it is important to see the relationship between the posture of the patella relative to the femur, the effect of hamstring tightness on patellofemoral compression, and the anatomic alignment of the lower extremity as these relate to patellar tracking dysfunction, patellar subluxation, and anterior knee pain.

In general, the patella is referenced to the femur in three positions (Fig. 13-29). A patellar posture that is more superior than normal is referred to as patella alta[28,34,46] and is associated with greater patellar instability.[34]

In addition to patellar posture, the **quadriceps angle (Q-angle)** is a significant clinical assessment that relates directly to patellar tracking deviations and variations in the line or angle of pull of the quadriceps on the patella.[46] The Q angle refers to a line drawn from the anterior superior iliac spine through the center or axis of

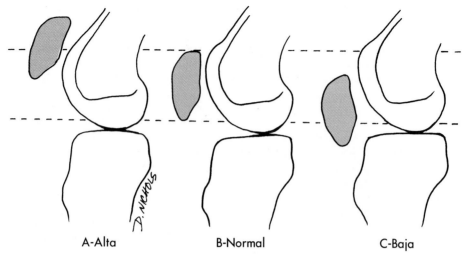

FIG. 13-29 Patella reference positions. **A,** Patella alta. **B,** Normal patella reference position. **C,** Patella baja.

the patella and distally to the insertion of the patellar tendon on the tibial tubercle (Fig. 13-30). The Q angle can be increased by proximal tibial external rotation or distal tibia varus.[28,46] Fig. 13-31 shows the various angles of muscular pull on the patella and how an increased Q angle can profoundly affect the tracking mechanisms of the patella during flexion and extension. Anatomic alignment of the lower extremity can also be a mechanism for patellar tracking dysfunction.

The **miserable malalignment syndrome** (Fig. 13-32)[26,28,34,46] is assessed with the patient in the standing position and provides objective data for the physician and physical therapist regarding the entire lower-extremity kinetic chain, patellar tracking dysfunction, and pain. This syndrome is characterized by femoral anteversion (internal femoral rotation), "squinting" patellae (patellae facing toward each other), proximal external tibial torsion (which results in what is called the "bayonet sign"), and foot pronation.[4,46] If the affected lower extremity demonstrates the miserable malalignment syndrome when the patient is in a standing position, it is easy for the physical therapist assistant to understand how the extensor mechanism can be changed and result in lateral tracking of the patella.

In addition to mechanical malalignment, muscle forces can also contribute to symptoms of anterior knee pain or retropatellar compression. Excessive hamstring tightness can increase patellofemoral compression because patellar excursion through knee extension is resisted by the hamstrings, requiring more quadriceps force (Fig. 13-33).[28]

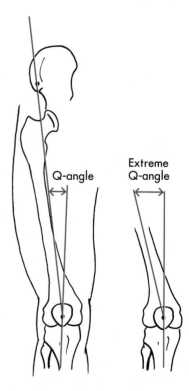

FIG. 13-30 The quadriceps angle (Q-angle) is measured from the ASIS, through the axis of the patella and distally to the insertion of the patellar tendon on the tibial tubercle.

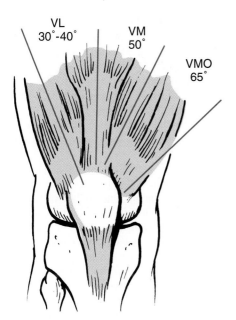

FIG. 13-31 Angles of muscular pull on the patella. Patellar reference positions and the Q-angle can affect mechanical tracking of the patella due to muscular angles of pull.

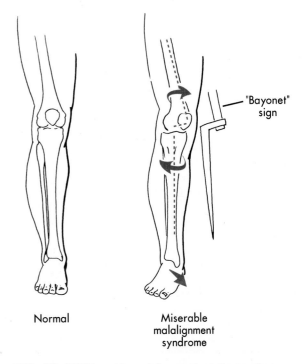

FIG. 13-32 Miserable malalignment syndrome. Anatomical alignment is assessed in the standing position. The miserable malalignment syndrome is characterized by combined femoral anteversion, "squinting patellae," external tibial torsion, and foot pronation.

In light of this information concerning patellar posture, Q angle, lower extremity malalignment, and muscle forces acting on the patella, the physical therapist assistant must recognize that the result of these abnormalities is pain and dysfunction related to femoral and retropatellar articular cartilage (hyaline cartilage) degeneration from excessive wear, buttressing, and compression of the patella that tracks abnormally.

Nonoperative rehabilitation of anterior knee pain. The initial course of treatment focuses primarily on controlling pain and swelling and initiating quadriceps strengthening exercises. Any activities that cause the patient discomfort are modified to accommodate pain and dysfunction. For example, stair climbing (descending more often than ascending) can reproduce symptoms of pain. The physical therapist assistant can counsel the patient to use the nonaffected limb in a straight-leg gait pattern when climbing or descending stairs. Ice packs, NSAIDs, and limb-elevation may be needed in the acute phase. However, the use of elastic compression bandages should be avoided to prevent continued patellofemoral compression.

Among the classic symptoms of retropatellar pain are signs of inflammation, crepitus (audible, palpable gritty sandpaper, cracking under the patella), pain, and a laterally tracking patella. The ultimate challenge for the

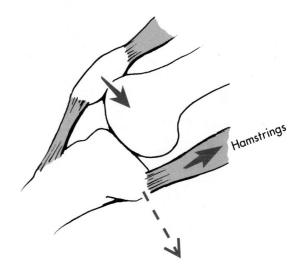

FIG. 13-33 Excessive hamstring tightness can contribute to increased patello-femoral compression.

rehabilitation team is the focused selection of appropriate and effective quadriceps strengthening exercises that act to counter the effects of tight lateral structures, a lateral tracking patella related to the Q angle and malalignment, and quadriceps weakness.

Strengthening of the quadriceps muscle group is initiated by introducing isometric sets that do not reproduce pain. In some instances submaximal isometric quadriceps sets are required at the beginning of the program to accommodate for any pain complaints the patient may have. The vastus medialis oblique (VMO) is the focus of attention when addressing quadriceps strengthening. Bennett[4] suggests that "these muscles are emphasized because of their ability to stabilize the patella superiorly and, more importantly, medially. The superior medial pull of the vastus medialis muscle complex directly counteracts lateral tracking syndromes." Therefore progressive quadriceps sets serve as the foundation of the initial rehabilitation program.

In conjunction with quadriceps strengthening, the tight lateral structures that act to pull the patella laterally must be addressed. Stretching the hamstrings, stretching the iliotibial band (ITB) (Fig. 13-34), and performing

manual patellar-stretching exercises (Fig. 13-35) are essential to counteract anterior knee pain that results from a lateral-tracking patella. Short-arc terminal knee extensions are gradually introduced in the early stages of rehabilitation to regain active quadriceps control. Care must be taken to begin this exercise with a very limited ROM (about 10 to 20 degrees of flexion) to avoid pain from lateral patellar compression and to accommodate the weakened quadriceps muscles, which cannot control the patella adequately.

In keeping with strengthening of the extensor mechanism, attention should also be turned to the hip adductors, which may influence a medially directed pull on the patella.[4] During quadriceps sets, short-arc terminal knee extensions, and straight-leg raises, the affected limb should be slightly rotated (approximately 10 to 15 degrees) externally to take advantage of the medial pull of the adductors and to minimize the potential for the patient to slightly internally rotate the affected leg to help substitute for the weakened quadriceps. Isometric hip adduction (Fig. 13-36) exercises are gradually advanced to isotonic hip adduction exercises (Fig. 13-37). As the strength of the quadriceps improves and as pain allows in the early stages of rehabilitation, isometric static holds can begin.

Functional CKC quadriceps strengthening exercises are introduced to the program as pain and strength allow. In some instances, patients may tolerate limited ROM leg presses, wall squats, and step-ups as well as open-chain quadriceps isolation exercises. Shallow step-ups using biofeedback (Fig. 13-38) over the VMO are excellent CKC functional quadriceps strengthening exercises. Limited ROM leg presses using elastic tubing to

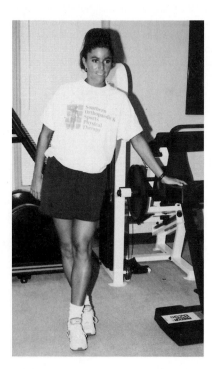

FIG. 13-34 Standing iliotibial band (ITB) stretching. Stretching the lateral structures of the hip and knee can aid in minimizing lateral tracking of the patella and lateral compressive forces.

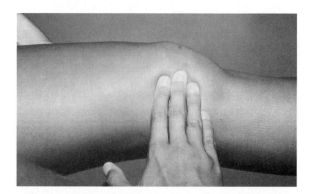

FIG. 13-35 Manual lateral patella stretching. The patient is instructed in "auto-stretching" of the patella. If the lateral retinaculum of the knee is tight and is causing the patella to track laterally, the patient can gently stretch the patella medially in order to stretch tight lateral structures.

strengthen the hip adductors can further facilitate quadriceps strengthening (Fig. 13-39).

Supportive devices can help dynamically stabilize the patella. Commercially available patellar stabilizing sleeves provide a lateral buttress support to the patella to minimize lateral tracking. Dynamic patellar stabilization is also aided by adhesive taping techniques.

Postoperative rehabilitation of anterior knee pain. The basic goal of operative management for anterior knee pain related to lateral patellar tracking

disorders (patellar subluxation) is to reestablish appropriate extensor mechanism function and to reduce patellofemoral contact forces.[20]

Surgical management of patellofemoral disorders can be classified as proximal realignment procedures, distal realignment procedures, various patellofemoral articular cartilage shaving procedures, and perforation or abrasion chondroplasty.[46]

Proximal realignment procedures involve lateral retinacular release with VMO advancement (Fig. 13-40).[45] Rehabilitation after proximal realignment procedures is essentially the same as for nonoperative treatment of anterior knee pain. However, pain and swelling after surgery as well as specific tissue healing and time constraints must be carefully addressed. Therefore the initial course of management after proximal realignment procedures is focused on the use of ice, a lateral patellar compression and buttress pad, limb elevation, temporary immobilization and weight-bearing as tolerated, and NSAIDs as prescribed by the physician. Control of pain

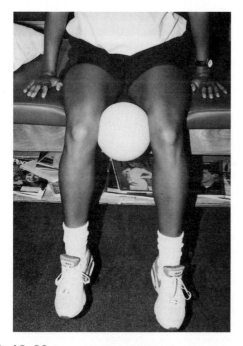

FIG. 13-36 Seated isometric hip adduction.

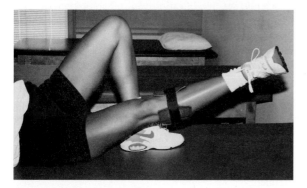

FIG. 13-37 Hip adduction strengthening exercises can be progressed from isometrics to side lying concentric and eccentric loading.

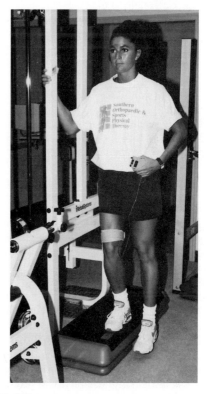

FIG. 13-38 Shallow step-ups with portable bio-feedback or EMS over the vastus medialis obliques (VMO) is an excellent closed chain functional drill to enhance control of the quadriceps.

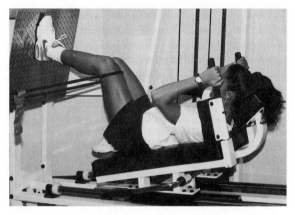

FIG. 13-39 Closed-chain leg-press exercise with elastic tubing to simultaneously enhance hip adduction control with concentric and eccentric loading of the quadriceps.

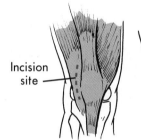
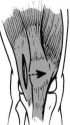

Incision site

Patella shifts medially for better alignment

FIG. 13-40 Lateral retinacular release surgical procedure is designed to "free-up" or release tight lateral structures and to allow the patella better anatomical alignment.

and swelling is essential to reduce the quadriceps inhibition produced by pain and swelling.

Temporary immobilization is specifically related to management of the lateral retinacular release procedure. Because the rationale behind this procedure is to reduce the pull of the vastus lateralis muscle and related lateral structures by surgically cutting (releasing) portions of their attachment on the superolateral aspect of the patella, long-term immobilization of the patellofemoral joint and tibiofemoral articulation helps "scar in" and reattach the release of these tissues and counteract the desired surgical goal of reduced lateral pull. Therefore in this specific procedure, early lateral patellar stretching exercises and early knee flexion ROM exercises are needed to ensure that the lateral structures are maintained in an "opened" or released position. In some cases the VMO is surgically cut and advanced to a more

mechanically advantageous angle on the patella to help produce a more midline pull of the patella. Early flexion exercises may stretch the advancement of the VMO, so extreme caution is needed when encouraging motion after lateral retinacular release with advancement of the VMO. When the VMO has been advanced, early active quadriceps-strengthening exercises must be delayed to allow for appropriate scarring and healing at the suture site.

As pain and swelling allow, supine wall slides, stationary cycling, prone leg flexion, and manual patellar stretching exercises are introduced. Quadriceps strengthening is the foundation for a successful outcome after this surgical procedure. Open-chain remedial exercises (quadriceps sets, short-arc terminal knee extensions, straight-leg raises, hip adduction exercises) give way to CKC functional exercises as soon as pain and tissue healing allow.

Step-ups with biofeedback over the VMO, wall squats, leg presses, stair-steppers, and normalized gait mechanics are encouraged during the early stages of postoperative rehabilitation. As with nonoperative management, hip abduction exercises are avoided initially to minimize the lateral pulling influence of this muscle group on the patella.

Distal realignment procedures are also termed *radical surgeries* by Bennett.[4] The goal behind these surgeries is to reduce severe patellofemoral compression loads and significant patellar subluxation by surgically removing the extensor mechanism's insertion (patellar tendon attachment on the tibial tubercle) and elevating and reattaching the tibial tubercle to a more mechanically advantageous site to improve the pull of the quadriceps.[4] The physical therapist assistant will encounter such procedures as the Hauser, Maquet, and Elmslie-Trillat (Fig. 13-41) surgical procedure. Each is a variation designed to realign the distal extensor mechanism.

Significant modifications in rehabilitation are required with distal realignment procedures based on bone and soft-tissue healing and promotion of quadriceps strength. Generally, immobilization in plaster or a hinged range-limiting brace is used for 4 to 6 weeks.[4,46] Crutches are encouraged for about 6 weeks,[46] with initial non–weight-bearing progressing to touch-down weight-bearing and then to full weight-bearing over the full 6 weeks of immobilization.[4,46] Advancing ROM measurements to approximately 100 degrees of knee flexion for the first 2 weeks and progressing to 120 degrees of knee flexion by 6 weeks is advocated by Bennett.[4]

Individual circumstances, surgical procedures, and the wishes of the physician dictate variations in this

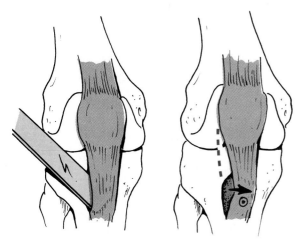

FIG. 13-41 Elmslie-Trillat surgical procedure for radical distal extensor mechanism realignment.

initial management plan. Isometric quadriceps sets, straight-leg raises, and short-arc quadriceps exercises are encouraged once pain, swelling, and tissue healing allow. With extensor mechanism repair as well as radical distal realignment procedures, a few weeks' delay is required before initiating quadriceps sets and straight-leg raises so as not to endanger the surgical repair site.

Many remedial quadriceps strengthening exercises can be performed in the brace during the early phases of recovery. ROM, CKC strengthening, and proprioception exercises are progressed according to the proximal realignment plan previously discussed.

Occasionally, arthroscopic procedures are used to directly address the condition of the articular cartilage on the undersurface of the patella and the femoral condyles in cases of anterior knee pain. The term *chondromalacia* describes retropatellar articular cartilage degeneration or softening. The diagnosis of chondromalacia can only be made at the time of surgery[34,46] because visualization of the articular surfaces is required.

Various surgical procedures are used to smooth rough articular surfaces and to stimulate an inflammatory response to enhance healing. Perforation or abrasion of subchondral bone (chondroplasty and abrasion arthroplasty)[4,7] stimulates a communication between the damaged articular surface and the vascular supply of subchondral bone. Pain and swelling after these procedures are a significant concern and require ice, compression dressings (being careful to avoid excessive patellofemoral compression), limb elevation, and antiinflammatory medications prescribed by the physician. Limited weight-bearing (non–weight-bearing progressing to

touch-down weight-bearing) is encouraged[4] for 4 to 6 weeks to accommodate the pain and healing of the articular cartilage surface. Regaining quadriceps strength by using isometrics, straight-leg raises, short-arc terminal knee extensions, hamstring stretching, manual patellar stretching, and stretching of the iliotibial band begins during the early recovery stages of rehabilitation. The physical therapist assistant must pay close attention to complaints of pain and objective signs of swelling and articular cartilage degeneration (crepitus) during all stages of recovery, particularly with knee extension exercises. The angle of short-arc knee extension may need to be reduced to eliminate pain. Modifying the angle of the leg press may also limit pain and articular wear. Occasionally, a change from open-chain exercises to limited ROM CKC exercises is appropriate (in consultation with the physical therapist) to minimize patellofemoral compression loads and encourage continued quadriceps strengthening.

FRACTURES

This section will briefly introduce management and rehabilitation programs associated with fractures of the patella, distal femur (supracondylar femur fractures), and proximal tibia (tibial plateau).

Fractures of the Patella

Fractures of the patella can occur with direct or indirect trauma.[46] The most common injury involves the patella making contact with a hard surface. Less frequently, the patella can be fractured by a violent contraction of the quadriceps.[33,46] In either case, if a transverse fracture occurs, avascular necrosis (AVN) can result, since the vascular supply to the patella is reserved for the central portion and distal pole, leaving the proximal segment of the transverse fracture prone to AVN.[33] Generally, nondisplaced patellar fractures are treated conservatively with immobilization of the affected limb in full extension.[31,33,46]

Some controversy exists concerning the recovery of motion and duration of immobilization.[33,46] Some authors advise plaster immobilization for 6 weeks. Other authorities[46] report: "There is no place in modern practice for the traditional 6 weeks immobilization of a nondisplaced patellar fracture."

Rehabilitation management of nondisplaced patellar fractures treated with immobilization is primarily supportive throughout immobilization and limited weight-bearing. The nonaffected limb can maintain strength and flexibility using quadriceps strengthening exercises (such as knee extensions, leg presses, leg curls), and aerobic fitness can be enhanced with the use of single-leg stationary cycling or an upper body ergometer (UBE). Ankle pumps are encouraged for the affected immobilized limb throughout immobilization. Quadriceps sets, short-arc knee extensions, and straight-leg raises are gradually introduced, once sufficient bone healing has occurred. If quadriceps strengthening exercises and knee flexion exercises are begun too soon, the force of muscle contraction and knee flexion stretching may separate and stress the fracture site, slowing the healing process and leading to fracture displacement.

The treatment of displaced patellar fractures is based on ranges of acceptable fracture fragment separation exceeding 3 to 4 mm.[31] Stabilization of displaced patellar fractures is best accomplished with an open reduction and internal fixation (ORIF) procedure. Fig. 13-42 portrays various patellar fracture patterns.

The most common fixation devices are tension band wiring and cerclage wiring (Fig. 13-43). The tension band wire is a dynamic compression device that approximates and compresses the patellar fragments. The additional use of cerclage wiring adds to the stability of the repair and allows early joint motion without redisplacing the fracture fragments.[46]

When tension band wiring is used with cerclage wiring, the immediate postoperative positioning of the patient calls for the prevention of full passive knee extension to maintain tension and compression of the patellar fracture fragments. Generally, the knee is immobilized in 20 degrees of knee flexion to support dynamic compression of the tension band wiring procedure. One week after surgery, active knee extension, submaximal quadriceps sets, and straight-leg raises can be initiated. Flexion of the knee out of the immobilizer is usually limited to approximately 100 degrees for at least 6 weeks to allow for proper bone healing. Weight-bearing as tolerated with assistive devices is encouraged during the first few weeks after surgery, then progressed to full weight-bearing by the third week. The long progression of quadriceps-strengthening exercises and the advancement of full knee flexion correlate with normal bone

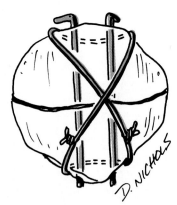

FIG. 13-43 Transverse fracture of the patella. Stabilization is achieved with tension band wire and cerclage wiring.

healing and individual tolerance. Care must be taken not to force aggressive knee extension strengthening exercises with heavy isotonic loads too early in the program. Isokinetic quadriceps and hamstring strengthening at submaximal effort with fast to moderate speeds of contraction can be used when immobilization is discontinued and the patient demonstrates good quadriceps control, improved knee flexion motion, nonpainful performance of the rudimentary quadriceps strength program (quadriceps sets, straight-leg raises, short-arc quadriceps exercises), and appropriate bone healing.

Supracondylar Femur Fractures

Distal femur fractures are classified generally as extraarticular, unicondylar, or bicondylar[33,34] (Fig. 13-44). These fractures are usually managed with an ORIF procedure, immobilization, and non–weight-bearing to allow for healing. Various internal fixation devices are used, depending on the position and severity of the fracture. Fig. 13-45 demonstrates fixation devices used for transverse **supracondylar fractures,** unicondylar fractures, and type C (T- and Y-pattern) fractures. Because of the location, pattern, and severity of supra-

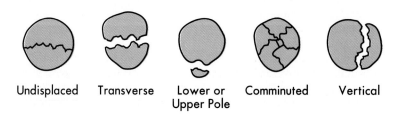

| Undisplaced | Transverse | Lower or Upper Pole | Comminuted | Vertical |

FIG. 13-42 Types of patellar fractures. (From Wiessman, Sledge: *Orthopaedic radiology,* Philadelphia, 1986, WB Saunders).

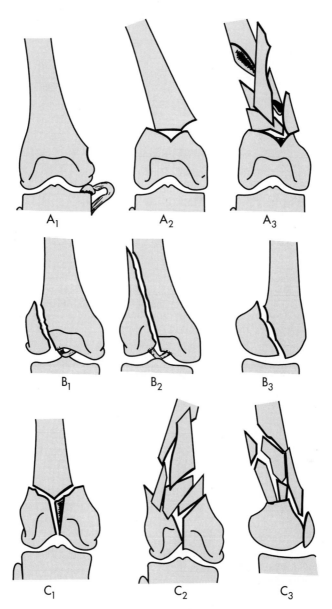

FIG. 13-44 AO/ASIF classification of supracondylar fractures. (From Johnson KD: *Ortho-paedic knowledge update* III, Rosemont, Ill., 1990, American Academy of Orthopaedic Surgeons).

condylar femur fractures, the quadriceps, hamstrings, and gastrocnemius muscle groups contribute to posterior angulation and fracture displacement.[31,33] Therefore the method of fixation focuses on fracture site stabilization and fragment apposition while minimizing the pull on the fracture site by the quadriceps, hamstrings, and calf muscles.

Fractures of the distal femur can create vascular injury to the popliteal fossa secondary to swelling and significant forces.[31] Displaced supracondylar fractures can be treated nonoperatively at the discretion of the surgeon. Physicians usually treat nondisplaced distal femur fractures nonoperatively with closed reduction of the fragments and tibial traction for approximately 8 to 12 weeks.[31]

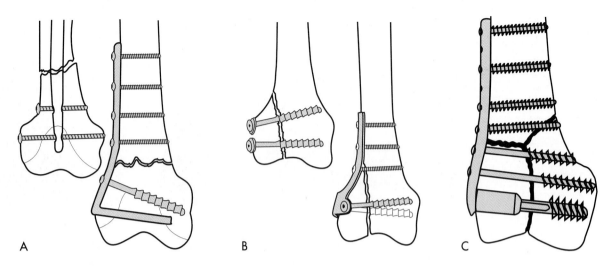

FIG. 13-45 Various methods of open reduction and internal fixation ORIF for **A,** Transverse supracondylar fractures, **B,** Unicondylar fractures, and **C,** T and Y condylar fractures. (From McRae R: *Practical fracture treatment,* ed 3, New York, 1994, Churchill Livingston).

Physical therapy management of supracondylar fractures is guided extensively by the healing process of bone and associated soft tissue. Generally, patients have limited weight-bearing for 10 to 12 weeks. Non–weight-bearing is followed strictly until subsequent radiologic assessment determines secure bone healing. With significant bleeding and associated tissue damage in distal femur fractures, arthrofibrosis and quadriceps adhesion to the bone are frequent problems.

Early postoperative management therefore focuses on patellar mobility (within the confines of the knee brace or immobilizer), active quadriceps strengthening exercises (quadriceps sets, straight-leg raises), and active knee flexion to minimize knee contractures. It is imperative to encourage strengthening and flexibility exercises for the non-involved limb and to instruct the patient in a general fitness program that does not compromise the healing of the injured limb. As bone healing progresses, appropriate normalized gait mechanics are encouraged and CKC-strengthening exercises are added cautiously. Throughout the course of healing, all fundamental quadriceps, hamstring, hip, and calf exercises are maintained, including quadriceps sets, straight-leg raises (all four positions), short arc terminal knee extensions, leg curls, ankle pumps, gluteal sets, and knee flexion ROM exercises.

When to begin CKC strengthening and proprioception exercises is determined by the healing of the stabilized fracture site, pain, swelling, improved ROM, improved quadriceps strength, and physician and physical therapist judgment.

As with many fractures about the knee, associated soft tissue injuries (ligaments, tendon, cartilage, muscle) are common. Thus the use of various exercises and the rate of healing are strongly influenced by bone and soft tissue healing.

Proximal Tibia Fractures (Tibal Plateau Fractures)

The general treatment of nondisplaced **tibial plateau fractures** (Fig 13-46) is described by Loth[31] as follows:

> These patients should be treated with early motion and protected weight bearing to prevent displacement. Traction, a knee immobilizer with intermittent motion, or a fracture brace with protected weight bearing may be appropriate for various fracture patterns. . . .

Associated knee ligament damage may be present,[31] so rehabilitation must address bone healing and repair of associated soft tissue structures. Quadriceps strengthening exercises (quadriceps sets, straight-leg raises in all four positions) in an immobilizer can commence as soon as the patient can tolerate them. Knee flexion motion is progressed as bone healing, swelling, and pain allow. Weight-bearing activities, proprioception, and CKC-strengthening exercises are deferred until secure bone healing and stabilization occur.

Displaced proximal tibial fractures are treated with an ORIF procedure. Fig. 13-47 illustrates various internal fixation devices used with different fracture patterns.

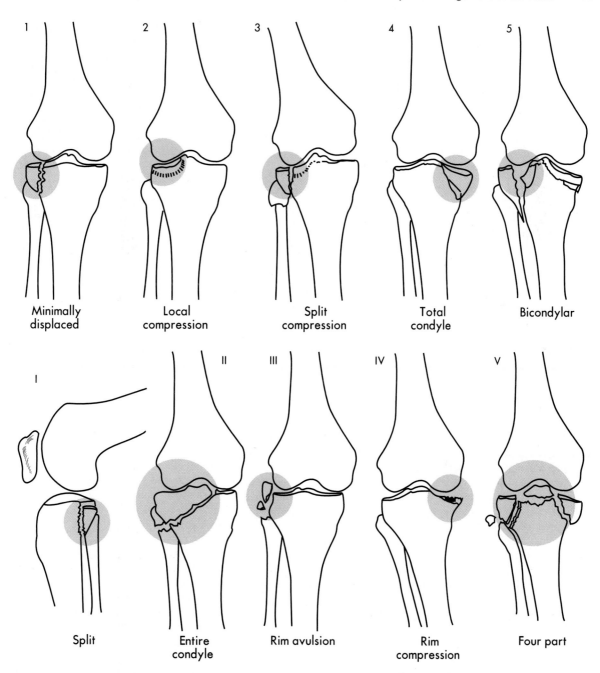

FIG. 13-46 Classification of proximal tibial plateau fractures. (From Loth T: *Orthopedic boards review,* St. Louis, 1993, Mosby).

Postoperative management and rehabilitation of tibial plateau fractures follow the course of bone and soft tissue healing.

First, the patient is placed in a leg immobilizer or fracture brace in full extension. Active quadriceps sets

are performed and the patient is generally non–weight-bearing or partial weight-bearing, depending on the severity of the fracture. After initial surgical wound healing has occurred, knee flexion exercises can begin, based on the patient's tolerance.

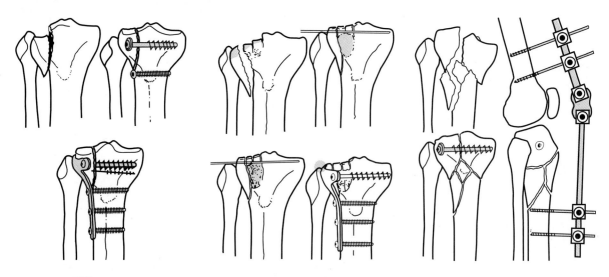

FIG. 13-47 Various methods of internal fixation of tibial plateau fractures. (From McRae R: *Practical fracture treatment,* ed 3, New York, 1994, Churchill Livingston).

Straight-leg raises can be taught during the first week postoperatively. Active ankle ROM and pumping are encouraged immediately, and hamstring stretching exercises are safely taught with the limb immobilized. A general conditioning program is advocated early, with specific strengthening exercises for the noninvolved limb and single-leg stationary cycling for aerobic fitness. As bone healing progresses (10 to 12 weeks), verified by radiographic examination by the physician, increased weightbearing, and normalized gait mechanics are encouraged.

Advanced strengthening exercises using isotonic knee extension and leg curl exercises, CKC functional exercises (stair steppers, short-arc step-ups, wall squats, leg presses), and proprioception exercises (balance boards, minitrampoline) are cautiously added as the patient demonstrates improved quadriceps strength, increased knee flexion motion, and reduced pain and swelling, and as the necessary healing of bone and soft tissue occurs.

KNEE JOINT RECONSTRUCTION

This section will introduce terminology consistent with total knee joint replacement (TKR) surgery, prosthetic design, and rehabilitation after surgery. In addition to discussing physical therapy management as it pertains to the physical therapist assistant, tibial osteotomy procedures and recovery are addressed.

Knee Arthroplasty

The indications for TKR are primarily to eliminate or reduce pain and to improve functional activities in severely disabled patients.[19,21,34] Osteoarthritis (degenerative joint disease [DJD]) and rheumatoid arthritis contribute significantly to unicompartmental (medial or lateral), bicompartmental (both medial and lateral joint compartments), and tricompartmental (medial, lateral, and patellofemoral components)[44] pain and dysfunction.[19,21,34]

Authorities define basic contraindications for TKR as active or recent septic arthritis, a "nonfunctioning extensor mechanism or severe neurologic dysfunction that prevents extension or control of the knee," and a neuropathic joint.[31,34] The age of many patients with rheumatoid arthritis who undergo TKR is less than 60 years.[21] Patients with osteoarthritis who seek the same procedure are usually over 60 years of age.[21]

TKR generally involves removing the degenerated articular surfaces of the tibia, the femur, and occasionally the articular surface of the patella, and replacing these structures with metal, plastic, or a combination prosthesis. The goals are to relieve pain, uniformly transmit forces across the joint, create a horizontal joint in the stance phase of gait, restore anatomic and mechanical axes, provide adequate stability, and improve function.[21,31,34,44]

The physical therapist assistant must be aware of common prosthetic designs as well as methods for securing these devices to bone because this information will affect the rehabilitation program. Two types of implants are used:

- **Constrained** or *conforming implants*—sacrifice the cruciate ligaments (ACL, PCL, or both) but rely on the "complete conformity between the components" for stability.[21,34,44]

- **Nonconstrained** *(cruciate-sparing) or resurfacing implants*—retain the soft-tissue stabilizing restraints (ACL and PCL).[21,34,44]

Miller[34] suggests that the nonconstrained implant is "rarely used due to exacting surgical technique and soft tissue balancing. . . ." Surgical techniques that sacrifice the cruciates (particularly the PCL) may cause problems with stair climbing.[34] Depending on the severity of joint degeneration involving the patellofemoral joint, the surgeon may elect to perform a nonconstrained procedure on the articular surface of the patella. With patellofemoral compression forces 1 to 1.5 times body weight while walking on level ground and 3 to 4 times body weight while ascending or descending stairs,[31] it is easy to appreciate the rationale for replacing a painful, degenerated retropatellar surface during TKR. One study[6] recommends that "the patella be resurfaced when an unconstrained prosthesis of this type is used in patients who have inflammatory arthritis or osteoarthritis. Failure to resurface the patella in patients who have these diagnoses may result in an increased rate of revision, including early revision, for the treatment of chronic patellar pain." Additionally, improved stair climbing can be expected after patellar resurfacing because of the reduced patellofemoral pain.[34] Patellar resurfacing components are plastic materials because metal-backed implants lead to wear fracture and create metallic debris particles in the joint.[34]

Securing the various components (tibial, femoral, and patellar) to bone has a direct effect on the progression of weight-bearing status after surgery.[21] The prosthesis can be secured with bone cement, usually polymethylmethacrylate (PMMA),[19,34] or a porous-coated cementless prosthesis can be inserted, in which the surrounding bone actually grows into and adheres to the prosthesis, creating a "direct biologic fixation."[21]

Cemented components may loosen over time in more active patient populations[21] whereas the noncemented prosthesis has no cement debris and a highly organized fibrous ingrowth adhering to the implant.[44] However, some authorities[31] suggest that uncemented knee prostheses are associated with a higher reoperation rate than cemented components. In addition, Loth[31] reports that total implant loosening is more frequent in noncemented prostheses.

Rehabilitation after TKR. Weight-bearing may be restricted longer in the noncemented group to allow for firm bone growth to the component.[21] Cemented components demonstrate a more secure fit earlier than the noncemented group, thereby allowing earlier progression in weight-bearing.

Immediate postoperative care uses a compression dressing with a knee immobilizer in full extension with the involved limb elevated 30 to 40 degrees to minimize swelling. The maximum-protection phase of recovery focuses on reducing unwanted stresses that may loosen the prosthesis, while stimulating muscle strength, increasing ROM, and reducing pain and swelling. Remedial exercises that are initiated immediately after surgery include quadriceps isometrics, ankle pumps, gluteal sets, active assisted straight-leg raises, and short-arc terminal knee extensions out of the immobilizer. As the surgical wound heals (2 to 3 days postoperatively), it is imperative to regain active control over knee flexion. Some authors report that continuous passive motion (CPM) may be beneficial in regaining knee flexion immediately after TKR surgery.[19,21] However, there appears to be no significant difference in the rate of wound healing and the incidence of thromboembolism in patients not receiving CPM during the immediate postoperative period.[31] The knee immobilizer can be removed to perform supine heel slides and supine hip- and knee-flexion exercises (Fig. 13-48). The appropriate time to begin weight-bearing will depend on the fixation used, but generally the patient is instructed in a partial weight-bearing gait with a walker or crutches.[19] Supine wall slides and active assisted wall slides (Fig. 13-49) can be added as pain allows. Usually, by 4 weeks the knee immobilizer is discarded, but an ambulatory assistive device is retained for support until strength and a normalized gait are achieved.

The moderate-protection phase described by Timm[43] extends over 7 to 12 weeks postoperatively and is characterized by enhanced gait mechanics for patients with a cemented prosthesis. Timm[43] recommends 50% weight-bearing by the eighth week, 75% weight-bearing by the tenth week, and full weight-bearing without an assistive device by the twelfth week for patients with noncemented components.

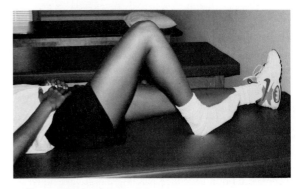

FIG. 13-48 Active supine knee-flexion range-of-motion exercises are performed daily with the immobilizer removed.

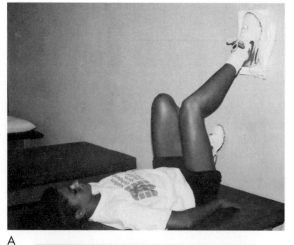

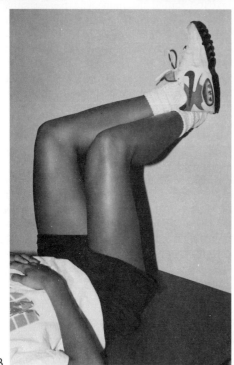

FIG. 13-49 A, Supine wall slides and **B,** Supine active-assisted wall slides for gaining knee flexion.

Patellar mobility must be allowed during the early phases of recovery. As the midline surgical incision heals, the patella should be mobilized in a caudal-cephalic motion to reduce patellofemoral adhesions.

Generally, by 13 weeks after surgery, the patient can progress to isotonic knee-extension exercises, isokinetic

knee flexion and extension,[43] stationary cycling for improved knee ROM, stair climbers, treadmill walking, and various CKC functional activities (balance board, mini-trampoline) as long as pain, swelling, quadriceps strength, joint stability, and tissue healing improve.

Commonly, the elderly population receiving TKR demonstrates reduced cardiovascular fitness and strength; therefore a general conditioning program should be started as soon as the patient can tolerate it. Early single-leg stationary cycling or UBE can be safely and effectively used to maintain or improve cardiovascular fitness. Since a TKR was performed to reduce pain and dysfunction related to osteoarthritis and/or rheumatoid arthritis, care must be taken to protect other affected joints during the initiation of a general conditioning program. In some cases, a swimming program may be more appropriate than either open-chain or closed-chain resistive exercises.

Throughout the course of recovery, the judicious use of ice, compression, whirlpool, and electrical stimulation may help control pain and swelling before and after the prescribed exercise program.

HIGH TIBIAL OSTEOTOMY (HTO)

A tibial **osteotomy** procedure can be performed on patients who demonstrate advanced osteoarthritis (DJD) of one compartment of the knee.[34] Most commonly, this is the medial joint compartment and is characterized by a varus (bow-legged) deformity that creates abnormal loads on the medial aspect of the tibiofemoral joint.[35] Less frequently, the lateral compartment is involved and creates a valgus deformity (knock-knees) (Fig. 13-50). Although this procedure is commonly performed on elderly patients (average age 60), one study[35] reports a mean age of 32 years, with a range of 16 to 47 years. This procedure is generally considered a temporary solution, lasting 7 to 10 years, before a TKR is considered.[34]

HTO attempts to realign the tibiofemoral joint by surgically creating a wedge in the proximal tibia or distal femur, depending on varus or valgus deformity, and redistributing the forces and compressive loads more evenly across the joint (Fig. 13-51). In valgus deformity associated with lateral tibiofemoral compartment destruction (see Fig. 13-50), a distal femur (supracondylar) closing-wedge osteotomy is performed and is stabilized with a plate.[34,41] Depending on the wishes and training of the surgeon, some patients use CPM immediately postoperatively to facilitate early flexion motion.[41]

Usually the knee is placed in an immobilizer in full extension with a suction drain inserted to help evacuate the excessive accumulation of blood. Initially, strengthening exercises (quadriceps sets, straight-leg raises in

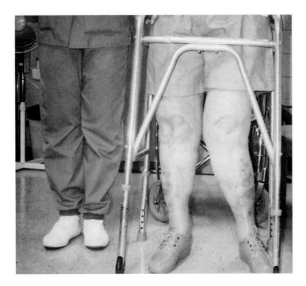

FIG. 13-50 Severe degenerative joint disease (DJD) of the lateral compartment of the knee. Note the severe valgus deformity of the knee.

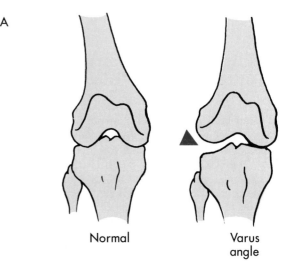

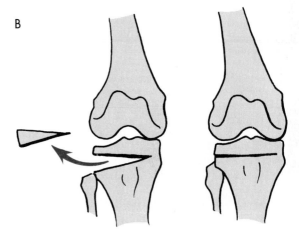

FIG. 13-51 High tibial osteotomy surgical procedure to redistribute compressive loads more evenly across the joint. **A,** Normal and abnormal varus angle. **B,** Wedge removed to change the angle of joint.

the splint, gluteal sets) are performed and advanced from the first day postoperatively. Manual patellar stretching is encouraged once initial surgical wound healing has occurred, especially with distal femoral wedge osteotomy (preoperative valgus deformity caused lateral joint compartment disease) because the procedure involves extensive invasion of the quadriceps.[41] If CPM is not used, the patient is allowed out of the immobilizer a few times a day to perform active knee flexion exercises. As patellar mobility (caudal-cephalic motion) improves, progressive knee flexion ROM exercises are added with the patient in a sitting position to allow gravity to influence the flexion range of the affected limb. Care must be taken to manually assist the affected limb from sudden flexion and to encourage quadriceps relaxation. Weight-bearing status after HTO is guided primarily by the mechanism and time constraints of bone healing as well as the type of fixation used to secure the bone.[41] Sisk[41] reports that blade or plate fixation "improves the rigidity of fixation of both tibial and femoral osteotomies, making supplemental casts unnecessary." Usually touch-down weight-bearing is allowed after surgery with the aid of crutches or a walker. Progressive ambulation follows bone-healing constraints, so protective weight-bearing is encouraged for up to 12 weeks.[41] Progressive resistive exercises for the quadriceps and hamstrings are initiated gradually within the first 3 to 4 weeks after surgery. Usually ankle weights, Thera-band resistance, seated isotonic quadriceps and hamstring exercises, and cables and pulleys can be cautiously added during the moderate-protection

phase of recovery (7 to 12 weeks), as described by Timm.[43] Knee flexion ROM improvement is encouraged by using supine wall slides, seated knee flexion, prone knee flexion, and stationary cycling.

The initiation of functional CKC resistance exercises is deferred until the physician receives radiographic confirmation of secure bone union. Assistive devices for ambulation are discontinued once a minimum of 8 to 12 weeks has passed, fixation of the bone has occurred, and the patient demonstrates good quadriceps strength, improved knee flexion ROM, and confidence in a normalized gait pattern.

COMMON MOBILIZATION TECHNIQUES FOR THE KNEE

Depending on which specific knee condition is present, the amount of pain, and which motions are limited, the physical therapist may prescribe appropriate directions of force and amplitude as well as specific mobilization techniques (see Chapter 11, Basics of Clinical Application of Joint Mobilization). The patient must be placed in the most comfortable position that allows for maximum relaxation of the affected limb. Patient relaxation and compliance can be enhanced through thermal agents and positioning before applying mobilization techniques.

The techniques presented here are generally safe, effective, and easily performed by the physical therapist assistant. It is very important to recognize that there are many techniques used to modulate pain and improve motion of the knee. The following examples demonstrate the most common techniques used for the patellofemoral and tibiofemoral joints.

Mobilization of the Patellofemoral Joint

With the patient supine on an examination table, mobilize the patella in a caudal direction by firmly grasping the proximal or superior pole of the patella with an open palm or fingertips (Fig. 13-52). Being careful to avoid patellofemoral compression, gently push or glide the patella in an inferior direction (caudally). When teaching the patient this technique, instruct him or her to use the thumbs of both hands to stretch the patella "toward the foot."

To achieve a superior glide motion (cephalic), place one hand at the inferior pole or distal border of the patella as just described. Taking care to avoid patellofemoral compressive load, gently stretch the patella superiorly (Fig. 13-53). Both medial and lateral glides of the patella can be achieved by placing the fingers on either the medial or lateral aspect of the patella and gently pushing either medially or laterally (Fig. 13-54). Avoid a compressive force to the patellofemoral joint.

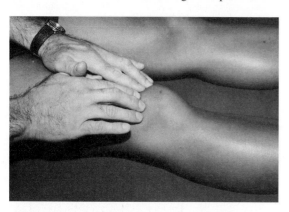

FIG. 13-52 Manual caudal glide of the patella.

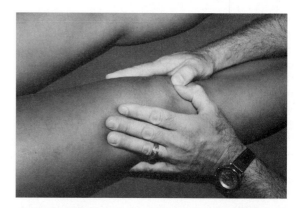

FIG. 13-53 Manual cephalic glide of the patella.

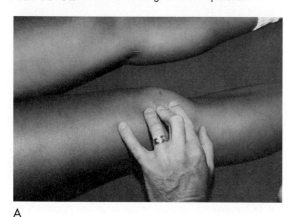

A

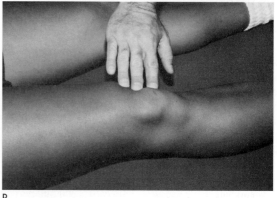

B

FIG. 13-54 A, Medial glide of the patella. **B,** Lateral glide of the patella.

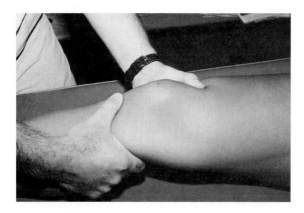

FIG. 13-55 Manual anterior-posterior glide of the tibiofemoral joint with the affected knee flexed approximately 30 degrees. This position parallels the Lachman exam position.

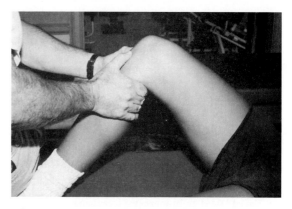

FIG. 13-56 Manual anterior-posterior glide of the tibiofemoral joint with the knee flexed 90 degrees. This position parallels the anterior-posterior drawer exam.

Mobilization of the Tibiofemoral Joint

Anterior and posterior glide motions described by Wooden[48] are similar to the Lachman examination and the anterior and posterior drawer tests previously described. To perform an anterior and posterior glide motion directed to the tibiofemoral joint, hold the patient's affected limb in approximately 30 degrees of flexion. Stabilize the distal femur with one hand, while using the other hand to firmly grasp the proximal tibia. Apply gentle anteriorly and posteriorly directed force (Fig. 13-55).

An anteriorly and posteriorly directed mobilization force can be performed with the affected limb held at approximately 90 degrees of flexion. Stabilize the foot of the affected limb by sitting on the dorsum of the foot. Use both hands to grasp the proximal tibia, with the thumbs of the hands directly on the anteromedial and anterolateral joint lines of the tibiofemoral joint. Apply gentle anteriorly and posteriorly directed force to the tibia (Fig. 13-56).

In another common mobilization technique, the patient is prone on an examination table with the affected limb flexed 60 degrees to 90 degrees. Place the foot of the affected limb on your shoulder and firmly grasp the proximal posterior tibia with open palms over the proximal calf muscles. With a very gentle anterior "scooping" motion of the hands, rock the tibia forward and away from the femur (Fig. 13-57).

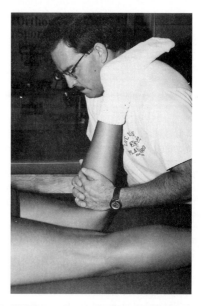

FIG. 13-57 Prone "scooping" of the tibiofemoral joint.

REFERENCES

1. Abbott LC, et al: Injuries to the ligaments of the knee joint, *J Bone Joint Surg* 26:503-521, 1944.
2. Arnoczky S, et al: Meniscus. In Woo SL-Y, Buckwalter JA, editors: *Injury and repair of the musculoskeletal soft tissues,* Park Ridge, Ill., 1988, American Academy of Orthopaedic Surgeons.
3. Barrack RL, Skinner H, and Buckley SL: Proprioception in the anterior cruciate deficient knee, *Am J Sports Med* 17:1-6, 1989.
4. Bennett JG: Rehabilitation of patellofemoral joint dysfunction. In Greenfield BH, editor: *Rehabilitation of the knee: a problem solving approach,* Philadelphia, 1994, FA Davis.
5. Beynnon BD et al: Anterior cruciate ligament strain behavior during rehabilitation exercises in vivo, *Am J Sports Med* 23, (1):24-34, 1995.
6. Boyd AD et al: Long-term complications after total knee arthroplasty with or without resurfacing of the patella,

Update, a Bi-monthly newsletter of the American Society of Orthopaedic Physicians Assistants, Nov/Dec, 1994.

7. Buckwalter J, et al: Articular cartilage: injury and repair, In Woo SL-Y, Buckwalter JA, editors: *injury and repair of the musculoskeletal soft tissues,* American Academy of Orthopaedic Surgeons Symposium, American Academy of Orthopaedic Surgeons, 1987.

8. Carlson TJ: The rationale behind meniscus repair, postgraduate advances in sports medicine, 1987, Forum Medicus, Inc. Course Outline.

9. Clancy WG, Shelbourne DK, and Zoellner GB: Treatment of knee joint instability secondary to rupture of the posterior cruciate ligament, *J Bone Joint Surg* 65A:310-322, 1983.

10. Daniel DM et al: Instrumented measurement of anterior knee laxity in patients with acute anterior cruciate ligament disruption, *Am J. Sports Med* 13:401, 1985.

11. Daniel DM, Fritschy D: Anterior cruciate ligament injuries. In DeLee JC, Drez D, editors *Orthopaedic sports medicine: principles and practice,* vol 2, Philadelphia, 1994, WB Saunders.

12. DeLee JC et al: The posterior cruciate ligament. In DeLee JC, Drez D, editors: *Orthopaedic sports medicine: principals and practice,* Vol 2, Philadelphia, 1994, WB Saunders.

13. Drez D, editor: Knee braces, Seminar report, American Academy of Orthopaedic Surgeons, 1985.

14. Einhorn AR, Sawyer M, Tovin B: Rehabilitation of intra-articular reconstructions. In Greenfield BH, editor: *Rehabilitation of the knee: a problem solving approach,* Philadelphia, 1993, FA Davis.

15. Engle RP, Meade TD, Canner GC: Rehabilitation of posterior cruciate ligament injuries. In Greenfield BH, editor: *Rehabilitation of the knee: a problem solving approach,* Philadelphia, 1993, FA Davis.

16. Fetto JF, Marshall JL: Medial collateral ligament injuries of the knee: a rationale for treatment, *Clin Orthop* 132:206-217, 1978.

17. Frank C et al: Medial collateral ligament healing: a multi-disciplinary assessment in rabbits, *Am J Sports Med,* 11:379-389, 1983.

18. Fu FH, Baratz M: Meniscal injuries. In DeLee JC, Drez D, editors: *Orthopaedic sports medicine: principals and practice,* vol 2, Philadelphia, 1994, WB Saunders.

19. Goldstein TS: Geriatric orthopaedics, rehabilitative management of common problems, In Lewis CB, editor: *Aspen series in physical therapy,* Gaithersburg, Md., 1991, Aspen Publications.

20. Grana WA, Kriegshauser LA: Scientific basis of extensor mechanism disorders. In Larson RL, Singer KM, editors: *Clin in Sports Med, The knee,* 4 (2):247-257, 1985.

21. Greene B: Rehabilitation after total knee replacement. In Greenfield BH, editor: *Rehabilitation of the knee: a problem solving approach,* Philadelphia, 1993, FA Davis.

22. Hammesfahr R: Surgery of the knee. In Donatelli R, Wooden MJ, editors: *Orthopaedic physical therapy,* New York, 1989, Churchill Livingstone.

23. Henning CE, Lynch MA: Current concepts of meniscal function and pathology, *Clin Sports Med* 4 (2):259-265, 1985.

24. Holden DL, Eggert AW, Butler JE: The nonoperative treatment of grade I and II medial collateral ligament injuries to the knee, *Am J Sports Med* 11(5):340-344, 1983.

25. Hughston JC: Patellar subluxation In: *Patellofemoral problems, Clin in Sports Med,* 8(2):153-162, 1989.

26. Hughston J: *Knee ligaments: injury and repair,* St Louis, 1993, Mosby.

27. Hughston J: Posterior cruciate ligament instabilities. In Hughston J, editor: *Knee ligaments: injury and repair,* St. Louis, 1993, Mosby.

28. Jacobson KE, Flandry FC: Diagnosis of anterior knee pain. In Henry JH, editor: *Patellofemoral problems, Clin in Sports Med,* 8(2):179-195, 1989.

29. Jensen JE et al: Systematic evaluation of acute knee injuries. In Larson RL, Singer KM, editors: *Clinics in Sports Medicine,* Philadelphia, 1985, WB Saunders.

30. Linton, RC, Indelicato PA: Medial ligament injuries. In DeLee JC, Drez D, editors: *Orthopaedic sports medicine,* vol 2, Philadelphia, 1994, WB Saunders.

31. Loth TS: *Orthopaedic boards review,* St. Louis, 1993, Mosby.

32. Malone T: Rehabilitation of the surgical knee: the therapist's view of surgery. In Davies G. editor: *Rehabilitation of the surgical knee,* Ronkonkoma, N.Y., 1984, Cybex.

33. McRae R: *Practical fracture treatment,* ed 3, Ronkonkoma, N.Y., 1994, Churchill-Livingstone.

34. Miller M: *Review of orthopaedics,* Philadelphia, 1992, WB Saunders.

35. Noyes FR, Barber SD, Simon R: High tibial osteotomy and ligament reconstruction in varus angulated, anterior cruciate ligament-deficient knees, *Am J Sports Med* 21(1), 1993.

36. O'Donoughue DH: Surgical treatment of injuries to the ligament of the knee, *JAMA* 169:142-151, 1959.

37. Parolie JM, Bergfeld JA: Long-term results of non-operative treatment of isolated posterior cruciate ligament injuries in the athlete, *Am J Sports Med* 14:35-38, 1986.

38. Paulos LE, et al: Knee rehabilitation after anterior cruciate ligament reconstruction and repair, *Am J Sports Med* 9:140, 1981.

39. Paulos LE, Payne FC, Rosenburg TD: Rehabilitation after anterior cruciate ligament surgery. In Jackson DW, and Drez D, editors: *The anterior cruciate deficient knee: new concepts in ligament repair,* St. Louis, 1987, Mosby.

40. Schenck RC, Heckman JD: Injuries of the knee, Presented at clinical symposia, Ciba-Geigy, 1993.

40a. Seto JL, Brewster CE: Rehabilitation of meniscal injuries. In Greenfield BH editor: *Rehabilitation of the knee: a problem-solving approach,* Philadelphia, 1993, FA Davis.

41. Sisk TD: Knee realignment and replacement in the recreational athlete. In DeLee JC, Drez D editors:

Orthopaedic sports medicine: principals and practice, vol 2, Philadelphia, 1994, WB Saunders.

42. Tenuta JJ, Arciero RA: Arthroscopic evaluation of meniscal repairs: factors that effect healing, *Am J Sports Med* 22 (6):797-802, 1994.

43. Timm K: Knee. In Richardson JK, Iglarsh ZA, editors: *Clinical orthopaedic physical therapy,* Philadelphia, 1994, WB Saunders.

44. Tippett SR: Total knee arthroplasty: An overview, physical therapy implications and rehabilitation concerns. In: *Advances in clinical education continuing education course notes,* p 248 -260, 1994, Course notes.

45. Turba JE: Formal extensor mechanism reconstruction. In: *Patellofemoral problems, Clin in Sports Med* 8 (2):297-317, 1989.

46. Walsh WM: Patellofemoral joint. In DeLee JC, Drez D, editors: *Orthopaedic sports medicine: principles and practice,* vol 2, Philadelphia, 1994, WB Saunders.

47. Wilk KE: Rehabilitation of medial capsular injuries. In Greenfield BH, editor: *Rehabilitation of the knee: a problem solving approach,* Philadelphia, 1993, FA Davis.

48. Wooden MJ: Mobilization of the lower extremity, In Donatelli R, Wooden MJ, editors: *Orthopaedic physical therapy,* New York, 1989, Churchill-Livingstone.

Orthopedic Management of the Hip and Pelvis

LEARNING OBJECTIVES

1. Identify common hip fractures.
2. Outline and discuss common methods of management and rehabilitation of common hip fractures.
3. Identify and describe common methods of management and rehabilitation following hip arthroplasty.
4. Identify and describe common soft tissue injuries of the hip.
5. Outline and describe common methods of management and rehabilitation of soft tissue injuries of the hip.
6. Identify common fractures of the pelvis and the hip.
7. Discuss methods of management and rehabilitation for fractures of the pelvis and acetabulum.
8. Describe common mobilization techniques for the hip.

CHAPTER OUTLINE

The practicing physical therapist assistant is exposed to many orthopedic problems involving the hip and pelvis. This chapter focuses attention on the more common classifications, management, and rehabilitation of hip fractures, joint reconstructive surgery (total hip arthroplasty), rehabilitation after hip replacement, and management of various pelvic fractures and soft tissue injuries of the hip.

HIP FRACTURES

The clinical significance of hip fractures is reflected in the annual rate of fractures and the financial burden to the economy that hip fractures produce.[4,8] Goldstein states that over 300,000 fractures occur annually with an associated cost of $10 billion. Other authorities[2,8] report that 267,000 fractures occur annually, with a price tag of $33.8 billion.[2] Although fractures in general occur to all age groups, hip fractures are most common among elderly women.[2,8,9] Hip fractures in women can be attributed in part to the higher incidence in this group of osteoporosis;[9] with regard to age, hip fractures represent the most common acute orthopedic injury in the geriatric population.[8]

The classification of hip fractures is clinically significant for the physical therapist assistant because the severity and location of the fracture profoundly affect surgical management and physical therapy interventions. The vascular supply to the femoral head and neck may be significantly compromised with certain fracture patterns and levels of severity (Fig. 14-1).[9] LeVeau[9] states, "The extent of the supply of blood to the head of the femur determines remodelling and healing after femoral neck fracture or hip dislocation."

Generally, hip fractures can be classified by location and described by severity (simple or comminuted).[3] Fractures of the hip can be located in the following areas:

- Extracapsular or trochanteric[3,4,13] (Fig. 14-2)
- Femoral neck or subcapital areas[5] (these are intracapsular) (Fig. 14-3)
- Proximal femoral shaft or subtrochanteric areas[5] (Fig. 14-4)

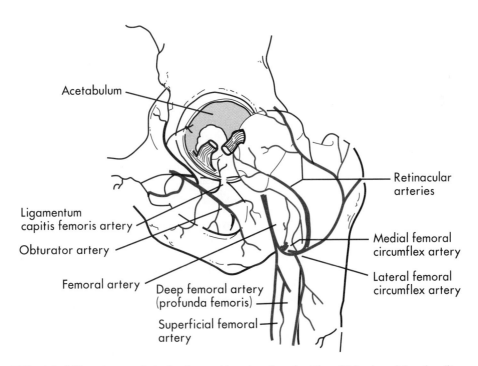

FIG. 14-1 Vascular supply to the femoral head and neck. (From Richardson, Iglarsch, editors: *Clinical orthopedic physical therapy,* Philadelphia, 1994, WB Saunders).

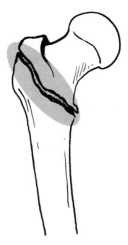

FIG. 14-2 Intertrochanteric hip fracture.

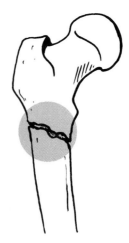

FIG. 14-4 Subtrochanteric hip fracture.

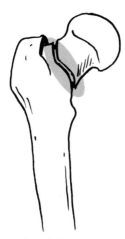

FIG. 14-3 Femoral neck fracture.

Secondary to the location and severity of hip fracture, the most significant complication is related to osteonecrosis and the loss of blood supply to the femoral head leading to **avascular necrosis (AVN).** Gross et al[5] found that "any fracture of the neck (femoral) can disrupt this tenuous blood supply. As a result, there is an exceedingly high incidence of avascular necrosis of the femoral head following hip fractures." LeVeau[9] states "avascular necrosis may occur after hip fracture in about 65% to 85% of the patients."

Three main clinical complications are noted with subtrochanteric fractures: malunion, delayed union, and nonunion.[10] Two factors are associated with malunion and nonunion of subtrochanteric hip fractures:
- The subtrochanteric area of the proximal femur is cortical bone, which has a decreased blood supply.
- The subtrochanteric area is prone to large biomechanical stresses that can lead to loosening of various fixation devices.[10] This complication must be considered by the physical therapist assistant when treating patients with this type of fracture.

Many options are available in treating hip fractures and the choice depends on the patient's age, location of the fracture, quality of bone, severity of the fracture (simple, displaced, or comminuted), activity level of the patient, associated soft tissue injuries, and specific goals for the patient's return to activity. Generally, hip fractures are managed surgically with an **open reduction and internal fixation (ORIF)** procedure that secures the fracture fragments with various rods, nails, pins, screws, and plates.[3,4,8] Some hip fractures can be managed conservatively with bed rest, traction, and protected weight-bearing.[10] For example, in a fractured greater trochanter where the displaced fracture fragment is less than 1 cm (as evaluated by the physician radiographically), the treatment could be bed rest for several days, ROM exercises, and limited weight-bearing for 4 weeks.[10]

With an isolated lesser trochanteric fracture (most common in adolescents), the physician bases treatment

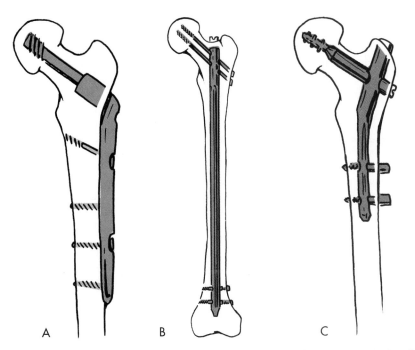

FIG. 14-5 Various methods of internal fixation for hip fractures. **A,** Screws and sideplate **B,** Rod **C,** Nails.

on the amount of fragment displacement. If the fracture is displaced more than 2 cm, the physician could perform an ORIF procedure; if the fragments are in closer apposition, the physician may elect rest, protected weight-bearing, and limited exercise for 3 to 4 weeks.[10] Fig. 14-5 depicts common fixation devices used to secure fracture fragments using an ORIF procedure.

While treating patients with hip fractures, the physical therapist assistant must also be aware that venous thrombosis is a potentially critical complication after hip surgery. Without prophylactic medications to minimize thrombosis, statistics show that 40% to 90% of patients develop thrombosis after hip surgery.[10] In an elderly population of patients, venous thrombosis is the most common complication after hip fracture.[10]

In addition to hip fractures and dislocations occurring as isolated events, they can occur in combination. Usually hip dislocations are either anterior or posterior (Fig. 14-6). Isolated hip dislocations are generally treated conservatively with bed rest, traction, and protected limited weight-bearing for up to 12 weeks.[10] For example, with an anterior hip dislo-

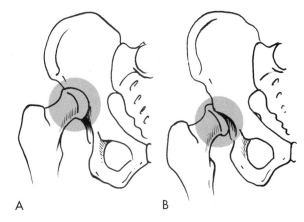

FIG. 14-6 Dislocation of the hip. **A,** Anterior dislocation **B,** Posterior dislocation.

cation, bed rest with traction is prescribed, with specific precautions to strictly avoid extreme hip abduction and external rotation to avoid redislocation. Usually protected weight-bearing is allowed when the patient can achieve painless hip ROM around 3 to 4 weeks after the incident.[10] Conversely, an isolated posterior hip dislocation is treated with bed rest and traction in abduction with precautions to avoid hip abduction, flexion, and internal rotation to protect the joint from dislocation.[10]

Rehabilitation After Hip Fractures

Any rehabilitation program used to treat hip fractures is highly individualized. The nature of the fracture type, classification, location, and method of internal fixation (if any) are considered, and the treatment program is adjusted to the patient's ability to cope with specific identified criteria. These criteria are established by the physical therapist and carried out by the physical therapist assistant.

The progression from maximum to minimal protection closely follows the rate of bone healing. However, other factors are considered in safely and effectively providing an environment for the return to functional activities. In the maximum-protection phase of recovery (phase 1—to 21 days postoperatively, as described by Goldstein)[3] the fracture site is protected; pain and swelling are reduced; and isometric exercises, gentle protected ROM, and limited weight-bearing begin.[3,9]

The general goals of recovery are to increase muscular strength specific to the surgery, improve overall conditioning, increase ROM of the affected hip, enhance aerobic fitness, increase local muscular endurance, reduce pain and swelling, reestablish normalized gait mechanics, and protect the healing structures from internal and external forces that can impede healing.[3,9]

During the maximum-protection phase the exercises used include active ankle pumps for both lower extremities, isometric quadriceps sets, gluteal sets, heel slides, hip abduction and adduction, and supine internal and external hip rotation. These exercises must be done at submaximal levels at first, then progressively made more difficult according to the patient's tolerance.

Goldstein[3] identified a few major complications that occur, particularly during the maximum-protection phase of recovery. Generally, no combined diagonal or rotary forces are used in exercises during this phase. If increased torque is placed through the healing fracture site by excessive unwanted forces, hardware loosening and delayed healing may occur.[3] No active straight-leg raises or supine hip bridges should be performed during the first 6 to 8 weeks after surgery. Goldstein[3] states "The power generated by the massive hip muscles is so great during those exercises that there is a danger of displacing the fractured segments."[3]

In addition to rudimentary isometric quadriceps sets, gluteal sets, ankle pumps, and gentle hip-motion exercises, authorities advocate adding the exercises described in Fig. 14-7 progressively during the first 3 weeks after surgery.[3]

Early protected weight-bearing is encouraged soon after surgery. Generally, touch-down weight-bearing (TDWB) or partial weight-bearing (PWB) is allowed by the second day postoperatively. Weight-bearing status increases as dictated by the rate of bone healing (over 8 to 12 weeks), which should be verified radiographically by the physician. Avoiding torque through the affected limb during standing minimizes loosening of the fixation device.

More demanding exercises are added as the bone and associated soft tissues heal. Closed-chain functional exercises are added as full weight-bearing is achieved. Partial wall squats and step-ups are usually initiated to regain concentric and eccentric muscle control of the quadriceps and hip extensors. A restorator or bike ergometer can be used during the early recovery phase if the patient can tolerate sitting, and depending on restrictions regarding hip flexion, ROM, and precautions.

The moderate-protection phase, defined as 3 to 6 weeks after surgery,[3] provides for more challenging exercises directed at regaining hip and knee motion, improving quadriceps and hamstring strength, and increasing strength to the hip extensors, abductors, and adductors. Standing four-position hip strengthening can be achieved using a cable system (Fig. 14-8). The initiation of limited ROM leg presses can commence during this phase as well.

The late healing phase (after 6 to 8 weeks) is characterized by normalized gait mechanics and reduced use of assistive devices for ambulation. A treadmill can be used, with step cadence and stride length adjusted, to enhance gait as well as to provide a stimulus for greater hip and quadriceps strength.

More advanced hip strengthening exercises can be added cautiously for more active patients. The stair stepper stimulates hip extension strength and local muscular endurance, but extreme caution must be used when initiating various opened-chain and closed-chain exercises after surgery for hip fractures. A fine line must be applied to avoid excessive forces (as in straight-leg raises or hip bridges), torque, and weight-bearing while stimulating hip and knee motion and improving strength and function.

Sitting
1. Knee extension (kicking)
   Slowly extend knee fully, hold for 1 second, and return slowly to flexed position under control.

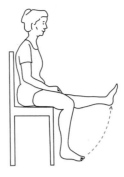

2. Hip flexion (marching)
   Lift alternate knees to chest, as if slowly marching in place while sitting.

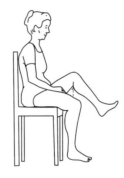

3. Forward bending of trunk
   Slowly reach hands down along the insides of the legs. Stop at the first pulling sensation. Return slowly to erect posture.

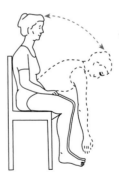

4. Armchair push-ups
   Place hands on armrests (or push-up blocks) and extend both elbows, lifting torso from chair seat. Feet should be placed on floor for balance, support, and assist.

FIG. 14-7 Progressive hip exercises are employed during the first 3-4 weeks following surgery. (From Goldstein T: *Geriatric orthopaedics*, Gaithersburg, Md., 1991, Aspen).

Continued

Supine Lying
 5. Hip rotations
      With hips slightly abducted and knees
      extended, slowly roll legs in and out.

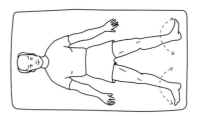

 6. Heel slides
      Slide heel along mat toward the buttocks
      and slowly return to original position.

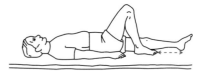

 7. Knee to chest
      Flex hip, bringing knee toward the chest,
      and slowly return limb to extended posi-
      tion.

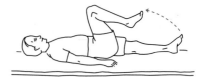

 8. Hip abduction/adduction
      Slowly spread legs apart and pull them
      together, keeping the knees extended and
      the toes pointed upward.

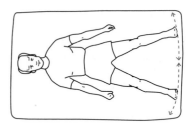

 9. Terminal knee extension

Prone Lying
10. Hip flexor stretch
      Lie prone for up to 20 minutes daily. Place pillow or bolster under ankles for comfort.

FIG. 14-7, cont'd. For legend see opposite page.

11. Knee flexion
   Flex knee and bring heel toward buttocks.
   Return to extended position.

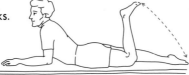

12. Hip extension
   With knee flexed to 90°, lift knee slightly
   off mat without rotating pelvis and slowly
   lower knee to mat.

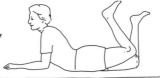

FIG. 14-7, cont'd. For legend see p. 193.

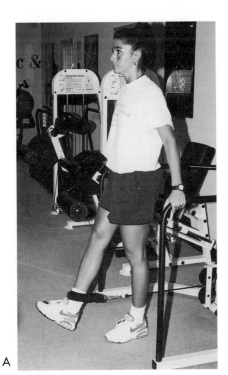

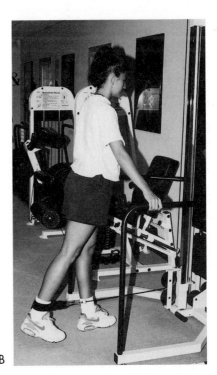

A

B

FIG. 14-8 Standing 4-way hip strengthening exercises using a cable column system. **A,** Hip flexion straight-leg raise **B,** Hip extension.

Continued

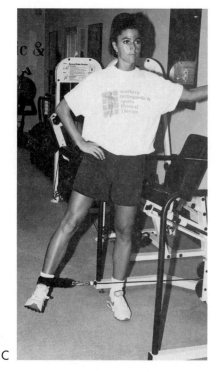

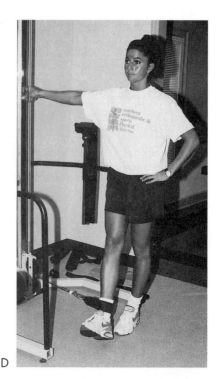

FIG. 14-8, cont'd. C, Hip abduction. **D,** Hip adduction.

PROXIMAL FEMORAL OSTEOTOMY

When **degenerative joint disease (DJD)** is extensive and results in hip pain associated with subchondral bone erosion, articular cartilage fibrillation and fissuring, and hip joint incongruity,[7] *intertrochanteric osteotomy* may be performed. The goal of this surgical procedure is to reduce pain and improve function related to advanced osteoarthritis by surgically changing the femoral neck-shaft angle so that healthy cartilage is exposed, thereby "improving joint surface congruity."[7] Fig. 14-9 illustrates this procedure and shows the changed neck-shaft angle relationship, reduced ligamentous and muscular tension, and improved joint articulation occurring after surgery.[7]

Rehabilitation After Proximal Femoral Intertrochanteric Osteotomy

Because a **proximal femoral intertrochanteric osteotomy** is performed to reduce symptoms related to advanced osteoarthritis (DJD) of the hip, the rehabilitation program must focus on joint protection principles (unloading forces through the hip) and postsurgical bone healing precautions. During the maximal-protection phase of recovery, avoiding unwanted forces, managing pain (with thermal agents and/or pain medication), using protected weight-bearing (to unload the hip from repetitive articular cartilage destruction), restoring hip motion, and improving strength are stressed. Quadriceps setting exercises, gluteal sets, ankle pumps, and gentle active hip ROM exercises are allowed from the first day after surgery.

Weight-bearing status is highly individualized but generally is progressed according to the rate and quality of bone healing. Typically, a walker or crutches reduces compressive loads through the hip during TDWB, PWB, and non-weight-bearing (NWB) gait techniques. In most cases, protected weight-bearing is strictly enforced for 8 to 12 weeks after this procedure.[7]

The contralateral hip, bilateral knee joints, and spine are targets of joint protection related to osteoarthritis. The physical therapist assistant must fully recognize that the whole person—not just the affected joint—should be addressed during all phases of recovery. In keeping with joint protection, once the surgical incision has healed and the patient is allowed PWB status, an underwater treadmill is quite useful to enhance normalized gait mechanics in a protected weight-bearing environment;

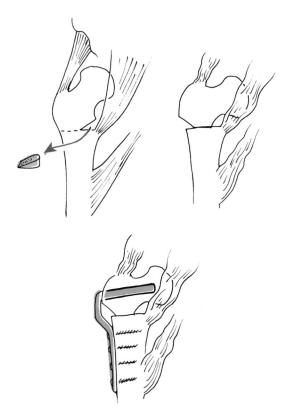

FIG. 14-9 Proximal femoral osteotomy.

the buoyancy of the water allows reduced compressive loads through the hip.

Once radiographic evidence suggests secure bone healing, more challenging and intense strengthening exercises are gradually added. Isotonic knee extensions, leg curls, and standing hip abduction, adduction, flexion, and extension motions are strengthened using a cable system or wall pulleys. Extreme caution must be used with closed-chain strengthening exercises. Minimizing joint compressive loads, which may contribute to articular cartilage degeneration, is the cornerstone in the long-term care of severe osteoarthritis. Therefore functional weight-bearing exercises must be added judiciously and without increased pain.

A limited ROM leg-press exercise can be used as the first closed-chain activity. As healing progresses, mini step-ups, short-arc wall squats, and treadmill walking are added. A general conditioning program that encourages weight control, specifically using aerobic exercise (unloaded, upper body ergometer, or recumbent or semi-recumbent stationary cycle ergometer), strengthen-

ing (while minimizing joint compressive loads and shearing joint motions), and flexibility should be implemented as soon as the patient can tolerate these activities.

HEMIARTHROPLASTY OF THE HIP

For femoral head osteonecrosis or severe femoral head fractures, **hemiarthroplasty** is used to eliminate pain and improve function. This procedure replaces the damaged femoral head with a bipolar prosthesis. Because hemiarthroplasty requires a normal acetabular surface,[7,14] it is rarely used for arthritis.[14] This is considered a "conservative" procedure[7] when compared with a total hip replacement. Hemiarthroplasty can be converted at a later date to total hip replacement if symptoms persist and the joint degenerates.[14] The term *bipolar* refers to two separate snap-fit components of one femoral prosthetic unit. A bipolar prosthesis is usually a large-diameter femoral head component that snap-fits snugly onto a smaller diameter femoral head, which is part of the total prosthetic unit.[3,7] A unipolar femoral prosthesis is a self-contained femoral head and shaft without additional components. The bipolar prosthesis usually produces less wear caused by friction and reduced impact loading of the acetabulum.[12]

FIXATION OF PROSTHETIC HIP COMPONENTS

As discussed in Chapter 13, the method of fixation of various prosthetic components directly effects the short-term and long-term course of rehabilitation after hip arthroplasty. Both femoral and acetabular components can usually be secured to the bone with a cement, polymethylmethacrylate (PMMA), which is not actually an adhesive, but rather provides a strong interference fit between the prosthesis and the bone,[12] or with a noncemented biologic tissue ingrowth prosthesis. Miller[14] recommends that cemented femoral stems be used only for patients over age 65, and that noncemented prosthesis be used for younger patients.[14] Weight-bearing precautions are related to the specific type of fixation procedure used to secure the prosthesis. Weight-bearing is generally deferred for longer periods of time with a noncemented biologic tissue fit prosthesis so that the bone can grow into the porous coated femoral stem. Weight-bearing with cemented devices can progress at a slightly faster rate. However, in either case, rotational forces (torque) must be strictly avoided to minimize the loosening of components.

TOTAL HIP REPLACEMENT

Total hip arthroplasty (**total hip replacement, [THR]**) involves replacing both the femoral head and the acetabulum, as contrasted with a hemiarthroplasty, which replaces only the femoral head. Indications for the use of THR include the following:

- Rheumatoid arthritis
- Osteoarthritis (both femoral head and acetabulum)
- Osteonecrosis
- Fractures
- Juvenile rheumatoid arthritis (the most common indication for THR in adolescents)[12]
- Pain
- Reduced ambulation
- Significant alterations in activities of daily living (ADLs)[14]

Before discussing rehabilitation procedures, it is exceedingly important to review pertinent complications and component design related to THR because these issues influence specific physical therapy interventions and precautions to be observed.

Surgeons must select a proper femoral head size for each patient. In theory, a large diameter femoral head may provide for greater ROM and inherent stability.[12,14] This makes sense because greater forces are required to dislocate a large diameter head from the acetabulum.[12,14] In practice, large diameter femoral head components do not reduce the incidence of dislocation after surgery.[12] Therefore the most commonly-used head size is moderate (26 to 28 mm)[14] rather than overly large (32 mm).[14]

One of the most common complications related to THR, using a noncemented femoral stem component, is persistent thigh pain with an antalgic gait (painful limp-gait) pattern. This thigh pain may last for 1 or 2 years after surgery and has been reported in approximately 20% of all patients with this fixation type.[12,14]

The most significant complication after THR, with the highest mortality, is thromboembolic disease.[12]

Because the method of fixation is directly related to the initiation and progression of weight-bearing after surgery, with uncemented components, some authorities recommend TDWB on the second day postoperatively, gradually progressing to full weight-bearing (FWB) by 8 weeks postoperatively.[3] With a cemented (PMMA) prosthesis, Goldstein[3] suggests TDWB 2 days after surgery, progressing to FWB by the third week postoperatively. These timetables for weight-bearing are directed by the biologic rate of bone healing as well as the wishes of the physician and are applied under the direction of the physical therapist. A cemented component generally allows earlier motion and weight-bearing than an uncemented prosthesis.

Loosening of the components has been estimated at 10% to 40% by 10 years postoperatively.[14] Loosening is more common among younger, more active patients, obese patients, patients with rheumatoid arthritis, and patients with previous hip surgery.[14] The physical therapist assistant must be acutely aware of these factors when treating THR patients and recognize the increased potential for component loosening.

Postoperative dislocation of the hip following THR is another clinically significant complication occurring at rates between 1% and 4%.[14] These dislocations are multifactorial, requiring an awareness of the basic concepts of hardware design, fixation procedures, and surgical approaches as well as patient compliance with specific total hip precautions to avoid dislocation. The most immediate concern during the recovery from THR is teaching and reinforcing precautions to the patient, nursing staff, family, and other care givers.

The physical therapist assistant should also be familiar with the surgical approach used to gain exposure to the hip. Universal **total hip precautions** are intended to avoid the exact position the surgeon used to expose and dislocate the hip in order to carry out the procedure. Usually these precautions are as follows:

- Avoid hip adduction. This is usually accomplished by using an abduction wedge or pillow.
- Avoid hip internal rotation. The affected limb can be supported medially with pillows or a wedge to maintain the limb in neutral or slight external rotation.
- Avoid hip flexion greater than 90 degrees.
- Avoid the combination (simultaneous performance) of hip flexion, internal rotation, and adduction for up to 4 months[3] after surgery.

The above precautions apply when a posterolateral or lateral approach is used. If an anterior surgical approach is used, combined hip extension and external rotation should be avoided.[3] Again, this variation is needed because the surgeon had to extend and externally rotate the limb to dislocate the hip and gain exposure for replacement.

Rehabilitation After THR

Recovery from the significant trauma of THR requires extensive bone and soft tissue healing. Following THR precautions, recovery may take up to 4 months in some cases.

The rehabilitation program can be divided into maximum-protection, moderate-protection, and minimal-protection phases of recovery. The time frames associated with each phase depends on the individual patient's ability to achieve certain criteria of improved motion (being careful not to compromise THR precautions), increased strength, weight-bearing status (taking into account whether the replacement has been secured with cement or with a porous coated biologic ingrowth component), reduced pain, compliance with THR precautions, bed mobility, transfers, and improved confidence.

In the maximum-protection phase of recovery, the patient is instructed in bilateral ankle pumps, isometric quadriceps sets, gluteal isometrics, and active knee flexion (being careful to avoid excessive hip flexion) exercises. The contralateral limb can be exercised with active straight-leg raises, quadriceps sets, hamstring sets, ankle pumps, and full knee and hip mobility exercises. To ensure primary healing, all universal hip precautions must be enforced (avoid hip flexion, adduction, and internal rotation with a posterolateral or lateral surgical approach, and avoid hip extension and external rotation with an anterior approach). In addition, the patient should be strongly cautioned to avoid the following positions and actions, as outlined by LeVeau:[9]

- Do not sit in low chairs.
- Do not cross your legs.
- Do not sleep on your side.
- Do not bend forward at your hip (causes excessive hip flexion).
- Do not squat.

Transfer training and bed mobility must be addressed immediately after surgery. The affected limb should be maintained in a stable, secure position during all transfers from bed to commode or wheelchair. A raised toilet seat is a basic requirement during the early phase of recovery. In addition, a raised and rigid (although padded) seat cushion is needed to eliminate the sling effect of the wheelchair seat, which places the hip in an internally rotated position.[3]

The use of crutches or a walker is advocated for TDWB or PWB, depending on how the prosthesis is secured. A cemented prosthesis requires TDWB on the second day after surgery, with the patient gradually progressing to full weight-bearing by 3 weeks. An uncemented THR can begin with PWB, then the patient can progress to full weight-bearing up to 8 weeks after surgery.

The moderate-protection phase can begin when the patient has demonstrated improved quadriceps control, active knee flexion, reduced pain, compliance with all precautions and exercises, independent bed mobility and transfers, and improved gait (with necessary weight-bearing precautions). Moderate protection does not in any way imply reduced THR precautions. During this phase, more challenging exercises are added to more closely approximate functional activities. Light resistance exercises for quadriceps strengthening in a semirecumbent position and elastic tubing (Thera-band) can

also be used to strengthen the hamstrings and hip extensors in a semirecumbent or seat-elevated position (Fig. 14-10). Standing exercises stress active hip motion (straight-plane motions, no combined rotational forces, THR precautions strictly enforced) and strengthening.

To enhance aerobic fitness, a recumbent bucket-seat bicycle ergometer or an upper body ergometer (UBE) can be used. The addition of increases in weight-bearing is determined by component fixation, tissue healing constraints, and the wishes of the physician. Closed-chain functional activities begin between 3 and 8 weeks, postoperatively[4] for cemented prostheses, with increased weight-bearing orders by the physician. These activities can include sit-to-stand exercises with an elevated seat, partial supported knee bends (for concentric and eccentric quadriceps control), weight-shifting exercises, treadmill walking, mini step-ups, and standing resisted hip and knee extension (Fig. 14-11A,B). For an uncemented prosthesis, closed-chain functional activities are deferred for 2 or 3 weeks longer than with cemented prostheses. However, standing straight-plane resistance exercises (hip extension, hip adduction, abduction, and flexion) are allowed between 3 and 8 weeks postoperatively.

The minimal-protection phase of recovery is initiated between 12 and 16 weeks after surgery. Depending on individual cases, the physician may elect to discontinue THR precautions during this phase. A great deal of soft tissue and bone healing must take place and muscular strength must improve dynamic stability before THR precautions are relaxed.

The minimal-protection phase is classically characterized by a return to normalized gait patterns without assistive devices, and by instruction in balance, coordination, proprioception, and advanced closed-chain functional activities that duplicate the patient's specific ADLs. The majority of patients recover most of their hip

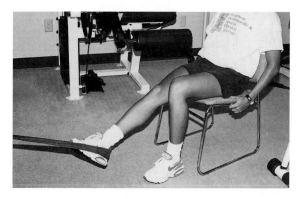

FIG. 14-10 Seated hamstring strengthening using elastic band.

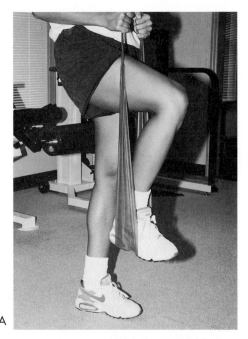 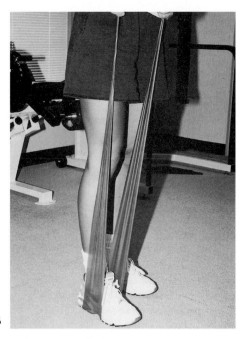

FIG. 14-11 Standing hip and knee extension press-down using elastic band. **A,** Starting position. **B,** Finish.

motion during the first year after surgery.[12] Therefore at this phase of recovery (approximately 4 months after surgery) the patient may still demonstrate decreased motion, but must be reassured that more time is needed before assessing the ultimate degree of hip motion attainable.

While addressing proprioception, coordination, and balance after either knee or hip replacement (single-leg standing, eyes open and eyes closed, single-leg standing on a mini-trampoline or balance board), the assistant must recognize that certain afferent neural input mechanoreceptors (type I—Ruffini; type II—pacinian; types III and IV—free nerve endings) will be lost because of the removal of the articulating joint surfaces. However, the joint capsule surrounding the joint replacement remains essentially intact and well supplied with mechanoreceptor feedback organs, which can be retrained and enhanced via appropriately applied weight shifting activities, balance board exercises, and closed-chain functional strengthening exercises.

LEGG-CALVÉ-PERTHES DISEASE

In 1910, three researchers identified a hip condition that usually affects children between the ages of 4 and 8 years[5] (according to LeVeau,[9] the range is 2 to 12 years

of age with the most common age being 6 years). This condition, which is referred to as **Legg-Calvé-Perthes (LCP) disease** or *coxa plana,* is characterized as a noninflammatory, self-limiting (can heal spontaneously with or without specific treatment) syndrome in which the femoral head becomes flattened at the weight-bearing surface[5] as a result of disruption of the blood supply (AVN) to the femoral head in the growing child.[5,9] The long-term complications of the flattened femoral head lead to an incongruous joint surface and advanced DJD (Fig. 14-12).[5,9,11]

Throughout the management of this disease, the primary focus is on maintaining the femoral head within the confines of the acetabulum, regaining motion, and reducing pain and dysfunction.[5,9,11] In the acute or maximum-protection phase, reducing pain and dysfunction is generally accomplished using physician-prescribed nonsteroidal antiinflammatory drugs (NSAIDs), bed rest, and traction to take the load off the hip and restore motion in abduction.

Keeping the femoral head seated within the acetabulum can be accomplished using an abduction orthosis (Fig. 14-13).[5,9] To aid healing and reduce unwanted stress on the affected hip, the abduction orthosis can be worn as long as 2 years.[9] During this time, the brace can be removed for short periods each day to exercise the

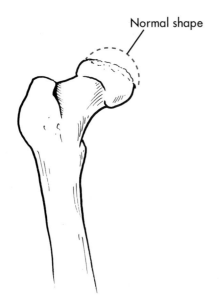

FIG. 14-12 Legg-Calvé-Perthes disease.

limb and attend to personal hygiene.[9] With the brace removed, the patient must maintain hip abduction during ROM exercises for the knee (flexion and extension), internal rotation of the hip, quadriceps strengthening, hip abduction, and hip extension strengthening exercises (gluteus medius and gluteus maximus).[9]

SOFT-TISSUE INJURIES OF THE HIP (BURSITIS, STRAINS, AND CONTUSIONS)

Trochanteric bursitis is a common soft tissue injury affecting the hip in an active population of patients. The greater trochanter of the femur is most commonly affected. The trochanteric bursa may become irritated and inflamed because of excessive compression and repeated friction as the iliotibial band snaps over the bursa while lying superior to the greater trochanter (Fig. 14-14).

Treatment for greater trochanteric bursitis is centered on relieving pain and inflammation while addressing the underlying cause of the condition. Rest, ice, and antiinflammatory medications are commonly used first to arrest the symptoms of pain and swelling. Any specific motions or activities (i.e., running) that may exacerbate the pain must be modified or eliminated. Typically, a program of stretching is essential to reduce the compression and friction from the iliotibial band (ITB) over the greater trochanter. After ice is applied directly over the affected hip, either standing or sidelying ITB stretches should be used slowly as long as the patient does not complain of pain. In addition, hamstring, quadriceps, and hip adductor stretching can be used as a total

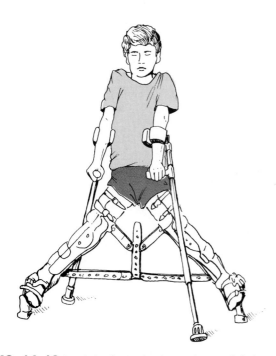

FIG. 14-13 An abduction orthosis can be used during the treatment of Legg-Calvé-Perthes disease to help maintain the femoral head seated within the acetabulum.

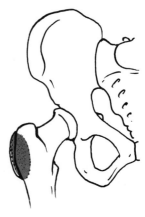

FIG. 14-14 Greater trochanteric bursitis.

program to improve hip flexibility in all planes and to maintain proper balance among these muscle groups.

A comprehensive program of care focuses on all aspects of the disorder. Strength must be addressed, taking care not to stress the affected hip and reproduce the symptoms of pain, swelling, and tightness of the lateral hip structures. Specific strengthening exercises include quadriceps strengthening, hamstring curls, hip adduction, hip extension exercises (partial squats, leg press), and hip abduction exercises. Aerobic fitness can be maintained using a stationary cycle, UBE, treadmill, or stair climber. In any case, the ROM must be modified to limit hip and knee motion and avoid repeated snapping of the ITB over the trochanter. Ultrasound and hydrotherapy may also be useful during the acute phase of recovery.

Two other areas of bursitis commonly affecting the hip are ischial bursitis and iliopectineal bursitis. *Ischial bursitis* (Fig. 14-15) is characterized by pain over the ischial tuberosity underlying the gluteus maximus. It can be caused by direct contusion of the ischial tuberosity or by extended periods of sitting.[5,15] Occasionally, this condition can mimic a hamstring strain at the origin of the muscle at the ischial tuberosity.[5,15] Management is similar to other forms of bursitis: rest from the aggravating activity, ice packs, NSAIDs, and a judiciously applied program of stretching exercises that do not aggravate the symptoms. Generally, hamstring stretches are encouraged along with quadriceps strengthening exercises. Occasionally, conservative care fails and the physician may elect to inject the area with corticosteroids.[5]

Iliopectinal bursitis is characterized by either local tenderness over the iliopsoas muscle and tendon or diffuse radiating pain into the anterior thigh (Fig. 14-16).[15]

Because the iliopectinal bursa lies deep to the tendon of the iliopsoas muscle, tightness of the iliopsoas alone and in conjunction with excessive hip extension can cause compression and frictional wear of the iliopectineal bursa. Specific care centers on reducing pain and irritation using a program of rest, ice, antiinflammatory medications, and physical therapy interventions such as thermal agents, stretching, and strengthening exercises.

Unfortunately, in some cases of iliopectinal bursitis, stretching the tight iliopsoas muscle group increases pain over the bursa. Stretching of the psoas muscle may need to be deferred in cases where pain is exacerbated by such activity. The use of ice, hydrotherapy, ultrasound, and physician-prescribed NSAIDs can minimize the pain and allow for the initiation of quadriceps strengthening exercises, hamstring stretches, ITB stretches, hip adductor stretches, and the beginning of an aerobic fitness program, as long as the symptoms do not increase. Once initial healing has occurred and the acute inflammatory process is arrested, specific stretching of the iliopsoas is indicated.

Most acute injuries affecting the hip are musculotendinous **strains** of the hamstrings, iliopsoas, adductors, and rectus femoris.[5,15] Injuries to the hamstrings at the origin (ischial tuberosity) can be caused by sudden, forceful contraction of the hamstrings or by decelerating the lower leg against the concentric contraction of the quadriceps during running as the hamstrings contract eccentrically (Fig. 14-17).

Initial injury management involves the application of cold packs for 20 minutes, 3 to 5 times daily. Wrapping the affected limb with a compression bandage can also help relieve stress on the limb. Motions that produce pain and interfere with the healing process should be

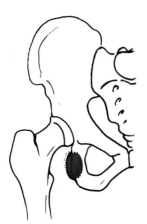

FIG. 14-15 Ischial bursitis.

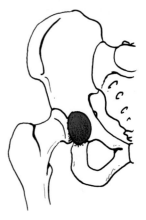

FIG. 14-16 Iliopectineal bursitis.

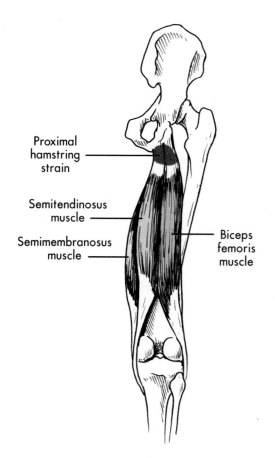

Proximal
hamstring
strain

Semitendinosus
muscle

Semimembranosus
muscle

Biceps
femoris
muscle

FIG. 14-17 Anatomy of posterior thigh musculature. Note proximal hamstring strain just inferior to the origin at the ischial tuberosity.

avoided. Two motions should not be attempted during the acute or maximal-protection phase of recovery: (1) full knee extension combined with forward trunk flexion and (2) full leg flexion.

The use of crutches may be indicated during this phase to limit stress on the hamstrings. The physical therapist assistant can significantly aid the patient in coping with a very difficult problem during the early recovery phase. Sleeping may be extraordinarily painful in some cases. The physical therapist assistant should counsel the patient to sleep supine with pillows under both knees to support the injured limb and to reduce passive nocturnal stretching by placing the hamstrings in a relaxed position. As pain and swelling are reduced, active knee extension and leg flexion are encouraged (if the patient remains pain free) to help influence the direction of immature collagen fibers (see Chapter 2, Stretching of Soft Tissue Contractures). The physical

therapist assistant must recall the intrinsic nature of muscle and tendon healing time constraints and avoid the temptation to encourage an aggressive stretching program for the hamstrings during the early maximum-protection phase of recovery. Sufficient time must be allowed for the torn tissue to scar and reorganize itself before subjecting the fragile immature collagen to excessive tensile loads that may impede healing. However, flexibility must certainly be addressed and will be the focus of long-term recovery during the moderate-protection and minimal-protection phases of recovery, as defined by the significance of the injury; the patient's ability to achieve improved motion; strength, and pain-free gait; the physician's wishes; and the physical therapist's direction.

Strength training proceeds according to the patient's individual situation and is strongly influenced by muscle and tendon healing constraints. Initially, isometric quadriceps sets and submaximal multiangle hamstring sets can be done as pain allows. Progressive strengthening can be achieved with prone manual resistive leg curls, ankle weights, or sitting Thera-band leg curls (this particular exercise strongly encourages slow eccentric hamstring muscle contractions). An excellent, dynamic, and fun exercise to perform is "scooting" with a rolling adjustable-height stool. This exercise encourages knee flexion against resistance at various controllable speeds. Supine hip bridges can be added as function increases.

An adductor muscle strain (usually the adductor longus) is termed a *groin pull*. A classic program of protection, ice, compression bandaging, the use of crutches, and protected weight-bearing during the acute or maximal-protection phase should be followed. As with other muscle and tendon strains, early aggressive stretching should be avoided. Once pain subsides, active hip flexion, gentle hip abduction and adduction motion, and knee ROM exercises should begin. Specific hip abduction stretching can be initiated, instructing the patient to perform the seated "butterfly" stretch, with a strong caution to proceed slowly without pain. Some authorities[5] suggest waiting 3 to 6 weeks before instructing the patient in progressive resistance exercises. However, resistance exercises can begin earlier depending on the severity of the strain. To specifically strengthen the hip adductors, submaximal isometrics (Fig. 14-18) can give way to proximally placed resistance in various positions (Fig. 14-19).

Progression to more dynamic strengthening exercises depends on the specific goals established by the patient and physical therapist. For example, in a young athletic population of patients eager to return to sports activities, a slide board can be an effective tool to introduce

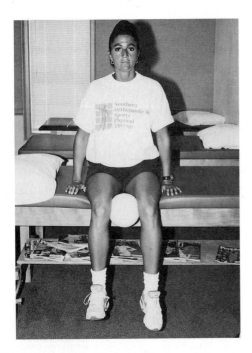

FIG. 14-18 Seated hip adduction isometrics.

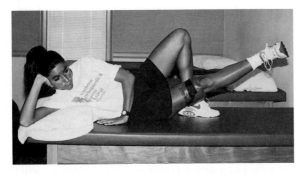

FIG. 14-19 Sidelying hip adduction concentric and eccentric contractions. Note the proximally-placed resistance.

dynamic hip adduction and abduction motions (Fig. 14-20).

An iliopsoas muscle strain is also referred to as a "hip flexor pull." This injury can occur from sudden, forceful extreme hip extension or by forced hip flexion against resistance.[15] A standard program of protection, rest, ice, and compression bandages with crutches and limited weight-bearing is encouraged in the acute phase. Sleeping comfort can be enhanced by sleeping supine with pillows under the knees to reduce hip extension. Gentle, active hip flexion and extension exercises are begun once the initial healing phase has ended and the

patient no longer complains of pain. A prolonged period of time may be needed to avoid hip extension (i.e., push-off during gait running or hip extension past neutral) and encourage healing. Gentle active stretching of the hip flexors can begin with the patient supine and the nonaffected knee and hip flexed. Additionally, a hurdler's stretch can be initiated once the patient demonstrates improved hip extension motion without pain. The physical therapist assistant should strongly encourage the patient to perform these stretches in a slow, static fashion without pain. Very close supervision is needed to guard against any ballistic, forceful, or violent motions that could impede healing and reinjure the affected limb.

The most common **contusion** affecting the hip and pelvis involves the subcutaneous tissues of the iliac crest and is commonly termed a *hip pointer.*[6] Typically, this injury can occur in one of two ways:

1. The iliac crest is contused by direct contact from an external force or by falling on the exposed iliac crest.
2. There is a sudden forceful contraction or overstretching of the muscles attached to the iliac crest.[6] This seemingly minor injury can be quite severe, causing extreme pain and dysfunction.

First, the patient is treated with protection, rest, ice, gentle compression wraps, crutches, and partial weight-bearing. Initial soft tissue healing must proceed without delay, so extreme caution is warranted to guard against unwanted forces or stress to the affected area. Stretching and strengthening of the affected hip commence once soft tissue healing has progressed and pain is controlled. Usually in the moderate-protection phase, ultrasound, hydrotherapy, electrical stimulation, phonophoresis, or iontophoresis can be used at the discretion of the physician and physical therapist to help control pain and swelling.

FRACTURES OF THE PELVIS AND ACETABULUM

General principles dealing with pelvic fractures and their classification with acetabular fractures dramatically show the physical therapist assistant the extensive and potentially life-threatening nature of these injuries.[5,13,14] This discussion will outline the profound complications that may occur with pelvic fractures, giving the physical therapist assistant a better understanding of the long-term rehabilitation needed in many cases of severe fractures.

The most basic classification of pelvic fractures refers to the injury as either stable or unstable.[5,13,14] *Stable fractures* include avulsion-type fractures of the anterior superior iliac spine, the anterior inferior iliac

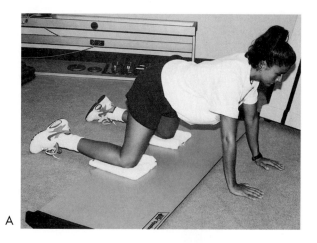

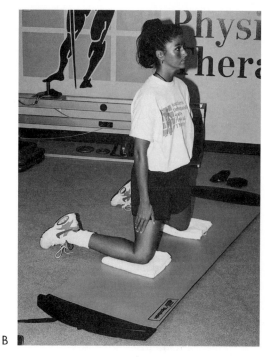

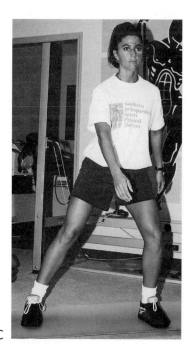

FIG. 14-20 Progressive slide board activities for dynamic closed-chain hip abduction and adduction. The series of exercises are begun **A,** On hands and knees for support; the patient then slowly abducts and adducts both hips, **B,** Kneeling position is slightly more challenging, and **C,** Standing position.

spine, the ischial tuberosity, and the iliac crest (Fig. 14-21).[5,13] Avulsion fractures of the pelvis can be treated conservatively with rest, protected weight-bearing, crutches, and avoidance of premature stretching and resistive exercises, which may delay bony union (usually within 6 weeks).[5]

McRae[13] advocates an ORIF procedure with avulsion fractures of the ischial tuberosity and fragment separation greater than 2 cm by saying: "Non-union is an appreciable risk, and if this occurs there may be problems with chronic pain and disability."[13] Usually avulsion fractures of the ischial tuberosity can be treated with rest, keeping the hip extended and externally rotated to avoid continued stress on the healing bone, and enforcing protected weight-bearing for approximately 6 weeks.[5] Once secure bone healing has been established, the physical therapist may direct the assistant to carry out a gentle, progressive flexibility program

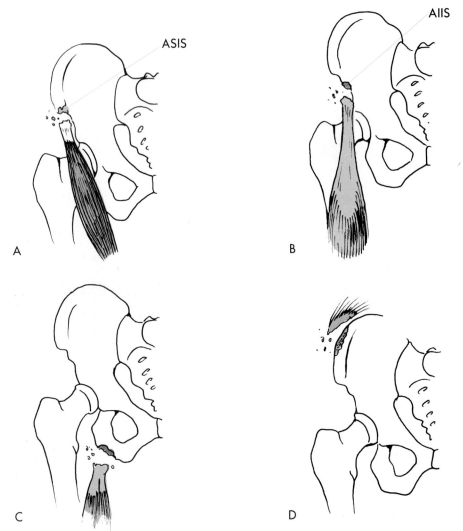

FIG. 14-21 A, Avulsion fracture ASIS. **B,** Avulsion fracture AIIS. **C,** Avulsion fracture ischial tuberosity. **D,** Avulsion fracture iliac crest.

to regain hip flexion. Strengthening exercises are added when the physician confirms radiographic evidence of secure union of the avulsion.

Other stable pelvic fractures include fractures of the superior pubic ramus, the superior and inferior pubic rami on one side, and the ilium (Fig. 14-22).[13] In general, stable fractures of the pelvis are treated nonsurgically with protection, bed rest (2 to 3 weeks),[13] and progressive motion and exercise once stable bone union has been confirmed.

Unstable pelvic fractures can usually be defined as either rotationally unstable but vertically stable, or rotationally and vertically unstable.[13] These severe injuries

can be treated with an external fixator, ORIF procedure, or extended convalescence involving bed rest.[5,13,14] The physical therapist assistant must be aware of complications after unstable pelvic fractures that can influence the time to begin rehabilitation procedures and can require protracted periods of recovery before physical therapy interventions. Box 14-1 outlines complications associated with these potentially life-threatening injuries.

The rehabilitation program employed after pelvic fractures is individualized and specific to the type and severity of fracture as well as the methods used to stabilize the fracture (ORIF, external fixator, long-term

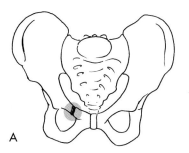 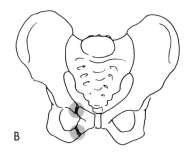 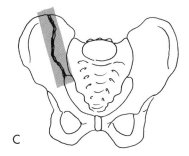

FIG. 14-22 A, Fracture of superior pubic ramus. **B,** Fracture of superior and inferior pubic ramus on one side. **C,** Fracture of the ilium.

BOX 14-1	Complications Following Pelvic Fractures

a. Hemorrhage (significant blood loss, shock)
b. Gastrointestinal injury
c. Diaphragm rupture
d. Bony malunion (limb length shortening)
e. Nonunion
f. Neurological damage
g. Degenerative joint disease (DJD)
h. Infection (sepsis)

From Miller M: Adult reconstruction and sports medicine. In: *Review of orthopaedics,* Philadelphia, 1992, WB Saunders.
From McRae R: *Practical fracture treatment,* ed 3, New York, 1994, Churchhill Livingstone.

---

convalescence). Because of the fragile hemodynamic nature of significant pelvic fractures, weight-bearing of any kind is deferred for 8 weeks or longer.[13]

Initially, the patient may be introduced to the vertical position using a tilt table. Pulse, respiration, and blood pressure are carefully monitored by the physical therapist assistant as directed by the physical therapist. Postural hypotension can be adequately addressed by gradually increasing the duration of elevation by small increments under the physical therapist's direction. Maintenance of joint mobility is addressed early after surgery and during long periods of immobilization.

Active bilateral upper-extremity ROM begins as soon as the patient's condition is stable. Lower-extremity motion is limited to bilateral ankle pumps, gentle knee motion, and limited hip motion, depending on the nature of the fracture, fixation techniques used, stabilization of

visceral damage (if any), and direction of the physician and physical therapist. By far, the most significant clinical features associated with pelvic fractures are the potentially life-threatening complications, which can be acute or arise during early recovery or just after the acute phase of the injury. The physical therapist assistant must closely supervise all vital signs before, during, and after all rehabilitation procedures. Once the physician has determined that the fracture site is stable and healed and the patient is medically stable, the physical therapist may direct the physical therapist assistant to follow a gradual program of general strength and fitness (a high priority with all patients requiring protracted periods of immobilization), quadriceps strengthening, hip motion, gait training, bed mobility, and transfer training.

The physical therapist assistant must be aware that fractures of the pelvis can also involve the acetabulum. The acetabulum has an articular cartilage surface that allows for articulation between the femoral head and acetabulum. Care of this area is extremely important because the hip joint is a major weight-bearing structure.

The classification system used to identify specific patterns of acetabular fractures is defined by Loth[10] as the Letornel classification model (Fig. 14-23). Generally, these fractures are treated according to the severity of the fracture, usually with an ORIF procedure or, conservatively, with bed rest and traction to reduce compression of the joint.[13] Conservative management of acetabular fractures is reserved for severely fragmented acetabular floor fractures in which surgery cannot realign the fragments to anatomically reconstruct the articular surface.[13] In all other cases, an ORIF procedure is used to stabilize the fracture.[10]

Protected weight-bearing is encouraged for 8 to 10 weeks; in cases of nonsurgical management, weight-bearing is permitted at 9 weeks. A lower-extremity

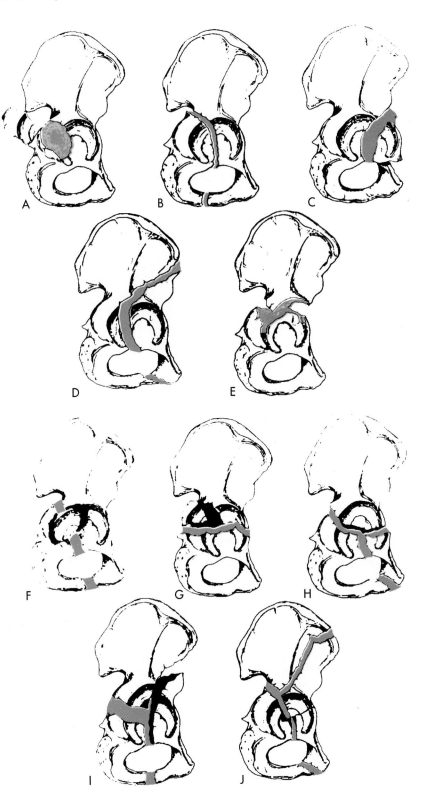

FIG. 14-23 Letornel classification of acetabular fractures. Simple: **A,** Posterior wall. **B,** Posterior column. **C,** Anterior wall. **D,** Anterior column. **E,** Transverse. Combined: **F,** Posterior column and post wall. **G,** Transverse and posterior wall. **H,** T fracture. **I,** Anterior column and posterior hemitransverse. **J,** Both columns. (From Loth: *Orthopaedic boards review,* St. Louis, 1993, Mosby).

strength program is initiated immediately after surgery and involves ankle motion, quadriceps sets, hamstring sets, gentle submaximal gluteal sets, and active knee and hip motion. As with all fractures, as bone healing progresses and the patient achieves individualized criteria (such as strength, motion, reduced pain, minimal swelling, increased weight-bearing, normalized gait), the rehabilitation program can be advanced, gradually incorporating more challenging functional exercises.

The physical therapist assistant must remember the nature of specific acetabular fractures, since these fractures involve articular cartilage as well as bone. Therefore the initiation of closed-chain functional activities, which naturally require vertical loads, may be deferred for longer periods to allow for appropriate articular cartilage healing. If premature loads are directed through the weight-bearing surface of the affected articular cartilage of the acetabulum, delayed union may result.

COMMON MOBILIZATION TECHNIQUES FOR THE HIP

Reduced motion secondary to pain and fibrosis after fractures, soft tissue injuries, and various hip arthroplasty techniques may warrant mobilization in conjunction with thermal agents, strengthening, stretching, and functional activities. The techniques presented here are identified by the physical therapist as appropriate techniques to use, based on pathology, the presence of pain, and/or defined limitations of movement. As with all mobilization techniques, the physical therapist selects which techniques to use and the direction of force, amplitude, grades, velocity, and distractions (see Chapter 11, Basics of Clinical Application of Joint Mobilization and Chapter 12, Common Mobilization Techniques for the Ankle, Foot, and Toe).

Most importantly, patient comfort and compliance with relaxation before and throughout the treatment are of paramount concern. Before each treatment session, the patient should be placed in the most comfortable position with attention paid to supporting the affected limb. The application of thermal agents (hot packs, ultrasound) to the affected limb and surrounding structures may be helpful to compose and relax the patient before treatment. If the patient has physician-prescribed pain medications and/or muscle relaxants, it may be helpful to consult with the physical therapist to suggest that the patient take these medications in a timely fashion before treatment to further enhance relaxation.

Long Axis Distraction

With the patient supine, place the affected limb in various degrees of abduction, depending on the specific

limitation of movement and the defined goals of the physical therapist. Place hands securely around the dorsum of the affected limb and the calcaneus. The knee of the affected limb should be flexed or held straight. The direction of applied force will be in a caudal direction, following the long axis of the femur (Fig. 14-24). The result is distraction of the head of the femur away from the acetabulum.

Lateral Distraction of the Hip

The patient is supine with the hip and knee of the affected limb flexed approximately 90 degrees.[1] Stand on the lateral aspect of the affected limb. Carefully support the affected limb against your chest. Place both hands around the proximal femur while applying a laterally directed force (Fig. 14-25).

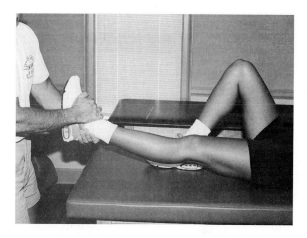

FIG. 14-24 Long-axis distraction of the hip.

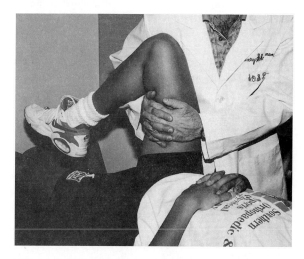

FIG. 14-25 Lateral hip distraction.

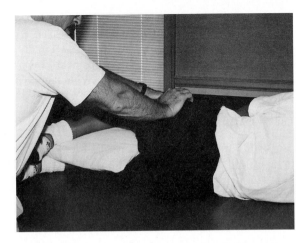

FIG. 14-26 Sidelying anterior-posterior (A-P) mobilization of the hip.

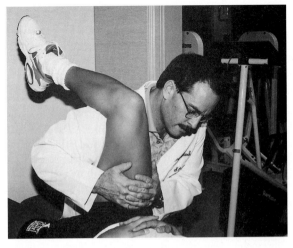

FIG. 14-27 Inferior glide of the hip.

Anterior and Posterior Mobilization

The patient is in a sidelying position on the unaffected side. The hips and knees are flexed with a pillow between the legs, supporting the thigh, knee, and lower leg. Stand in front of or behind the patient. Use both hands to firmly grasp the greater trochanter. In this position, apply an anteriorly and posteriorly directed force,[1] effectively translating the head of the femur away from the acetabulum (Fig. 14-26). Make certain that the force is applied directly anteriorly and posteriorly. If performed casually, the femur will be internally and externally rotated instead of appropriately translated forward and backward.

Inferior Glide of the Hip

The patient is supine with the affected hip flexed approximately 90 degrees. Place the knee of the affected limb over your shoulder. With both hands (in an open palm position), grasp the proximal femur and apply a "pulling" or "scooping" directed force. The head of the femur is glided from the acetabulum inferiorly (Fig. 14-27).

REFERENCES

1. Corrigan B, Maitland GD: The hip. In *Practical orthopaedic medicine,* Newton, Mass., 1992, Butterworth-Heinemann.
2. Cummings S, Nevitt M: A hypothesis: the cause of hip fractures, *J Gerontal Med Sci* 44(4):107-111, 1989.
3. Goldstein TS; Treatment of common problems of the hip joint. In Goldstein TS, Lewis CB, series editors: *Geriartric orthopaedics rehabilitative management of common problems,* Gaithersburg, Md., 1991, Aspen Publishers.
4. Goldstein TS: The adult and geriatric hip, continuing education course notes, 1994, Quest Seminars.
5. Gross ML, Nasser S, Finnerman GAM: Hip and pelvis. In DeLee JC, Drez D, editors: *Orthopaedic sports medicine: Principles and practice,* vol. 2, Philadelphia, 1994, WB Saunders.
6. Henry JH: The hip. In Scott WN, Nisonson B, Nicholas JA, editors: *Principles of sports medicine,* Baltimore, 1984, Williams & Wilkins.
7. Kozinn SC, Wilson PD: *Adult hip disease and total hip replacement,* Clinical symposia, 1987, Ciba-Geigy.
8. Lewis CB, Bottomley JM: Orthopaedic treatment considerations. In *Geriatric physical therapy: a clinical approach,* New York, 1994, Appleton & Lange.
9. LeVeau B: Hip. In Richardson JK, Iglarsh JK, editors: *Clinical orthopaedic physical therapy,* Philadelphia, 1994, WB Saunders.
10. Loth TS: Lower extremity. In *Orthopaedic boards review,* St. Louis, 1993, Mosby.
11. MacEwen GD, Bunnell WP, Ramsey PL: The hip. In Lovell WW, Winter RB, editors: *Pediatric orthopaedics,* Philadelphia, 1986, JB Lippincott.
12. McDonald D et al: Total joint reconstruction. In *Orthopedic boards review,* St. Louis, 1993, Mosby.
13. McRae R: *Practical fracture treatment,* ed 3, New York, 1994, Churchill-Livingstone.
14. Miller M: Adult reconstruction and sports medicine. In *Review of orthopaedics,* Philadelphia, 1992, WB Saunders.
15. Saudek CE: The hip. In Gould JA, editor: *Orthopaedic and sports physical therapy,* ed 2, St. Louis, 1990, Mosby.

Orthopedic Management of the Lumbar, Thoracic, and Cervical Spine

LEARNING OBJECTIVES

1. Outline and describe basic mechanics of the lumbar spine.
2. Discuss and apply the principles of fundamental mechanics of lifting.
3. Identify common sprains and strains of the lumbar spine.
4. Discuss common methods of management and rehabilitation of lumbar spine sprains and strains.
5. Identify and describe injuries to the lumbar intervertebral disc.
6. Discuss methods of management and rehabilitation for injuries to the lumbar intervertebral disc.
7. Define and describe methods of quantifying back strength.
8. Define and describe components of the back school model.
9. Define ergonomic and functional capacity evaluations.
10. Define spinal stenosis and describe methods of management and rehabilitation.
11. Define and contrast the terms *spondylolysis* and *spondylolisthesis.*
12. Describe methods of management and rehabilitation for spondylolysis and spondylolisthesis.
13. Identify common lumbar and thoracic spine fractures.
14. Define kyphosis, lordosis, and scoliosis.
15. Identify and describe methods of management and rehabilitation for kyphosis and scoliosis.
16. Identify and describe common cervical spine injuries and discuss methods of management and rehabilitation.

KEY TERMS

Disc
Annulus
Nucleus pulposus
Prone extension
Spine stabilization
Herniated nucleus
  pulposus (HNP)
Disc protrusion
Extruded disc
Sequestrated disc
Radicular signs
Peripherilization
Centralization
Spinal stenosis
Spondylolysis
Spondylolisthesis
"Back schools"
Ergonomics
Functional capacity
  evaluations (FCEs)
Kyphosis
Scoliosis
Cervical spondylosis
Thoracic outlet (inlet)
  syndrome

CHAPTER OUTLINE

In this chapter the physical therapist assistant is introduced to injuries that affect the spine. Common soft tissue injuries (muscle, ligament, disc) and fractures of the lumbar, thoracic, and cervical spine are listed, with specific therapeutic interventions, back testing procedures, functional (or physical) capacity evaluations, and injury prevention techniques (patient education through back school training).

THE LUMBAR SPINE

Perhaps no other medical condition draws as much attention from researchers and clinicians as the identification, treatment, and rehabilitation of lumbar spine injuries. The estimated aggregate financial burden to the United States economy ranges from 7.2 billion[1] to more than 40 billion[12] and as high as nearly 100 billion dollars[32] annually for the care of low back–related problems. Lumbar spine injuries also account for literally millions of lost work days per year in the United States and England.[14,32] The rate of disability from injuries to the low back was estimated over a 10-year period to be a staggering 14 times greater than the rate of population growth for that same period.[1,7] Overall, lumbar spine injuries are the second leading cause of all physician visits in the United States.[1]

Some studies suggest that nonspecific low back dysfunction may affect 80% of the adult population in the United States at some point in their lives.[33] While acute management and criteria-based rehabilitation programs for low back dysfunction can prove effective, some authorities point out that over half of the patients with back pain recover in 1 week and 90% improve within 1 to 3 months from the onset of injury.[27]

Currently there is no universally accepted philosophic agreement regarding the most efficient, effective, and economical method for treating low-back dysfunction. Historically, absolute bed rest, medications, thermal agents (hot packs, ultrasound), and a series of rudimentary lumbar flexion exercises (pelvic tilts, single knee-to-chest, double knee-to-chest, partial direct and oblique sit-ups) were the components of a typical protocol for lumbar sprains, strains, and disc-related pathologic conditions (Fig. 15-1). However, with sophisticated long-term studies and the development of advanced evaluation technology (computed tomography [CT], magnetic resonance imaging [MRI]), improved understanding of the mechanics of the lumbar spine has led to significant advances in the care of soft tissue and bony injuries to this area.

Basic Mechanics

Understanding the principles of intradiscal pressure and fluid mechanics related to motion of the disc helps to clarify the rationale for using specific therapeutic measures for individual low back conditions.

The lumbar spine is composed of five anterior convex segments and posterior concave segments that produce the recognizable lordotic curve. Between each vertebral body lies a **disc** (Fig. 15-2). The outer wall of the disc is called the **annulus** and comprises 12 to 18 concentrically arranged rings of fibroelastic cartilage.[14,30] Contained within the annulus is the **nucleus pulposus.** Nuclear material is a mucopolysaccharide gel[14] that transmits forces, equalizes stress, and promotes movement.[29] As well as containing the nucleus, the annulus provides stability, enhanced movement between vertebral bodies, and shock absorption.[29] The disc provides stability between the vertebral bodies, permits movement within each vertebral segment, and transmits motion.[30] The disc is an avascular and aneural[25] (although the outer fibers of the annulus are innervated)[14] structure that obtains nutrition by diffusion from the vascular supply of the vertebral bodies.[7,14,25,30]

Allman[1] describes lumbar motion and postural alterations as producing significant pressure within the disc (intradiscal pressure). The compressive forces that influence intradiscal pressure are as follows:[1]

- *Standing:* Disc pressure is equal to 100% of body weight
- *Supine:* Disc pressure is less than 25% of body weight
- *Side-lying:* Disc pressure is less than 75% of body weight
- *Standing and bending forward:* Disc pressure is approximately 150% of body weight
- *Supine with both knees flexed:* Disc pressure is less than 35% of body weight
- *Seated in a flexed position:* Disc pressure is approximately 85% of body weight
- *Bending forward in a flexed posture and lifting:* Disc pressure is approaching 275% of body weight

Intradiscal pressure can also be expressed in terms of pressure or load measured within the intervertebral lumbar disc. Cailliet[4] reports that isometric abdominal sets produce approximately 110 kg of pressure within the disc, while walking produces 85 kg, sitting 100 kg, bilateral straight-leg raises in supine position 120 kg, and lifting with a flexed torso and knees held straight an astounding 340 kg of intradiscal pressure. This information may help clarify the rationale for protective postures, lifting protocols, and appropriate body mechanics, as well as prescribed exercises for specific lumbar spine conditions.

The fluid mechanics of the disc (nucleus pulposus) itself are also strongly influenced by the motion of the lumbar vetebral segments. McKenzie[25] describes flexion

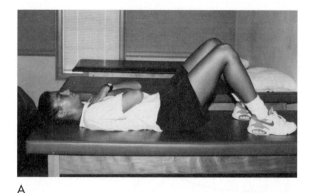

A

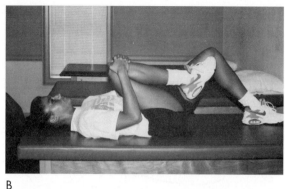

B

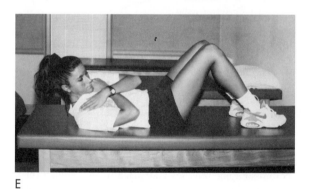

C

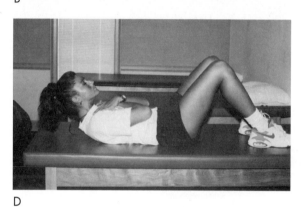

D

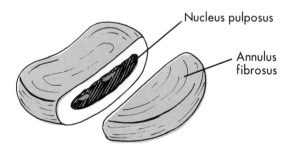

E

FIG. 15-1 Williams flexion exercises. **A,** Pelvic tilt, **B,** Single knee to chest, **C,** Double knee to chest, **D,** Partial direct sit-ups, **E,** Partial oblique sit-ups.

Nucleus pulposus

Annulus fibrosus

FIG. 15-2 Intervertebral disc.

and extension motion of the spine as having clinically significant effects on the nucleus' direction of movement. When positional changes occur in the lumbar spine, from flexion to extension, the nucleus moves anteriorly (Fig. 15-3).[25] Conversely, when the spine moves from extension to full flexion, the nucleus tends to displace or move posteriorly (Fig. 15-4). Thus it is necessary to fully understand the individual nature of each injury and to avoid or enhance certain motions and postures as directed by the physical therapist.

It is important to confirm or deny positive sciatic and femoral nerve-root tension signs seen during the initial

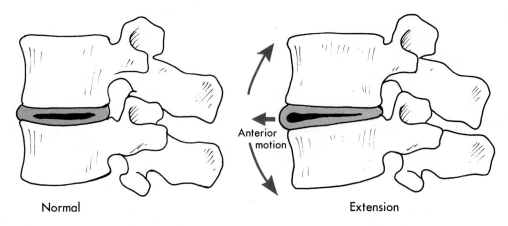

FIG. 15-3 Movement of the spine from a position of flexion into extension causes the nucleus to move in an anterior direction.

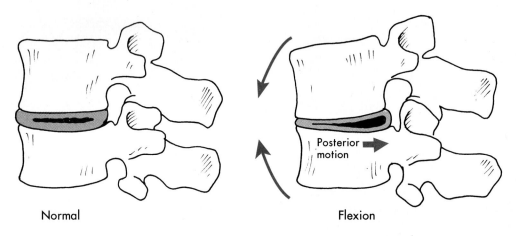

FIG. 15-4 Movement of the spine from a position of extension into flexion causes the nucleus to move in a posterior direction.

evaluation performed by the physical therapist.[37] Pain that radiates into one or both lower extremities early in the initial evaluation could signify nerve root compression from an adjacent herniated intervertebral disc. A sensitive test for nerve root compression requires the patient to be supine while one leg is raised passively with the knee completely extended (straight-leg test). The opposite leg is tested in the same manner. The test is considered positive only if radicular pain is increased,[11] which indicates stretching of the sciatic nerve. Anterior radiating thigh pain can be evaluated by the physical therapist as follows: Have the patient assume the prone position with one knee flexed to 90 degrees. Then passively extend the hip and document any increase in radiating anterior thigh pain.[11] This test (the femoral nerve tension sign) is not considered positive if back pain occurs.

Gould[14] suggests that muscle spasm in the thoracolumbar spine muscles may actually be a compartment syndrome in which swelling accumulates (after injury) within the defined series of compartments formed by the fascia and muscles of the spine. This occurs as the spine is straightened and the lordotic curve reduced.

Fundamental Mechanics of Lifting

Forces and stresses related to lifting, sitting, standing, walking, sleeping, and twisting are common to all activities of daily living (ADL). O'Sullivan, Ellis, and Makofsky[28] have identified a novel concept to instruct patients in proper lifting mechanics, listing the "five L's" of lifting: load, lever, lordosis, legs, and lungs.

The *load* to be lifted is central to all concepts of lifting mechanics. The amount of weight to be hoisted

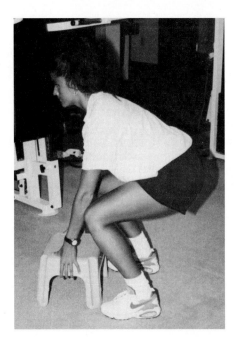

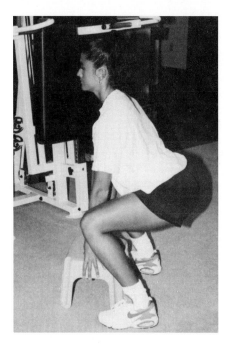

FIG. 15-5 In a flat back lifting position, the abdominals are shortened, lumbar paravertebral muscles show little or no EMG activity, the posterior ligaments are stretched, the nucleus is forced posteriorly, and the center of gravity is posterior to the base of support.

FIG. 15-6 Maintenance of lumbar lordosis during the lift. In this position the abdominals are in normal anatomical length, lumbar paravertebral muscles are contracted, posterior ligaments are relaxed, posterior annular wall is protected, nucleus is in a normal position, and the patient's center of gravity is over the base of support.

should be appropriate for the task and for the individual attempting to lift it. The *lever* refers to keeping the object as close to the body as is functionally possible throughout the lift. If the object is held away from the body, the increased force (both intradiscal pressure and muscle strain) may strain the lumbar spine. *Lordosis* refers to maintaining a normal anatomic lordotic curve while lifting any object. Teaching the patient (and the assistant) to lift with the *legs* is basic to all lifting procedures. The muscles of the legs should be conditioned to fully participate during the lifting of any object from the floor. If the legs are not used fully, the muscles of the back may be required to absorb increased stress. The *lungs* refer to the use of proper breathing techniques during lifting. The Valsalva maneuver (closed glottis during attempted expiration) should be avoided and instruction given on exhaling during the actual lift.

Kaiser, Rose, and Apts[20] have identified a lumbar stabilization model comparing two lumbar spine postures during lifting. In the first posture (tested electromyographically) the starting position is characterized by a posterior pelvic tilt. The abdominal muscles are in a shortened position, the lumbar paravertebral muscles show no electromyographic activity, the posterior ligaments and posterior annular wall are stretched, the

nucleus is forced posteriorly, the knees are in a position of decreased leverage, and the patient's center of gravity is posterior to the base of support.[20] In the second posture, the patient's lumbar lordosis is maintained during the lift. The abdominal muscles are in their normal anatomic length, the paravertebral muscles contracted, the posterior ligaments relaxed, the posterior annular wall protected, the nucleus in a "normal" position, the knees in an optimal leverage position, and the patient's center of gravity over the base of support. Figures 15-5 and 15-6 graphically describe these two contrasting lifting postures.

Quantifying Back Strength

Beginning with the initial evaluation process and continuing throughout rehabilitation and discharge from formal physical therapy, quantifying back function is paramount for developing an individualized recovery program. Usually the physical therapist directs the assistant to help in patient set-up, testing procedures, and data accumulation (the physical therapist is responsible for all data evaluation and interpretation) using various commercially available testing devices.

At present, there is great controversy concerning the most efficient, effective, meaningful, and economical method of isolating and quantifying lumbar strength. Tan[35] outlines and describes common lumbar testing devices, as follows:

- Isometric (cable tensiometers, strain gauge, Med-X lumbar extension)
- Isokinetic (Cybex, Lido, Kin-Com, Biodex)
- Isoinertial (Isotechnologies Isostation B-200)

Although isometric exercise in general provides appropriate stress as well as morphologic and functional changes in skeletal muscle, the advantages of isometric strengthening have been identified as follows:[6]

- Increases muscle strength
- Is position dependent, with strength gains (isometrically) that are joint-angle specific
- Reduces muscle atrophy
- Produces muscle hypertrophy

The negative aspects of isometric training are as follows:[6]

- Fatigues muscles rapidly
- Can profoundly increase blood pressure, heart rate, and cardiac output
- The hypertensive response can lead to a marked increase in left ventricular wall stress

Based on this information, isometric lumbar extension strength testing must be highly selective and must be applied to patients who can tolerate these activities. The advantages are simplicity of application and "ease of interpretation."[35] Some authorities point out that there are clinically significant strength gains realized by isolating, training, and testing lumbar extension.[12] Fulton[12] reports that "lumbar muscles will respond only to specific, isolated exercise ... with specific exercise, increases in strength of the lumbar muscles of more than 100% are below average, increases of several hundred percent are common, and increases of several thousand percent are not rare." Isometric testing may appear very attractive if the single, primary cause of dysfunction is muscle weakness. The fundamental disadvantage is the "poor correlation with real life dynamic activities."[35] The physician and physical therapist will determine if isometric strength testing is a safe and appropriate means of quantifying back strength for a particular patient.

Isokinetic training and testing have been validated by a select group of orthopedic surgeons[6] as (1) efficient to develop strength in a normal individual, (2) allowing for exercise throughout a velocity spectrum, (3) producing strength gains at high speeds that carry over to slower speeds, and (4) able to document and reproduce performance testing. However, Tan[35] suggests that there are inherent limitations with isokinetic lumbar strength testing, primarily that isokinetics "does not simulate real life because we do not move at constant velocity."

The only currently available isoinertial (defined by Tan[35] as a muscle exertion on a constant inertial mass) testing device is the Isostation B-200.* This device is a three-axis dynamometer that measures motion, velocity, and torque simultaneously in three planes.[33] Tan[35] suggests that isoinertial back testing may more closely duplicate functional real-life activities in which the load lifted remains constant.

Regardless of which type of device is available (isometric, isokinetic, isoinertial), the physician and physical therapist must identify specific patient candidates who are appropriate for testing. Not all patients should be tested isometrically, nor do all spinal dysfunction pathologies require isolated lumbar extension strength testing. The criteria for using the various lumbar spine testing procedures have been identified as follows:[35]

1. Clinical use (objective findings, measure groups, reinforcement)
2. Medicolegal use (identify maximum effort, consisting of effort, documentation, and assessment of physical impairment)
3. Occupational use (ergonomic and rehabilitation guidelines, job screening, work site evaluations)
4. Research use (standardization)

The physical therapist assistant must become familiar with a wide variety of testing implements as well as indications (objective documentation of strength, ROM, local muscle endurance, fatigue resistance) and contraindications (acute injury, unstable fractures, spondylolisthesis, sequestrated nucleus pulposus) for static (isometric) or dynamic (isokinetic, isoinertial) lumbar extension strength testing.

Muscle Strains

Injury to the muscles of the lumbar spine can be caused by sudden, violent contraction (as in attempting to lift a heavy object), rapid stretching, combined lumbar extension and rotation (torque), eccentric loading, and repetitive overuse resulting in microscopic damage to the muscle. Although some authorities[12] point out that most low-back–related dysfunction results from soft tissue injury, many other structures are involved with back pain (ligaments, disc, nerve tissue, bone) and many other causes of nonspecific lumbar spine dysfunction are possible. The function of the lumbar spine muscles contributes to dynamic stability.[29] Panjabi and coworkers[29] have identified the need for specific low back strengthening to reduce injury and "to stabilize the spine within its normal physiologic motions."

---

*Isotechnologies, Hillsborough, NC.

Muscle strains of the lumbar spine are exceedingly common and treatment goals are as follows:[37] reduce or eliminate inflammation (pain, swelling), restore muscle strength, restore flexibility, enhance aerobic fitness (weight management), restore function, and protect the affected area from further injury through education and supervised practice of proper lifting mechanics.

In general, the initial care of muscle strains focuses on the control of pain and swelling. In addition to any physician-prescribed medications (nonsteroidal anti-inflammatory drugs [NSAIDs], analgesics, muscle relaxants), the physical therapist can employ a wide range of agents to reduce pain and swelling. Therapeutic heat, cold (cryotherapy), electrical stimulation, pharmacophoresis (iontophoresis and phonophoresis), and massage are common agents used to control symptoms of inflammation after soft tissue injury.[31] The affected area must also be protected from unwanted stresses. Through a detailed and comprehensive evaluation, the physical therapist identifies the most comfortable resting position for the patient and attempts to place the affected muscles in this shortened position.

Submaximal isometric exercises are generally well-tolerated once the acute phase of healing has ended. The physical therapist assistant may instruct the patient to perform gluteal sets (possibly while pain control modalities are applied), quadriceps sets, hamstring sets, and abdominal sets. The quality (intensity) of the muscle contraction is increased as the patient develops tolerance. The use of gentle lumbar stretching exercises must be approached cautiously. Although improved low back flexibility may be indicated after muscle strains, if stretching is attempted too soon, initial healing and scarring of the muscle may be delayed. Gentle low back stretching can usually proceed once the patient can tolerate increased intensity isometric exercises. With the patient supine, single knee-to-chest and double knee-to-chest motions can be performed. Pelvic tilt exercises are considered appropriate early motion, stretching (lower back), and strengthening (isometric abdominal set with simultaneous gluteal set) exercises.

Prone extension exercises are added once the patient can perform pain-free isometric exercises and flexibility exercises, and once the acute phase has been achieved. The progression of prone extension exercises can be viewed in three phases or positions. Prone lumbar extension necessarily involves thoracic extension and scapular retraction. By strengthening the lumbar extensors (thoracic and scapular muscles as well) with prone active extension exercises, functional strength is restored to the affected muscle groups.

The first position of prone lumbar extension requires the patient to be prone with the arms resting at the sides

of the body. The head and neck must be maintained in a midline position to reduce the risk of torquing the cervical spine. In addition, some therapists advocate the use of an abdominal bolster or support when the patient is in a prone position. This issue depends largely on the specific nature of the injury, the comfort of the patient, and the wishes of the physical therapist. In the figures in this chapter, an abdominal bolster is used. Lumbar extension exercises in the first position (with arms at the sides) involve limited pain-free extension with an emphasis on slow, controlled motion, both concentrically and eccentrically (Fig. 15-7). As the patient's condition improves, greater motion is allowed.

The second position increases the intensity of effort for the back extensors. While the patient is prone, his or her hands are placed palm open on the back of the head. The patient must not push the hands hard on the back of the head but rather let the open hands gently rest on the head. Again, the back is extended while pulling the scapulae together (retraction). Nonballistic, controlled concentric and eccentric motions are encouraged (Fig. 15-8).

The third position involves even greater intensity than the second. The patient extends both arms overhead (elbows straight) while extending the trunk in a prone position (Fig. 15-9).

Although this series of prone extension exercises is employed safely to strengthen lumbar and thoracic extension, other, more demanding exercises can be used judiciously if the patient is an active athlete. For example, prone bilateral leg lifts can be incorporated at the discretion of the physical therapist to further strengthen the low back, gluteals, and hamstrings. Initially, the patient is prone with the arms and trunk stabilized. First, he or she

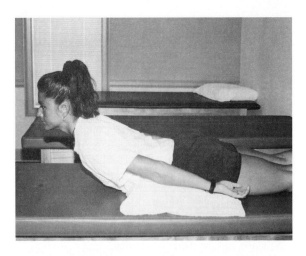

FIG. 15-7 Prone lumbar and thoracic extension with arms at the sides.

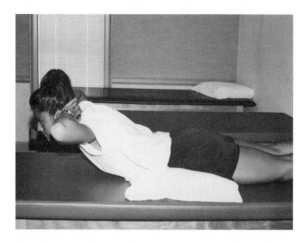

FIG. 15-8 Lumbar and thoracic extension with hands behind the head. In this position the lever arm is extended, requiring greater strength of the lumbar paravertebral muscles and scapular adductors to lift the trunk.

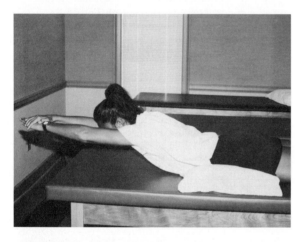

FIG. 15-9 Prone lumbar and thoracic extension in the arms extended position.

performs a single-leg lift, alternating between legs. Then the patient performs bilateral elevation of the legs throughout a pain-free ROM. Finally, the legs are lifted from a flexed knee position up to a neutral position.

A strong word of caution: Other symptoms may develop during the treatment of muscle strains. For example, if a patient complains of radicular pain into one or both lower extremities during or after the performance of any trunk flexion exercise (recall that trunk flexion produces posterior movement of the nucleus that can involve nerve root irritation), the exercise must be terminated and the therapist notified.

Generally, local muscle soreness[11] and postexercise stiffness are anticipated consequences and the patient

must be reassured that these are normal. However, burning, numbness, tingling, and radiating pain are not normal responses and must be recognized early.

A general conditioning program should be encouraged as soon as possible after the acute phase of muscle strain has passed. Addressing functional gait mechanics early in the recovery phase, by advocating walking as both exercise and treatment, is highly effective.[10] As articulated by Edgelow,[10] walking has a rather broad impact on recovery from low back dysfunction. Walking:[10]

- Stimulates circulation
- Enhances cardiovascular and cardiorespiratory fitness
- Stimulates the mechanoreceptor system
- Improves the coordination and strength of the muscles needed to control the movement of the mobile segment

All this is accomplished through the reciprocal contraction and relaxation of muscles engaged in walking.[10] Walking can be initiated on a treadmill to control cadence, stride length, and speed of gait. Usually patients can adapt more easily to a treadmill because the hand rails provide added support and comfort when beginning a walking program. Also, although stationary bicycle ergometers can be used as a form of aerobic fitness after acute lumbar muscle strain, a standard saddle seat may be uncomfortable for many patients. A semirecumbent cycle with a large bucket seat, where a lumbar extension roll can be used, is generally well tolerated.

The general conditioning program must also focus attention on abdominal muscle support during dynamic functional activities. Abdominal isometrics can be encouraged along with partial direct and oblique sit-ups. With all abdominal exercises after low back muscle strain, emphasis must be placed on limited flexion during the performance of the partial sit-ups. Limited ROM trunk flexion during sit-ups (with knees flexed) are effective and minimize excessive flexion of the trunk, which can potentially aggravate an underlying disc condition.

Throughout the course of recovery from lumbar muscle strain, patients must be directed to perform functional, dynamic back strengthening and abdominal exercises to protect the low back during ADLs. Dynamic back strengthening exercises can be viewed as end stage or functional recovery exercises initiated once the patient can demonstrate improved static or isometric strength, increased walking without complaints of pain, improved lumbar motion, increased lumbar extension strength (through the three positions of prone lumbar and thoracic extension exercises), and improved awareness and demonstration of appropriate, safe lifting mechanics to protect the spine.

Watkins and Dillon[37] strongly advocate trunk strengthening and dynamic support exercises in the treatment and prevention of muscle strains of the lumbar spine. The concept of isometrically holding a neutral lumbar spine position during all functional activities is the cornerstone for recovery from and prevention of low back muscle strains.[37] Watkins and Dillon[37] report: "The key to safe strengthening is the ability to maintain the spine in a safe, neutral position during the strengthening exercises." In addition, "Trunk strength also prevents back injuries and is an important treatment method for back pain."[37] Therefore dynamic functional strengthening of the lumbar spine after muscle strain focuses on isometric cocontractions of the abdominals, erector spinae, and gluteals, as well as challenging the lumbar and abdominal muscles to contract synergistically during functional exercises.[32]

A Physio-ball is an extremely effective and efficient tool to use in developing dynamic lumbar and abdominal strength. A Physio-ball is a large (3 to 4 feet in diameter) sturdy rubber ball that is safe to sit on. Dynamic strengthening using the Physio-ball can proceed in sequential fashion progressing from a seated position to the prone and supine extension positions. Seated trunk stabilization is initiated by simply sitting on the ball while maintaining correct back extension posture and equilibrium (Fig. 15-10). The patient can be effectively challenged to maintain support by gently rolling the ball slightly from side to side, front to back, and diagonally. The patient's abdominal and back extensor muscles must quickly contract to stabilize the spine and maintain proper balance. As the patient demonstrates improved trunk control, partial sit-ups while seated on the Physio-ball can be added for most patients (Fig. 15-11). This progression effectively challenges the patient to maintain support during dynamic muscle activity. Prone extension exercises can begin once the patient demonstrates good balance, trunk control, and strength in the seated position. The patient maintains trunk support and balance in a neutral position while lying prone across the ball (Fig. 15-12). Initially, the patient may need to use hand support. Gradually, as control improves, the hands are lifted while the physical therapist assistant supports the legs (Fig. 15-13).

Ligament Sprains

The spinal ligaments[41] (anterior longitudinal ligament, posterior longitudinal ligament, interspinous ligament, ligamentum flavum, supraspinous ligament) can be injured by a sudden violent force or from repeated stress. The physical therapist will conduct a comprehensive evaluation of the patient to (1) confirm or deny the

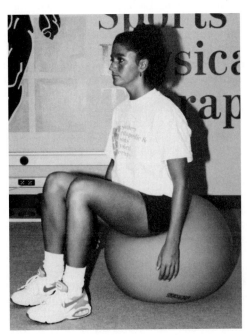

FIG. 15-10 Seated dynamic trunk stabilization while seated on a physio-ball.

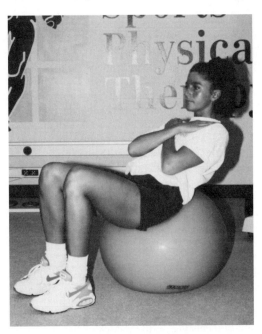

FIG. 15-11 Seated partial direct sit-ups on a physio-ball. This is a challenging exercise to maintain balance while performing dynamic exercise.

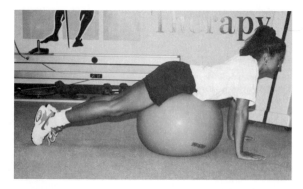

FIG. 15-12 Lying prone across a physio-ball with foot and arm support.

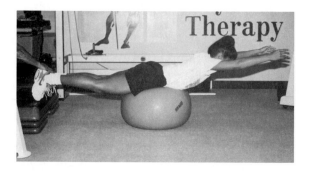

FIG. 15-13 Progressively more challenging dynamic prone extension on the physio-ball. The patient attempts to maintain balance while elevating one arm then both arms as the clinician provides support at the feet.

presence of segmental instability (hypermobility resulting from ligament sprain) and (2) evaluate the degree of pain with or without active or passive movement of the lumbar spine in general or in individual segments. In addition to isolated ligament sprains, muscle strains can be superimposed, making the identification of specific single-ligament sprains exceedingly difficult.

The management of lumbar ligament sprains essentially parallels the care of muscle strains. In general terms, recovery from muscle strains, ligamentous sprains, and various degrees of disc herniations can be divided into four phases.[5] In each phase, the cornerstone of care is patient education and pain-free appropriate lifting, posture, sitting, standing, and bending body mechanics.

Phase I focuses on healing and pain control. During this phase, rest, restricted activity, pain medications, physical agents to control swelling and pain (ultrasound, ice packs, moist heat, electrical stimulation, massage, etc.), and patient education principles regarding body mechanics are introduced.

Phase II of recovery is characterized by the initiation of mobilization involving early active and passive motion. Therefore attention is centered on increasing the patient's activity level without undue complaints of pain, initiating motion and flexibility exercises (defined by Chappuis, Johnson, and Gines[5] as "nondestructive movement") consistent with and conducive to tissue healing, performing specific muscle-strengthening exercises (isometrics, **spine stabilization,** neutral spine strengthening, lumbar extension strengthening, and abdominal strengthening), and continuing education and reinforcement of body mechanics information.

Phase III focuses on the prevention of reinjury. A total body conditioning program is encouraged that emphasizes overall strength, flexibility, aerobic fitness (weight management, body composition, endurance), proprioception exercises, and advanced, more challenging neutral spine stabilization exercises.

The return to normalized activity is characteristic of phase IV. During this phase, the patient is gradually introduced to work site activities, ADLs, and sports activities, with particular attention paid to movements, loads, positions, and frequency of activity.[5]

The four-phase recovery program just outlined is offered only as a general guide and is not intended to describe a comprehensive rehabilitation plan for all spinal dysfunction. Each patient will have specific, identified needs and goals that must be addressed individually through the initial evaluation performed by the physical therapist.

Immediate attention is directed at alleviating pain and inflammation with the use of physician-prescribed NSAIDs, oral analgesics, muscle relaxants, and various agents (heat, ice, electrical stimuli, ultrasound, massage, etc.). Protection of the affected area must coincide with pain-relieving physical agents. The assistant, under the direction of the physical therapist, must identify which specific positions are contraindicated by carefully reviewing the initial evaluation data. Both the short-term and the long-range goals for recovery from lumbar strains and sprains emphasize protecting the spine from unwanted forces and positions. As with other ligament sprains, those positions that stretch the affected ligaments must be avoided. Therefore neutral spine stabilization (maintenance of pain-free posture with a normal lordotic curve during exercise) is particularly important during all phases of recovery from ligament sprains. Once the pain-free position is identified, the course of recovery focuses on isometrically strengthening the abdominals, gluteals, and lumbar extensors throughout functional activities. This does not mean that specific lumbar extension strengthening exercises (three-position prone extension) should be strictly avoided. On the contrary, these exercises, if well-tolerated after the acute stage of healing, should be introduced to specifically isolate the lumbar and thoracic extension muscles. In many cases, trunk flexion stretches the affected ligaments, so flexion should be minimized.

The abdominal muscles can be effectively conditioned with isometric sets while the lordotic curve is maintained. Paris[30] identifies sitting as a characteristically uncomfortable position for many patients suffering from lumbar sprains. The sitting posture may be enhanced and the flexed lumbar posture while seated minimized using a lumbar extension roll placed in the small of the back. While maintaining a pain-free neutral spine, the patient is encouraged to walk; perform isotonic strengthening exercises that do not compromise lumbar flexion, rotation, torque, or vertical compressive loads; and do flexibility exercises, carefully avoiding all unwanted lumbar spine motions. Muscle and ligament tissues heal and effect repair at different rates, so while some mild muscle strains heal quickly, a prolonged period may be needed with ligament injuries. To avoid further injury, the patient must be educated thoroughly about lifting mechanics that do not reproduce pain, protective sitting postures, and maintenance of a general conditioning program to increase strength, flexibility, and endurance while maintaining a neutral, pain-free lumbar spine.

Injuries to the Lumbar Intervertebral Disc

The physical therapist assistant is strongly encouraged to thoroughly review the anatomic relationship between the lumbar vertebral bodies, the disc, the spinal canal, and the nerve roots. DeRosa and Porterfield[7] state: "The intervertebral disc is the largest avascular structure in the human body." Without an intense vascular response to injury, the disc has a limited capacity to heal and repair. The vascular supply to the disc is provided by diffusion from the vertebral bodies above and below the disc.[7,14,25,30] Neurologic innervation is reserved for the outer fibers of the annulus,[14] while the remainder of the disc is aneural. Also, the disc itself is wedge shaped, with a thick anterior portion and a thin posterior portion.[7] Understanding this relationship helps in understanding specific disc injuries and in choosing which therapeutic maneuvers are best.

Various terms are used to describe injuries to the disc. Although "slipped disc" is a common expression used to describe various ailments of the low back among the general population, a disc does not "slip" from within its confines between the vertebral bodies. The generally accepted term, **herniated nucleus pulposus (HNP),** is rather broad and should be clarified by

specific nomenclature to more precisely describe the injury. Miller[27] describes the three categories of HNP as protrusion, extruded, and sequestrated. In a **disc protrusion,** the nucleus bulges against an intact annulus (Fig. 15-14). An **extruded disc** is characterized by the nucleus extending through the annulus, but the nuclear material remains confined by the posterior longitudinal ligament (Fig. 15-15). Finally, in a **sequestrated disc,** the nucleus is free within the canal (Fig. 15-16).

Macnab[24] offers a variation of this classification model:
Disc protrusion:
Type I: Peripheral annular bulge
Type II: Localized annular bulge
Disc herniation:
Type I: Prolapsed intervertebral disc
Type II: Extruded intervertebral disc
Type III: Sequestrated intervertebral disc
Thus in a disc protrusion the annular fibers are intact, although the annulus bulges. A prolapsed disc has the nucleus contained only by the outer fibers of the bulging annulus.

Regardless of the exact nature of the injury, HNP remains primarily a disease of young to middle-age adults.[27] Age-related changes include decreased hydration, with a decreased water content from 70% to 88% by the third decade; biochemical changes in the glycosaminoglycans of the nucleus; and increases in collagen. These changes make disc herniations rare in the elderly.[27,30] Burkus[3] has identified five separate categories of low back pain that clarify the complex and interrelated nature of various organs and systems affecting low back pain. The five categories are defined as follows:

1. *Viscerogenic pain:* Pain that originates from the kidneys, pelvisacral lesions, and retroperitoneal tumors. "This type of pain is neither aggravated by activity nor relieved by rest. This differentiates it from back pain which is a result of spinal disorders."[3]

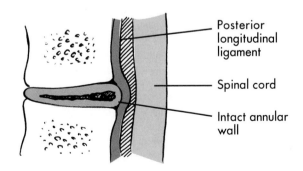

FIG. 15-14 Disc protrusion. The nucleus bulges against an intact annulus.

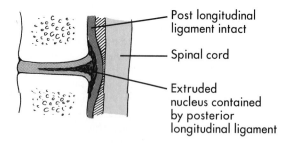

FIG. 15-15 Extruded disc. The nucleus extends through the annulus; however, the nuclear material remains confined by the posterior longitudinal ligament.

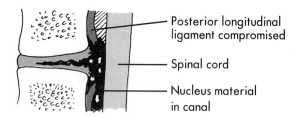

FIG. 15-16 Sequestrated disc. The nucleus is free within the spinal canal.

2. *Neurogenic pain:* Pain commonly caused by neurofibromas, cysts, and tumors of the nerve roots in the lumbar spine.
3. *Vascular pain:* Pain characterized by intermittent claudication from aneurysms and peripheral vascular disease.
4. *Psychogenic pain:* Pain that is quite uncommon and ascribed to nonorganic causes. The physician must completely rule out all organic factors before considering psychogenic pain as the primary cause of low back dysfunction.
5. *Spondylogenic pain:* Pain directly related to the pain originating from soft tissues of the spine and sacroiliac joint. This type of pain is classically characterized as aggravated by activity and relieved by rest.

Although their are many causes of low back pain, the physical therapist assistant directs attention at spondylogenic pain as it relates to the orthopedic conditions outlined in this chapter. However, other causes of back pain must always be considered and a high degree of suspicion maintained for all low back pain patients who do not demonstrate consistent objective changes after therapeutic interventions. For the physical therapist assistant, pain originating from any classification model of a herniated disc is defined as spondylogenic pain.

The criteria-based rehabilitation program used to treat HNP is directly and profoundly related to the precise data gained during the initial physical therapy assessment. Not all herniated discs are treated in the same manner. Depending on the extent of the herniation, the patient may demonstrate **radicular signs,** such as pain radiating into the buttocks or legs (sciatica), posterior thigh pain, and paresthesias (numbness or tingling radiating distally below the knee as a result of nerve root impingement).

With regard to radicular signs, during the initial evaluation process, the physical therapist will confirm or deny the presence of **peripheralization** or **centralization** phenomena.[22,25] As defined by Kisner and Colby,[22] during the initial evaluation, "When repeating the forward-bending test, the symptoms increase or peripheralize. Peripheralization means the symptoms are experienced further down the leg." Centralization is defined by McKenzie[25] as "the phenomenon whereby, as a result of the performance of certain repeated movements or the adoption of certain positions, radiating pain originating from the spine and referred distally, is made to move away from the periphery and toward the mid-line of the spine." The motion of the nucleus during lumbar spine flexion (nucleus moves posteriorly) and extension (nucleus moves anteriorly) must be abundantly clear because of three important exceptions to the centralization and peripheralization phenomenon identified by Kisner and Colby,[22] as follows:

1. If there is a lateral shift of the spinal column, backward bending increases the pain. Note that with posterolateral disc herniations and nerve root impingement, the patient may list or shift away from the painful side in an attempt to reduce pain by decreasing impingement. If the lateral shift is first corrected, then repeated backward bending lessens or centralizes the pain.
2. If the protrusion cannot be mechanically reduced, backward bending peripheralizes or increases the symptoms.
3. If there is an anterior protrusion, backward bending increases the pain and forward bending relieves the pain.

Therefore the evaluation data obtained by the physical therapist from the patient is essential to determining treatment.

The keys to managing HNP involve the following four basic objectives:[7]

1. Reduce pain via physician-prescribed analgesics and a combination of thermal and/or electrical modalities.

2. Protect the affected area from unwanted stress and forces (determined from the initial evaluation) while encouraging and promoting movement.
3. Increase muscle strength, endurance, and flexibility.
4. Counsel the patient concerning correct body mechanics.

Chappuis, Johnson, and Gines[5] elaborate on these goals by specifically identifying nine essential steps:

1. Reduce pain.
2. Increase flexibility.
3. Increase strength.
4. Education.
5. Increase cardiovascular fitness.
6. Decrease stress.
7. Improve posture.
8. Improve body mechanics.
9. Improve the sense of personal responsibility.

In addition, the nine components of a comprehensive nonsurgical rehabilitation regimen[5] are as follows:

1. Restrictions: Identify specific limitations that preclude involvement in all areas of recovery
2. Education: Anatomy and body mechanics
3. Symptomatic treatment: Thermal and/or electrical agents, medications, and posture
4. Posture adjustment: Body mechanics
5. Flexibility
6. Cardiovascular training
7. Balance training
8. Strengthening
9. Ergonomics instruction: Work site evaluation, ADLs, and sports activities.

The physical therapist determines if lumbar flexion or extension should be encouraged during recovery from HNP. Initial management can generally proceed with the patient prone on a mat or table while applying thermal and/or electrical agents. If the therapist has determined that lumbar extension reduces radicular symptoms (centralization), initially a small pillow can be placed under the patient's chest to achieve a small, pain-free degree of passive lumbar extension. McKenzie[25] advocates that, after the patient has rested a short while in this position, he or she should be encouraged to prop up on the elbows to further enhance the lordotic curve (Fig. 15-17). The therapist is attempting to reduce or relocate the herniated nucleus to a more anterior location and away from the impingement (Fig. 15-18). From this intermediate position, the patient now performs press-ups, which further enhance lumbar extension. Press-ups can be modified to be performed repeatedly (slow, continuous, reciprocal up-and-down motions) or held statically (maintained in a pain-free extended position) for short periods of time.

In many cases of true disc herniation with radicular signs, passive and active extension effectively relieve symptoms and provide a mechanical foundation for healing. The nucleus is reduced to a more anterior location and away from the impingement. However, for long-term care the patient must be counseled concerning proper lifting mechanics and sitting postures (using a lumbar extension roll while seated to maintain an appropriate anatomic lordotic curve) and to avoid positions that contribute to lumbar spine flexion and posterior translation of the nucleus. Occupational risks (lifting and prolonged sitting) as well as all ADLs must be modified to enhance appropriate mechanics and minimize the potential for repeated stress to the disc.

The physician and/or physical therapist may prescribe pelvic or lumbar traction to stretch muscles, enhance vertebral segment separation, reduce nerve root impingement, and decrease pain.[22] The clinical application of mechanical lumbar-pelvic traction is beyond the scope and intent of this text.

In addition to the use of passive extension procedures to relocate a posterior bulge of the disc, active prone extension exercises can be employed (three-position thoracic and lumbar active extension) once the acute phase has resolved as documented by centralization of radicular signs and control of pain. Some patients may be unable to perform various prone position exercises; standing back extension with hand support or the use of a supine back extension apparatus may prove more comfortable. During the early recovery phase, it is important to gradually add more challenging and functional exercises that also enhance normal lordotic posture while strengthening the posterior lumbar muscles.

The use of "all fours" postural extension exercises can begin once the patient effectively demonstrates improved passive extension (without symptoms), proper body mechanics (particularly with lifting), and increased lumbar extension strength. The patient does these exercises on hands and knees with the low back held in a normal lordotic posture. First, the patient elevates one arm to an overhead, outreached, and extended position (Fig. 15-19). This position is held for 6 seconds, then the arm is returned to the supported position and the other arm is raised reciprocally. This exercise effectively teaches the patient to maintain correct lordotic posture with strong abdominal isometrics to stabilize the pelvis, while performing active arm and shoulder-flexion exercises.

The next progression on all fours requires the patient to elevate one arm while simultaneously extending the contralateral lower limb (Fig. 15-20). Correct lumbar extension posture must be maintained. This exercise is

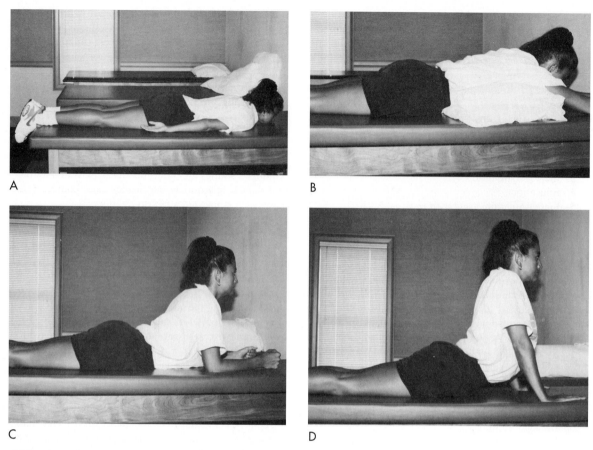

FIG. 15-17 Passive prone extension sequence. **A,** Patient lying prone without pillow for support. **B,** Patient prone with pillow under the chest for mild thoracic and lumbar extension. **C,** Patient propped up on elbows for improved extension. **D,** Prone, elbows extended for maximum extension.

intended to encourage shoulder flexion, lumbar extension, and hip extension (gluteals and hamstrings) while maintaining proper balance and posture on all fours.

Once the patient is comfortably demonstrating improved posture and control of pain, a general fitness program can begin. The goal in exercising is to improve overall body strength, aerobic fitness, and flexibility without compromising lumbar spine flexion.

Conservative management of HNP involves the introduction and continuous reinforcement of proper body mechanics (lifting, sitting, sleeping) to control unwanted forces and stresses that are not conducive to long-term healing. The physical therapist assistant educates patients as to the virtues of physical conditioning (with the use of protective postures) and the daily application of safe lifting principles to protect the spine from further injury.

Invasive Management of Lumbar Disc Herniation

When conservative physical therapy (including rest, medications, exercise, and postural counseling) fails to bring significant relief from symptoms, the physician may offer several invasive procedures designed to relieve pain and to remove its cause, which is presumed to be the disc.

For some patients whose persistent radicular pain (sciatica) cannot be controlled by conservative measures, the physician may prescribe an epidural steroid injection to relieve pain.[11,27] These injections are given only to relieve pain and reduce inflammation, and are not intended to be used as a curative procedure to correct any neurologic deficits.

When surgery is needed to correct a herniated disc, the physician will determine the exact nature of the

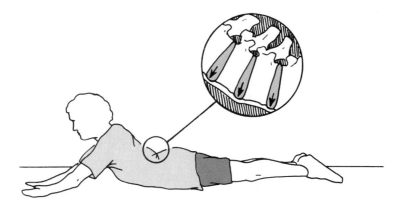

FIG. 15-18 Passive prone extension. The nucleus moves in an anterior direction.

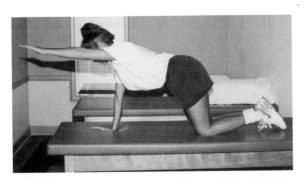

FIG. 15-19 All-fours postural extension. One arm elevated and extended while the patient maintains proper lordotic posture.

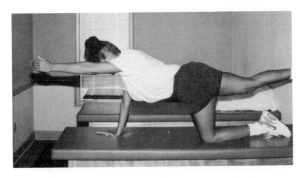

FIG. 15-20 All-fours postural extension. With one arm elevated and extended, the patient is instructed to extend the contralateral lower limb.

herniation (protruded, extruded, sequestered) and select the appropriate surgical procedure. As described by Miller[27] and Eismont and Kitchel,[11] the most common procedure is a laminotomy with a decompression discectomy. In this procedure the physician gains exposure to the herniated disc by cutting into the lamina and then removing all nonviable disc material, thereby decompressing the affected nerve root (Fig. 15-21). Miller[27] reports that with this particular surgical procedure, 95% of patients demonstrate good or excellent results. However, as many as 30% of these patients may have significant back pain at long-term follow-up.[8,27] Other procedures, such as microsurgical discectomy and automated percutaneous discectomy, also remove the cause of the nerve root impingement (disc).

Rehabilitation after any surgical procedure is highly patient-specific and directly related to the data obtained at the initial postoperative physical therapy evaluation. Generally, recovery closely parallels the criteria established with conservative management of a herniated disc. However, extensive surgical exposure is required to perform a laminotomy with discectomy, and tissue healing constraints will influence recovery.

After surgery, the patient is taught bed mobility and transfer training using the log-roll technique to move from a supine to sitting position. Ambulation with a walker or crutches is allowed 1 day after surgery. Ambulation distance and endurance activities are increased according to each patient's ability. Rudimentary bed exercises can be performed the day after surgery and include active ankle pumps, gentle hip and knee flexion, and isometric exercises (quadriceps and gluteals). The physical therapist will guide the assistant concerning whether or not the postoperative patient will be performing any isometric exercises. The assistant must instruct the patient in and reinforce proper breathing techniques if isometric exercises are done. The Valsalva maneuver is strictly avoided during all exercises.

For the first 3 days after surgery[5] the patient is limited to sitting for no more than 1 hour at a time and must maintain proper spinal position with no flexion.

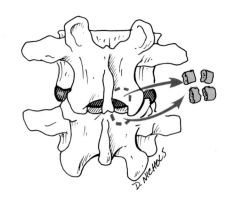

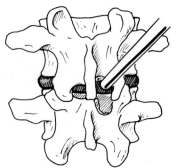

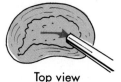

Suction probe removes
disc material

Top view

FIG. 15-21 Laminotomy with decompression discectomy.

The physical therapist assistant continually reinforces and encourages proper posture during the first week of recovery. The patient should be cautioned to avoid forward bending and trunk rotation.

More demanding and functionally relevant activities that do not stress the surgical site are gradually added. Transfers from supine to sitting and from sitting to standing must be demonstrated by the patient and observed by the clinician to be safe, efficient, and free from all unwanted stress. Throughout the first week, exercises can progress to include partial squats, which focus on functional closed-chain strengthening while maintaining proper neutral spine stabilization throughout the squat.

When initial wound healing is complete and pain is decreased, a more accelerated program of strengthening can begin. Extension is encouraged gradually, progressing to active lumbar and thoracic extension strengthening while avoiding lumbar flexion. ROM exercises for the spine are encouraged as soon as the patient can tolerate these motions. Gentle active extension exercises and pelvic tilts (which promote pelvic motion, control,

as well as limited-motion lumbar spine flexion and extension) begin early in the recovery phase.

The patient must achieve increased motion, controlled pain, improved endurance, and sufficient strength before beginning a general conditioning program after surgery. The longer recovery period is needed to allow for proper soft tissue healing, bone healing, and control of inflammation and pain before subjecting the affected area to stress. From 3 to 5 weeks after surgery, the goals of recovery are identified as restored lumbar motion, normalized upper and lower extremity strength, improved aerobic fitness, and decreased pain and swelling.[5] As the patient achieves these criteria, progressive functional exercises can be added. These include treadmill walking, balance activities, isotonic strengthening exercises, general flexibility exercises, and cardiovascular conditioning (via upper body ergometer, recumbent cycle ergometer, treadmill, stair stepper, and cross country ski machine).

Spinal Stenosis

Lumbar spinal stenosis is defined as a narrowing of the spinal canal, which constricts and compresses nerve roots (Fig. 15-22).[27] This gives rise to symptoms of neurogenic or spinal claudication, which are as follows:

1. Radicular ache into the thigh and less frequently into the calf[3]
2. Paresthesis into the lower extremity[13]
3. Disturbances in motor function[13]

This condition occurs in males "twice as often as females"[27] and typically is observed during late middle age and older.[13,27]

Lumbar **spinal stenosis** is most commonly acquired as a result of degenerative arthritic changes that encroach on the diameter of the canal, producing nerve root compression.[27] The patient with stenosis frequently complains of pain and increased symptoms with lumbar extension. Extension of the lumbar spine in a patient with stenosis further compresses the spinal canal, thereby increasing pain and paresthesias.[7,13,27]

During ambulation and gait training, an elderly patient typically demonstrates a forward-flexed trunk posture when using a walker. Under careful observation and questioning, the patient may suggest that leaning forward feels better and reduces back and leg pain. Unless this position is recognized as being appropriate for relieving pain in patients with stenosis, the clinician may encourage a less appropriate, erect extended trunk posture that may exacerbate the pain.

Management of spinal stenosis focuses on flexion exercises (Williams flexion exercises, including pelvic tilts, knee-to-chest exercises, and partial direct and oblique sit-ups) and avoiding lumbar extension. The physical therapist assistant also educates the patient and reinforces appropriate posture (flexed, in this case), body mechanics, lifting techniques, and sitting and sleeping changes as well as a general physical conditioning program and a weight management program, which Miller[27] identifies as an important adjunct in the care of spinal stenosis.

Spondylolysis and Spondylolisthesis

Spondylolysis is a bony defect (stress fracture or fracture) in the pars interarticularis of the posterior elements of the spine* (Fig. 15-23). **Spondylolisthesis,** on the other hand, describes a forward slippage of one superior vertebra over an inferior vertebra (usually L4-L5 and L5-S1)[8,11] as a result of instability caused by the bilateral defect in the pars interarticularis (Fig. 15-24).*

---

*References 3,4,7,11,27,30,37.

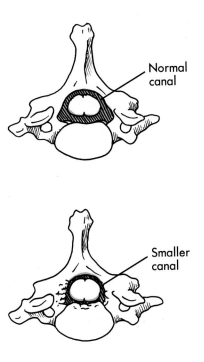

FIG. 15-22 Lumbar spinal stenosis. Narrow diameter of the spinal canal can lead to constriction and compression of nerve roots.

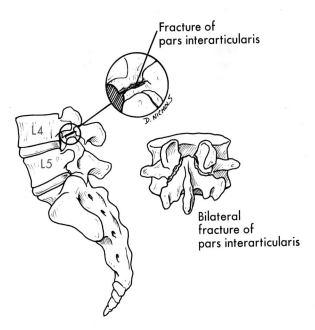

FIG. 15-23 Spondylolysis. Fracture of pars interarticularis of the posterior elements of the spine.

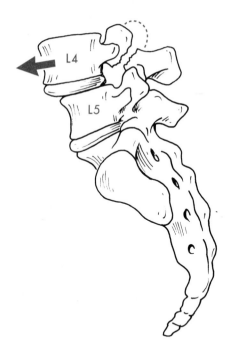

FIG. 15-24 Spondylolisthesis. The resultant forward slippage of one superior vertebrae over an inferior vertebra.

There are specific classification types as well as degrees of slippage or "migration" of the vertebrae in the disease process of spondylolisthesis.[11] Five types, or classifications, have been identified, as follows.[3,11,27]

Type I: Congenital or dysplastic. Results from a "congenital malformation of the sacrum or neural arch of L5, which allows forward slippage of L5 on the sacrum."[3] Most common in children.

Type II: Isthmic spondylolisthesis. The most common type, affecting persons from 5 to 50 years of age.[27] Usually a result of mechanical stress that causes a stress fracture at the pars interarticularis.[11,27]

Type III: Degenerative spondylolisthesis. Most commonly affects an older population. Characterized by a loss of ligament integrity (or stability) that results in forward slippage of the vertebrae. Generally associated with the normal aging process.[3]

Type IV: Traumatic spondylolisthesis. Caused by trauma that produces an acute fracture of the pars interarticularis. Casting is the most appropriate form of treatment.[3] Because of their generally high levels of physical activities, this type usually affects young patients.[27]

Type V: Pathologic spondylolisthesis. Characterized by bone tumors that affect the pars.

The degree or grade of slippage is determined radiographically by the examining physician and is defined as the amount of forward displacement of the superior vertebrae over the inferior vertebrae, as outlined here.[3,7,27]

Grade I: 0 to 25%
Grade II: 25% to 50%
Grade III: 50% to 75%
Grade IV: 75% to 100%

The cause of the defect in the pars interarticularis is in part a congenital weakness in this area. In addition, the pars is subjected to high levels of mechanical stress.[38,39] Authorities[39] also suggest that the primary initial cause of the most common type of spondylolisthesis (isthmic) is fatigue fracture of the pars interarticularis.

Patients primarily report pain with extremes of lumbar motion, especially extension. The pain generally follows the belt line.[19] During examination, the physical therapist may also identify a palpable step-off between the affected lumbar vertebrae (usually L4-L5) because of the forward slippage.[7]

The management of spondylolisthesis is dictated by symptoms as well as the degree of vertebral slippage (grades I to IV). For example, an adult with isthmic spondylolisthesis of radiographically determined grade I (0 to 25% slippage), may not experience significant symptoms with activity or extremes of lumbar extension. Thus treatment is aimed at preventing any progression to grade II (25% to 50% slippage). This is usually accomplished by instructing the patient to avoid ballistic lumbar extension as well as vertical loading while seated or standing, so as to minimize anteriorly directed shearing forces on the spine. In addition, abdominal strengthening exercises, neutral spine stabilization exercises (controlled lumbar extension strengthening, isometrics, rectus and oblique abdominal strengthening while in the neutral spine position), and stretching exercises for the trunk and lower extremities are encouraged.

When there is a greater degree of slippage with significant symptoms, the patient may require more specific attention. Generally, pain and muscle spasm are addressed with physician-prescribed analgesics, muscle relaxants, NSAIDs, and agents (heat, ice, ultrasound, electrical stimulation) to alleviate acute pain and swelling. If the pain is related to a fatigue fracture of the pars, initial treatment focuses on managing stress to the fracture site using a lumbosacral corset or orthosis positioned to create a slight amount of lumbar flexion, which reduces anterior shearing forces through the fracture site and allows for bone healing.[11,19]

The cornerstone in the care of spondylolisthesis is avoidance of extreme lumbar extension and application of abdominal muscle strengthening exercises to provide dynamic support for the spine during acitivity. A young athletic patient must modify activities that directly influence the course of this disease. For example, weight lifting contributes significantly to the occurrence of spondylolysis.[9] The young athlete must modify or avoid dynamic overhead lifting, which contributes to vertical compressive loads and anterior shearing forces of the lumbar spine, and he or she must critically examine other weight lifting activities.

Surgery is rare and is usually reserved for patients with radicular symptoms and high-grade slippage (grades III or IV), which compresses the nerve roots and causes neurologic signs.[3,27] The type of surgery advocated in these cases is a decompression laminectomy (to reduce compression of the nerve roots) with fusion to stabilize the vertebral segments.[3,27]

Rehabilitation after surgery for spondylolisthesis is deferred until solid bony union is determined radiographically. The patient is usually in a lumbosacral orthosis that does not permit lumbar extension. During immobilization, the patient can ambulate as tolerated and perform rudimentary ROM and strengthening exercises for the upper and lower extremities (ankle pumps, quadriceps sets, knee ROM). Once bone healing is confirmed, a gradually progressive program of abdominal strengthening (from isometrics to concentric and eccentric abdominal contractions), lumbar ROM (avoiding dynamic, ballistic, extreme lumbar extension), general conditioning, and a progressive return to function is advocated.[3,27]

Lumbar Spine Fractures

Fractures of the lumbar vertebrae generally occur after a profound traumatic event and can be classified according to the forces that produce the fracture. For example, compression, flexion, extension, flexion-distraction, flexion-rotation, and lateral flexion are forces that produce fractures.[27] Lumbar spine fractures can also be described in terms that graphically depict a specific fracture deformity, including crush, wedge, burst, shear, slice, and teardrop fractures.[27]

Perhaps the most clinically relevant spine fracture for the physical therapist assistant to consider is the vertebral compression fracture. These fractures occur at a rate of approximately 530,000 annually,[17] with many lower thoracic and high-level lumbar fractures caused by osteoporosis.[7,13,23] In an elderly population of patients with osteoporosis, many benign activities can produce compression fractures.[3,23] Care must be taken to ensure that no rapid deceleration occurs when an elderly patient transfers to a bedside commode or any other hard surface. This seemingly trivial activity frequently causes multilevel compression fractures in patients with osteoporosis. Compression fractures produce symptoms ranging from acute local pain to essentially no signs at all.[23] Thus subtle complaints of pain caused by typical daily activities, such

as bending, lifting, or rising from a chair, must be viewed with a high level of suspicion in elderly patients.[23]

Treatment of compression fractures focuses on relief of pain, with authorities[13,23] advocating bed rest, physician-prescribed analgesics, NSAIDs, heat, ice, massage, and electrical stimulation to control pain, swelling, and associated muscle spasm. During the acute and subacute phases of recovery, the patient with compression fractures must avoid thoracic or lumbar flexion activities.[13] Trunk flexion is contraindicated because it creates an anterior wedging of the vertebral bodies, producing greater stress and compression at the fracture site.[13]

As the symptoms of pain and swelling subside, the patient may be allowed out of bed for a few minutes each hour.[13,23] During this time, the patient performs isometric lumbar stabilization exercises (isometric abdominal sets, gluteal sets, scapular retraction) in a comfortable position. Extension activities are also allowed to reduce vertebral body compression and build up thoracic and lumbar extension strength. Walking short distances and sitting tolerance must be closely followed and progressed according to the individual. Endurance-type activities that do not create lumbar flexion are advocated as soon as the patient can tolerate prolonged periods of ambulation. Local muscular endurance activities help with the adaptation and preparation for ADLs that use the postural muscles.

If the patient is allowed adequate rest for healing and performs lumbar stabilization exercises while avoiding lumbar flexion, the return to function and normal activities can be expected 6 to 8 weeks after injury.[13] The identification and management of acute lumbar fractures is dictated by the physician, who must determine if the fracture is stable or unstable. The most common lumbar fracture is the compression fracture and it is treated as described earlier.[26] Unstable fractures may be accompanied by neurologic involvement that necessitates open reduction and internal fixation of the unstable spine segments as well as possible fusion of the segments.[26] McRae[26] has outlined the goals of treatment of unstable lumbar spine fractures as follows:

- To reduce displacement of the fracture segment
- To prevent any recurrence of displacement that may lead to catastrophic neurologic involvement

Stability can be achieved by either allowing the unstable segments to heal spontaneously through long-term conservative care, which facilitates the healing of bone and posterior longitudinal ligaments, or by open reduction and internal fixation with fusion of the unstable segments.[26] In either case, any detailed discussion of recovery after spine surgery with neurologic involvement is beyond the scope of this text. Generally, recovery time parallels the time required for healing of bone, muscle, and ligament.

A lengthy period of convalescence is needed with a gradual, progressive sequence of active lower-extremity ROM, isometric exercises, bed mobility, transfer training, sitting tolerance, gait training, endurance activities, upper-extremity strengthening, and a slow return to function once the spine is stable.

Prevention and Education for Back Dysfunction: The Back School Model

While understanding and managing low back dysfunction is the focus of this section, prevention of lumbar spine injuries is also pertinent to this discussion, because the physical therapist assistant is frequently directed to participate in and to carry out community-based back injury prevention programs under the supervision and direction of a physical therapist. These education programs are commonly referred to as **"back schools"** and are designed to provide an understanding of anatomy, causes of back pain, lifting mechanics, posture, self-care for back pain, exercise, nutrition (weight management), **ergonomics** (which involves lifting, posture, general body mechanics, job modifications, and work site protection and redesign to minimize back injury), and stress reduction for high-risk patients as well as the population at large.

Often patients with a history of back pain are identified as ideal candidates to participate in these programs. Also, persons at risk (identified by job responsibilities, repetitive lifting, overweight condition, poor posture, poor body mechanics, relative weakness, and poor general physical conditioning) may be referred to these programs.

Many back schools involve a 1-hour or 2-hour class (consisting of lectures, slides, demonstration, and participation) each week for 4 to 6 weeks. Each session or class builds on the previous lecture to convey the principles seen in spinal anatomy, causes of back dysfunction, risk factors, posture, body mechanics, and treatment approaches.[1] Back schools can be based in outpatient physical therapy clinics, hospitals, industrial health clinics, wellness programs at work, or community fitness centers. In every case, the program is under the direction and supervision of a physician and physical therapist.

Allman[1] has identified the outline in Box 15-1 as an appropriate general back school program.

BOX 15-1   Appropriate General Back School Program

Introduction to back dysfunction.

The primary purpose is to increase the patient's awareness of back care, posture, and body mechanics.
Basic spinal anatomy and physiology
Causes of back pain and dysfunction
1. Sprains and strains
2. Disc injuries (HNP)
3. Spinal stenosis
4. Spondylolisthesis

Risk factors associated with back injury

1. Poor general conditioning
2. Poor posture
3. Poor body mechanics and poor lifting style
4. Repetitive heavy lifting
5. Long-term sitting and driving
6. Stress (emotional)

Posture positioning and general body mechanics

1. Sitting
2. Sleeping
3. Standing
4. Lifting
5. ADLs, job assessment, recreational activities

Treatment approaches

1. Ice or heat
2. Stretching
3. Posture changes
4. Back support
5. Conditioning

General physical conditioning

1. Warm-up. Patients are introduced to the concept of a general warm-up preceding any physical activity.
2. Aerobic fitness. Patients are introduced to the methods, equipment, and implementation of general and specific endurance activities to improve cardiovascular fitness and control body weight.
3. Anaerobic power. Activities are outlined that develop intense physical effort of short duration.
4. Strength. Patients are instructed in methods to improve general body strength as well as in specific lumbar extension strength exercises.
5. Flexibility. Patients are introduced to the philosophy, design, and implementation of daily, full-body stretching exercises with specific emphasis on the trunk and lower extremities.
6. Nutrition. Direct attention is focused on reducing the number of calories consumed by overweight individuals. Usually this education is conducted by a registered dietitian.
7. Relaxation techniques, stress reduction, and recreational activities.

From Allman FL: Back school program In Introduction to Back Injuries, 1990, The Atlanta Sports Medicine Clinic.

The general back school curriculum described in Box 15-1 clarifies the rudimentary concepts of education and prevention for a wide variety of back-related problems. The physical therapist assistant who presents this information must be given specific information, evaluation data, indications, and contraindications for each patient participating in the back school program. In this way all phases of recovery as well as prevention can be individualized for each patient.

Ergonomics and Functional Capacity Evaluations

In concert with back injury prevention through education and in accordance with the back school model is the concept of ergonomics and the implementation of **functional capacity evaluations (FCEs),** which are also referred to as physical capacity assessments (PCAs), related to physical stress job analysis. The term *ergonomics* refers to a quantifiable system of job or ADL modification (or redesign) that allows for continued productivity while reducing work-related physical stress. As with the back school model, an FCE may require the assistant to prepare the evaluation area, set up all necessary testing equipment (see discussion of quantifying back strength), and assist the therapist with the collection, documentation, and storage of data. The implementation of an FCE is highly specific to the individual's job task. Its goal is to identify risk factors associated with a particular job or activity and then quantify the physical capacity of the individual being asked to perform the specific task in order to reduce the risk of back injury. In most cases an FCE is administered to a patient recovering from a back injury before he or she returns to the job. An FCE can also be used as a screening tool to acquire data related to preemployment risk assessment and management of back injuries. Certain job or activity risk factors have been identified[16] that directly relate to the FCE. A few ergonomic risk factors are outlined by Hebert[16] as follows:

- How much weight is lifted
- How often you lift
- How low you bend to lift the load
- How high you lift the load
- How far you carry the load
- How far you twist with the load
- How far you reach with the load
- How long you sit at your job
- What the specific design of your seat is
- If there is sustained or repeated bending, twisting, or reaching

Hundreds of factors may be related to job tasks. Each item to be tested in the FCE must be quantifiable and reproducible to enable the physical therapist to make

---

BOX 15-2   Testing Procedure that Identifies the Various Components of an FCE

Musculoskeletal profile

1. Blood pressure
2. Posture
3. Gait
4. Balance
5. Range of motion
6. Neurologic (reflexes)
7. Sensory
8. Muscle strength

Functional abilities screening

1. Push-pull
2. Dynamic lifting
3. Gross mobility
4. Hand strength (grip dynamometer)
5. Sitting and standing

From Work site Partners, Functional Capacity Evaluation System, Industrial Rehabilitation Solutions, U.S. Physical Therapy.*

---

recommendations for reducing the risk of back injury. General testing parameters may be divided into categories that attempt to duplicate the requirements of the task to be performed while evaluating the patient's physiologic responses and assessing his or her physical abilities to carry out the task.

Authorities[36] advocate a multiphase testing procedure that identifies the various components of an FCE, as shown in Box 15-2.

Within each FCE the aerobic end-point (heart rate exceeds 85% of maximum heart rate) as well as the biomechanical analysis of the patient's lifting-risk posture is assessed. In each section of the test, the parameters evaluated are performed directly as they relate to the specific job or task in question.

THE THORACIC SPINE
Thoracic Spine Muscle Injuries

Soft tissue injuries of the thoracic spine usually involve some type of direct contact (contusion during athletic activities) or indirect overstretching or contraction of the thoracic muscles. Muscle contusions and strains of the thoracic spine occur primarily in younger active patients. The primary focus of management for these self-limiting injuries is the control of pain and swelling.

---

*System Manual U.S.P.T., Houston, TX, 1994.

Generally, ice is applied directly over the involved area during the acute stage of injury. Physician-prescribed analgesics, NSAIDs, moist heat applications, ultrasound, electrical stimulation, and massage are used judiciously to help control pain. Once pain has been effectively limited, the patient is allowed to participate in active ROM activities and strengthening exercises. The assistant may instruct the patient to perform seated, postural-awareness exercises that focus on thoracic extension and scapular retraction.

Prone thoracic and lumbar extension strengthening exercises are employed as early as the patient can tolerate. These involve a three-position progression from hands at the sides, to hands behind the head, and finally to arms fully extended while performing prone thoracic and lumbar extension. As pain is reduced and strength increases, the patient can begin isotonic strengthening exercises that focus on the scapular and thoracic spine muscles (Fig. 15-25).

Thoracic Disc Injuries

Thoracic disc herniations are quite rare (less than 0.3% of the population) and affect both men and women equally from the fourth through the sixth decades of life.[3] The most common segments affected are between the ninth and twelfth thoracic vertebrae.[3]

The type of treatment employed for thoracic disc herniations depends on whether the disc is herniated laterally or centrally.[3,11] Central disc prolapse generally produces symptoms of "spastic paraparesis, increased deep tendon reflexes, and a positive Babinski response."[11] However, lateral thoracic disc protrusions produce signs more consistent with nerve root compression.

The assistant will be exposed to both conservative care and postsurgical recovery after thoracic spine disc herniations. Less severe lateral disc herniations can be treated effectively with periods of bed rest, analgesics, modalities to control pain and swelling, and epidural injections. More severe central disc herniations, which involve neurologic deficits, must be treated surgically to decompress the neurologic impingement and with fusion to help stabilize the affected segment.[3,11] Recovery after thoracic decompression and fusion closely follows the time required for healing of bone and soft tissue with extensive periods of recumbency, bracing to protect the affected spine from unwanted forces, and a progressive regimen of active motion, strengthening, and endurance activities, and a return to function with specific limitations caused by the fusion.

Kyphosis

Kyphosis is defined as an increase in the thoracic posterior convexity that is manifested by a rounded-back (and pro-

tracted scapulae) posture. Kyphosis can be subdivided into congenital, neuromuscular, and postural categories.[11] Osteoporosis, which can lead to multilevel thoracic compression fractures, causes anterior wedging of the involved segments and creates the kyphotic curvature.

The causes of pain associated with an increased thoracic convexity have been identified as stress originating from the posterior longitudinal ligaments, muscle fatigue resulting from stretched and weakened erector spinae and rhomboid muscle groups, and various postural and neurologic syndromes.[22]

The treatment of kyphosis depends on the degree of curvature, which is determined radiographically by the treating physician; any associated disc involvement; and the severity of symptoms.[2] In advanced cases of postural kyphosis with profound curvature and significant symptoms, the patient may require bracing of the thorax to minimize the compression associated with anterior wedging of the vertebral bodies. With less severe kyphosis, the physical therapist assistant plays a critical role in patient education, postural awareness, and the application of specific exercises to simultaneously stretch the anterior shoulder and pectorals and to strengthen the thoracic extension muscles.

To effectively strengthen the scapular retractors, rhomboids, middle trapezius and erector spinae of the thoracic region, a sufficient degree of freedom of movement in these areas is needed. Generally, the anterior shoulder muscles and pectorals are shortened and relatively weak in response to the increased thoracic convexity. Therefore to provide the needed stimulus for full ROM strengthening, the anterior aspect of the thorax must also be addressed. Stretching the anterior shoulder muscles can be done both actively by the patient and passively, where the clinician provides the stretching. An effective active assisted stretch can be performed with the patient facing the corner of a room or standing in an open doorway. Place both of the patient's hands in a comfortable position on either side of the doorway. Then have the patient slowly lean forward providing a slow, static stretch to the pectorals and anterior shoulder. This position can be held for a prolonged stretch and is usually performed for multiple sets.

A passive stretch can also be employed with the patient in a seated position. With both of the patient's hands placed behind his or her head, stand behind the patient and grasp both elbows. Deliver a slow, posteriorly directed stretch to the pectorals and anterior shoulder muscles. To be effective, stretching must be performed consistently each day. Therefore the patient must perform stretches 2 or 3 times daily as part of a home exercise program. In addition to stretching the thorax,

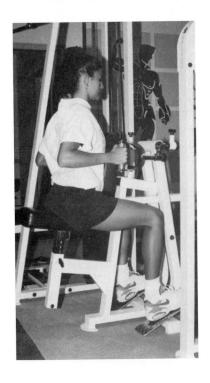

A

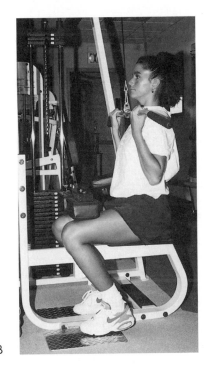

B

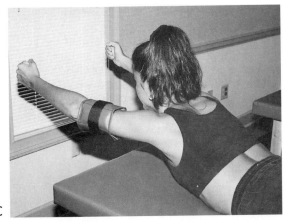

C

FIG. 15-25 Scapular and thoracic extension strengthening. **A,** Seated rowing machine to encourage scapular retraction. **B,** Lat bar pull-down in front. **C,** Prone lumbar and thoracic extension with scapular retraction using cuff weights. Notice the proximal placement of the resistance. As strength increases, the resistance can be moved to the patients hands.

posterior thoracic strengthening must be addressed. The patient performs seated active scapular retraction exercises with an emphasis on maintaining an isometric contraction or "set" of the scapular muscles with each repetition.

As previously described, the patient does the three-progression prone thoracic extension exercises. In addition, the patient performs scapular adduction while lying prone with both arms held straight at 90 degrees from

the shoulder. Both arms are elevated while adducting the scapulae and holding the contracted position isometrically for 10 seconds.[22] This position can be modified slightly by having the patient hold weights while performing scapular adduction with both elbows flexed, creating more of a prone rowing motion.

The patient must perform both stretching and strengthening exercises daily as part of a home program. As the patient's motion improves and where posterior scapular strength increases, isotonic resistance exercises should be encouraged to a greater degree to provide increased stimulus for strengthening. In the home program, latex tubing or Thera-band can be used in a seated rowing position to enhance scapular adduction. Commercially available isotonic rowing machines effectively provide greater resistance for the scapular muscles.

When treating postural kyphosis, the home exercise program must be carried out faithfully and the patient must develop an acute postural awareness at home and at work. If the patient performs tasks at work that contribute to a rounded-shoulder position, modifications of these tasks is necessary. In many cases, the cause of poor thoracic posture is an inefficient work station arrangement in which the patient must maintain poor posture to perform tasks such as typing, writing, assembly work, or computer data entry. A simple adjustment in the height of the work station so that it is closer to and centered midline with the patient encourages a more erect thoracic spine. Therefore the total care of the patient focuses on symptomatic pain relief using physician-prescribed analgesics, thermal agents, massage, and a comprehensive program of stretching, strengthening, education, and work site modifications.

SCOLIOSIS

Scoliosis can be identified as any lateral curvature of the cervical, thoracic, or lumbar spine.[21] Scoliosis is usually idiopathic (cause unknown), but it can also result from neuromuscular causes or can be related to degenerative disease, osteoporosis, trauma, and postsurgical factors.[27] Kisner and Colby[21] identify the incidence of idiopathic scoliosis as being as high as 75% to 85% of all recognized types of scoliosis. Generally scoliosis can be recognized as either structural or nonstructural.[21]

Structural scoliosis is defined as an "irreversible lateral curve of the spine with fixed rotation of the vertebrae."[21] During the physical therapist's initial evaluation of structural scoliosis, the assistant observes that with forward trunk flexion the identified lateral curve does not decrease. Therefore structural idiopathic scoliosis is not corrected by changes in the patient's position or during active voluntary activities.[21] Nonstructural scoliosis is classified as reversible, wherein the lateral curve dissipates with positional changes. In either case, pain is the foremost presenting feature of scoliosis,[27] although cosmesis is a great concern. Other complaints involve decreased cardiopulmonary function (usually with thoracic curves greater than 65 degrees) and neurologic symptoms associated with spinal stenosis.[27]

The nonoperative management of idiopathic scoliosis primarily involves the assistant in instructing the patient regarding therapeutic exercises outlined and prescribed by the physical therapist. Scoliosis treatment involves both stretching and strengthening much like kyphosis. Exercise by itself does not halt the progression nor correct scoliosis.[21] The effective use of therapeutic exercise is intended primarily to improve spinal motion, increase muscle strength, and reduce back pain.[21]

In addition to exercises, bracing has also been advocated in the treatment of scoliosis.[21,27] However, bracing is intended to halt progression of the curve and not to correct cosmetic deformity.[27] Perhaps the most commonly used brace for scoliosis is the Milwaukee brace.[21,27] Generally this brace is worn 23 or 24 hours a day.[21] However, Miller[27] suggests that part-time brace-wearing is as effective as the traditional long-term application.

A fundamental principle in managing idiopathic scoliosis is stretching of the tight muscles on the concave side of the curve, while simultaneously strengthening the muscles on the convex side of the curve. In addition, trunk axial elongation (stretching vertically) is quite important throughout exercise. As stated previously in the section on kyphosis, for strengthening exercises to be effective, some freedom of motion must be available.

Stretching exercises directed toward the concavity must address all of the spinal muscles (note that a right thoracic convexity results in a left lower thoracic concavity as well as associated right lumbar concavity with left lumbar convexity) (Fig. 15-26). Strengthening exercises are performed for all of the muscles affected on the convex side of each lateral curve.

Various stretching exercises can be performed in prone, side-lying, or heel-sitting position.[21] While prone, the patient places both hands behind his or her head while tilting the thorax away from the concave side of the curve (Fig. 15-27). In another prone stretching exercise, the patient reaches overhead and extends the arm on the concave side, thereby effectively stretching the thoracic concavity (Fig. 15-28). In the heel-sitting position, the patient places both hands forward and flat while emphasizing long-axis stretching. The lateral stretching component of this exercise is accomplished by having the patient slowly stretch both arms laterally away from the concave side of the curve (Fig. 15-29).

Static stretching can also be performed with the patient lying on the side. Place a small, soft rolled pillow or towel directly under the apex of the thoracic convex curve and support and stabilize the pelvis. For an advanced progression of side-lying stretching, the pa-

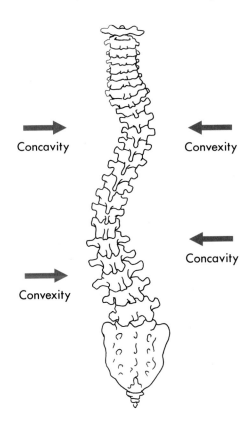

FIG. 15-26 Scoliosis. A right thoracic convexity will result in a left lower thoracic concavity as well as an associated right lumbar concavity with left lumbar convexity.

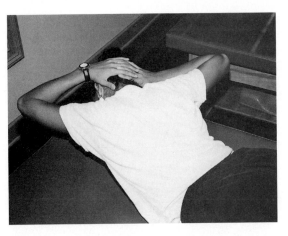

FIG. 15-27 Prone lateral trunk tilt. The patient is instructed to tilt (stretch) away from the concave side of the curve and towards the convexity.

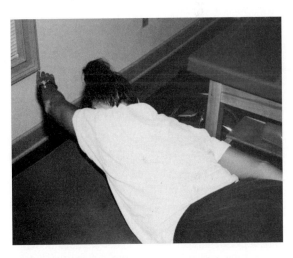

FIG. 15-28 Prone lateral trunk tilt with arm stretch. While prone the patient stretches (tilts) towards the convex side of the curve while extending the arm on the concave side, thereby effectively enhancing the thoracic stretch towards the concavity.

tient lies over the apex bolster toward the end of a treatment table (Fig. 15-30).

As alluded to earlier, trunk elongation (axial stretching) is also an effective stretching procedure used to treat scoliosis. Standing, the patient faces a wall and attempts to "walk up the wall" with both hands. The patient must reach as high as possible with both hands. A more progressive form of trunk elongation is to have the patient hang by both arms from an overhead bar.

Strengthening the thoracic and lumbar spine toward the convex side focuses on thoracic and lumbar extension strength as well as specific lateral strengthening maneuvers. Prone thoracic and lumbar spine active exercises were previously outlined and described. These are effective when used early to enhance the strength of the thorax.

Specific lateral strengthening can proceed with the patient in a side-lying position on the concave side of the curve. While you stabilize the trunk, have the patient lift the trunk up toward the convex side of the curve

(Fig. 15-31). This exercise can be viewed as a side-lying sit-up.

While this brief discussion has focused on a few rudimentary stretching and strengthening exercises for mild to moderate idiopathic scoliosis, an outline of surgical procedures to correct severe scoliosis is warranted. Surgery is reserved for severe symptomatic curves—those more than 50 to 60 degrees.[27] With surgery, curves of this magnitude can be improved by about 50%.[21] The exact surgery performed depends on

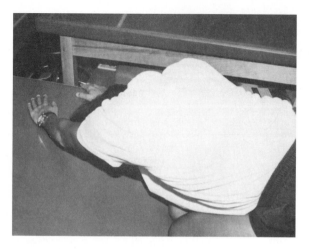

FIG. 15-29 Heel-sitting lateral trunk stretch with long-axis stretch and lateral stretch of both arms.

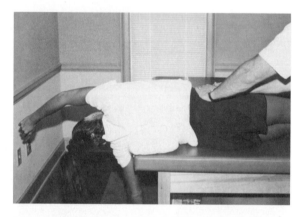

FIG. 15-30 Side lying apex stretch over the end of a table. A pillow is placed directly under the apex of the convex curve. With the patient's pelvis stabilized, the patient slowly stretches over the end of the table. Note the patient's arm position to enhance the stretch.

many factors. However, a spinal fusion with or without Harrington rod instrumentation[21] is designed to elongate and stabilize the spine and thereby reduce pain and improve appearance.

Physical therapy after spine fusion for advanced, severe scoliosis requires extensive convalescence, the application of a postoperative brace, and very limited activity for up to several months after surgery.[21]

THE CERVICAL SPINE

Without question, the most profound and catastrophic cervical spine injury is a fracture dislocation resulting in

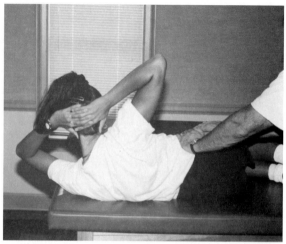

FIG. 15-31 Sidelying lateral trunk sit-up. With the patient's pelvis supported, the patient is instructed to lift the trunk towards the convex side of the curve.

quadriplegia. The description of these spinal injuries is beyond the scope of this chapter. This section will identify various soft tissue and bony injuries of the cervical spine common to orthopedic physical therapy.

Acute Sprains and Strains

Muscular strains of the cervical spine are fairly common among young athletes and in association with flexion-extension, lateral flexion, and acceleration-deceleration "whiplash" type automobile injuries.[34,40] The muscles involved in cervical strains appear to be the sternocleidomastoid, trapezius, scalenes, erectors, rhomboids, and levator scapulae.[40] The mechanism of injury producing cervical strains and sprains varies but includes hyperflexion, rotation, and lateral flexion of the head and cervical spine.[34]

Forces are usually great enough with automobile accidents that ligament injuries occur in conjunction with muscle strains. In fact, Stratton and Bryan's[34] experimental studies have demonstrated a rather wide range of tissue damage with hyperextension type automobile injuries:

1. Tearing of sternocleidomastoid muscle
2. Tearing of longissimus coli muscle
3. Pharyngeal edema
4. Tearing of anterior longitudinal ligament
5. Separation of cartilaginous end-plate of the intervertebral disc

With hyperflexion injuries as a result of automobile accidents, similar types of injuries occur:[34]

1. Tears of the posterior cervical muscles
2. Tears of the ligamentum nuchae

3. Tears of the posterior longitudinal ligament

4. Intervertebral disc injury

The treatment of traumatic cervical spine sprains and strains is symptomatic during the acute stage of recovery. The treating physician usually prescribes a course of analgesics, NSAIDs, or muscle relaxants; rest; and agents to control pain and swelling (heat, cold, ultrasound, electrical stimulation). The healing constraints of muscle and ligament tissues differ, and both must be addressed throughout recovery.

After the initial pain and swelling are controlled, the patient may be introduced to a series of active ROM exercises, cervical isometric strengthening exercises, and education in cervical posture mechanics. Initial ROM exercises must be approached cautiously to avoid reproducing the motion that caused the injury. As with all soft-tissue injuries, attention must be focused on protection of the affected area while striving to prevent further injury. If, for example, the mechanism of cervical sprain and strain was hyperflexion, care must be directed at avoiding the end range of head and neck flexion. Gentle active ROM exercises can proceed after moist heat application for 20 minutes to enhance muscle relaxation, relieve pain, and stimulate greater mobility.

An important practical matter to consider when instructing patients to perform cervical ROM exercises is how to stabilize the trunk and shoulders. With both muscle and ligament damage, the long-term effect of healing is fibrous tissue contraction, which results in stiffness, restriction, and limitation of motion.[40] Therefore to effectively direct the stretch to the affected area, the surrounding structures must be supported and stabilized. For example, assume a patient has a lateral flexion injury resulting in muscle and ligament damage. Without stabilizing the shoulders, if the patient is instructed to gently stretch laterally away from the side of the injury, the opposite shoulder would elevate (because of the shortened tissues), rendering the stretch ineffective. To stabilize the shoulder, the patient should perform the stretch while seated and use both hands to grasp under the seat. With the arms fully extended and secured under the seat, when the patient attempts to stretch the head and neck laterally, no shoulder elevation will occur.

Initial strengthening of the cervical spine after a muscle-tendon strain or ligamentous sprain is usually accompanied by isometric stabilization exercises. Submaximal contractions and precise techniques are exceedingly important, and they must be carefully explained and demonstrated to the patient. Before applying isometric exercises, the full cervical ROM must be achieved and pain controlled. For isometric stabilization exercises, the patient performs a series of four-way isometrics in an anatomically neutral cervical spine position.

The four-position isometric exercises are forward flexion, lateral flexion (right and left), and extension. In preparing to perform these exercises, the patient must demonstrate the ability to hold his or her head and neck in midline without excessive rotation, lateral flexion, forward flexion, or extension malalignment.

To begin, have the patient sit before a mirror to get visual feedback while maintaining proper head and neck alignment. Explain and demonstrate the proper execution of the first isometric position of forward flexion. With one hand placed on the midline of the forehead (the patient must bring the hand into the described position and not rotate the head toward the hand), have the patient direct a posterior force to the forehead with the hand while resisting head and neck flexion, thereby stimulating isometric strengthening of the anterior cervical muscles. Have the patient gradually and slowly "build" the resistance using the rule of tens (gradually initiate isometrics with 2-second submaximal contraction, then hold for 6 seconds, then slowly reduce for 2 seconds) rather than suddenly applying maximal force (Fig. 15-32).

For the second position, have the patient use both hands to support the occiput. The patient should maintain

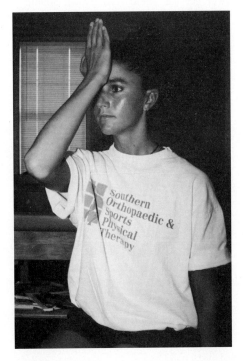

FIG. 15-32 Cervical isometrics for forward flexion. Notice the head must remain in midline and not be allowed to rotate.

the head and neck in the anatomical midline position and not allow the head to flex forward. Encourage the patient to gradually apply an anteriorly directed force with both hands while resisting extension of the head. This position effectively strengthens the head and neck extensor group (Fig. 15-33).

The next position is lateral flexion. While observing proper head and neck alignment in the mirror, have the patient bring one hand to the side of the head but do not allow the head to rotate or laterally flex to meet the hand. The patient then applies lateral pressure while resisting this force (Fig. 15-34). This position is repeated on the opposite side. In each position no head or neck motion must occur. Usually the patient carries out a series of 2 to 3 sets of 10-second isometric exercises two to three times daily. As strength improves, the patient gradually increases the intensity, but avoids sudden or ballistic contractions.

Educating the patient about cervical spine postural mechanics is as important as the actual management of any physical dysfunction. One of the most commonly recognized postural malalignment syndromes affecting the cervical spine is a forward head posture. Typically, this posture is characterized by a loss of flexion in the upper cervical spine region and a loss of extension in the lower cervical spine. The patient should perform axial extension or cervical retraction exercises. The physical therapist will determine which exercises are appropriate for each patient and will identify which patients are candidates for specific axial-extension exercises.

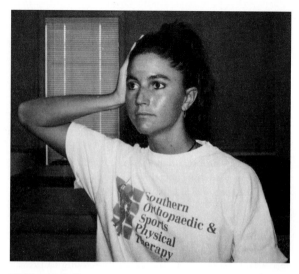

FIG. 15-34 Cervical isometrics for lateral flexion.

Retraction exercises require that the patient is able to demonstrate a midline neutral position. The patient may need to sit in front of a mirror initially to perform this exercise correctly. Have the patient imagine that his or her head is resting on a conveyor belt. The patient must be able to align the ears with the shoulders and move the head straight back on the conveyor belt (Fig. 15-35). If done correctly, as the patient moves the head back, a

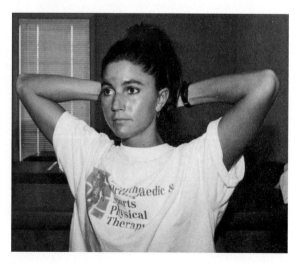

FIG. 15-33 Cervical isometrics for head and neck extension.

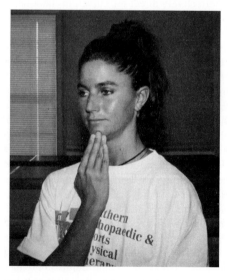

FIG. 15-35 Axial extension-cervical retraction. The head of the patient should move directly posterior. No head or cervical extension should occur. Attempt to produce a double chin without head or neck flexion.

"double chin" is produced. If done incorrectly, the head and neck move into extension. Encourage the patient to perform this exercise at home for multiple sets throughout the day or as prescribed by the physical therapist. Because this is a stretching exercise to improve motion restriction, each retraction of the head should be held for 10 seconds.

Full recovery from acute sprains and strains of the cervical spine involves the elimination of pain and swelling initially, appropriate rest from any aggravating positions, protection from unwanted stress, the return of normal cervical spine ROM, enhanced muscle strength through isometric stabilization exercises, worksite modifications, and postural-awareness activities (axial extension-retraction exercises).

Cervical Disc Injuries

The symptoms of peripheral pain, radicular signs, local cervical pain, and scapular pain are consistent with the symptoms of disc herniations observed in the lumbar spine.[34]

Iglarsh and Snyder-Mackler[18] define two types or positions of cervical spine motion that help alleviate the symptoms of disc herniations. In the first group, flexion activities improve the symptoms. In the second type, extension activities reduce symptoms.[18] As with lumbar disc herniations, the initial goals are to relieve symptoms, reduce pain and swelling, control muscle spasm, and work toward centralizing the symptoms. Iglarsh and Snyder-Mackler[18] define improvement in both categories as "a decrease in the extent and/or intensity of the peripheral symptoms."

The specific exercises for cervical disc herniation patients must be carefully identified by the physician and physical therapist. Once the appropriate category of relief is recognized,[18] the physical therapist organizes a comprehensive plan of pain relief, motion, strength, and postural education activities for the physical therapist assistant to follow and apply. In the flexion group, motion is slowly developed into flexion, with close observation and documentation of any changes in radicular signs. In the extension group, the initial activities focus on axial extension and retraction. In either case, the aim is to accurately identify which motions and positions exacerbate the pain. Once these are recognized, the patient is taught to avoid these positions. As the signs and symptoms of radicular pain begin to centralize, the physical therapist may initiate isometric stabilization exercises, with extreme caution to avoid positions or intensity of contractions that increase symptoms.

Cervical Spondylosis

In contrast to cervical disc herniations, **cervical spondylosis** involves chronic rather than acute degenerative disc, which results from "wear and tear on the weight-bearing structures of the cervical spine."[34] The symptoms are characteristic of spinal cord compression (myelopathy) or nerve root compression with radicular signs.[27] Cervical spondylosis is seen most often during the fourth and fifth decades of life and characteristically affects men more than women at the C5-C6 and C6-C7 segments.[27]

Sustained impact loading and repetitive microtrauma[34] are causative factors that can produce cervical cord impingement, nerve root impingement, osteophytes, bone sclerosis, loss of cervical lordosis, and central or posterolateral disc herniations.[27,34]

Initial physical therapy interventions focus on pain relief with thermal and electrical agents, physician-prescribed analgesics, and rest from aggravating positions. A semirigid cervical collar may be of some use in select cases. As with other disc conditions, the physical therapist provides a comprehensive evaluation to accurately determine which motions cause pain and radicular symptoms and which relieve pain. From this detailed initial evaluation, the physical therapist outlines and describes specific exercises consistent with these findings. Axial extension-retraction exercises are effective for patients who derive pain relief from extension. Flexion-type activities are reserved for patients who obtain relief from cervical flexion. In either case, traction is an effective tool to minimize joint compressive loads and reduce cord compression or nerve root irritation.[27] The physical therapist will determine if mechanical traction or manual cervical traction is more appropriate. Isometric cervical spine stabilization exercises (four-way isometrics) and ROM exercises are initiated once pain has been reduced and the appropriateness of these activities is determined by the physical therapist.

When cord compression (myelopathy) progresses and radicular pain persists, the physician can use various surgical interventions. Miller[27] describes an anterior cervical spine approach to accomplish a discectomy and fusion or a posterior approach for a foraminotomy or multilevel laminectomy to relieve cord and/or root compression.

Because cervical spondylosis is a chronic degenerative condition, long-term care involves protection from inappropriate and unwanted forces and instruction in cervical posture mechanics, flexibility exercises, and strengthening activities.

Thoracic Outlet Syndrome

Some texts cover **thoracic outlet (inlet) syndrome** within the subject matter affecting the shoulder.[41] Because of the anatomic proximity of the structures involved, this condition is discussed within the context of

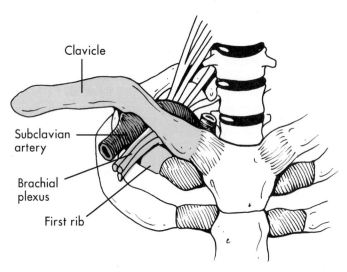

FIG. 15-36 Thoracic outlet syndrome. Note proximal compression of the subclavian artery and vein as well as the brachial plexus.

the cervical spine. Authorities[34,41] point out that the term *thoracic inlet syndrome*[34] is a more precise and anatomically-accurate term used to describe compression of vascular and/or neurologic tissues as they exit the "superior triangle opening of the thorax"[41] (Fig. 15-36). Specifically, proximal compression of the subclavian artery and vein as well as the brachial plexus is the most probable neurovascular factor involved with thoracic inlet syndrome.[34] Many structures can cause compression of these tissues. Foremost is the presence of a cervical rib, a shortened or hypertrophied anterior scalene muscle, or malunion of the clavicle and subluxed first thoracic rib.[15,34,41] Symptoms of this condition include radicular signs of pain, numbness, tingling, weakness, and skin and temperature changes consistent with neurovascular tissue compression.[15,34,41]

Typically, physical therapy management addresses specifically defined limitations of movement and affected bony or soft tissues during the initial evaluation performed by the physical therapist. Once the physical therapist has determined which specific tissues are affected and has also identified any underlying causes of postural variations, an individualized comprehensive program of stretching, strengthening, and education can commence.

Soft-tissue stretching focuses on the anterior scalene muscles. The patient is instructed to laterally flex and extend the head to the opposite side of the shortened muscle (Fig. 15-37). Thoracic kyphosis tends to accentuate the symptoms of thoracic inlet syndrome, so pectoral stretching (facing an open doorway with hands

on either side and leaning forward) and thoracic extension mobility and strengthening exercises are used to specifically address muscle weakness and soft tissue restrictions. A host of clinically applicable thoracic extension mobility exercises can be used. Examples include seated scapular retraction, prone scapular and thoracic extension, and seated rowing activities with elastic tubing.

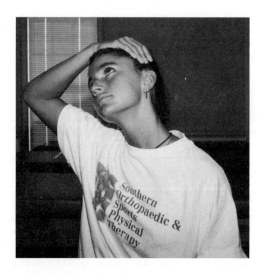

FIG. 15-37 Stretching of the anterior scalene muscles by laterally flexing and extending the head towards the opposite side of the shortened muscle. Note the gentle overpressure provided by the hand.

In addition to stretching and strengthening exercises, cervical posture correction is needed; poor cervical posture is a common problem in the workplace.[15] To address the forward head posture and tight anterior neck muscles, the patient can perform axial extension or cervical retraction stretching exercises, as previously described.

The effective management of thoracic inlet syndrome focuses on specific stretching of affected muscles, thoracic mobility, and extension strengthening, as well as education concerning proper cervical spine alignment and the performance of cervical retraction exercises.

MOBILIZATION OF THE LUMBAR, THORACIC, AND CERVICAL SPINE

Although peripheral joint mobilization is covered in this text, axial skeleton mobilization techniques for the lumbar, thoracic, and cervical spine are not addressed. The extraordinarily complex arrangement and intimate anatomic relationship between vertebral segments and surrounding neurovascular structures require intense, exhaustive study and precise application of techniques after detailed training and clinical practice to be safe, effective, and efficient. The scope of the physical therapist assistant's training is not consistent with the demanding working knowledge of neurovascular anatomy, biomechanics, and pathophysiology of the lumbar, thoracic, and cervical spine needed to provide mobilization techniques to these areas.

REFERENCES

1. Allman FL: Back school program, The Atlanta Sports Medicine Clinic, PC, Introduction to Back injuries, 1990.
2. Brashear HR, Raney RB: Affections of the spine and thorax in: *Handbook of orthopaedic surgery,* ed 10, St. Louis, 1986, Mosby.
3. Burkus JK: Spine. In Loth T, editor: *Orthopaedic boards review,* St. Louis, 1993, Mosby.
4. Cailliet R: Low back pain syndrome, ed 3, Philadelphia, 1981, FA Davis.
5. Chappuis JL, Johnson GD, Gines AM: A source guide for spine care, Atlanta, Ga., 1994, Greater Atlanta Spine Center.
6. DeLee JC et al: Therapeutic exercise modalities. In Drez D, editor: *Therapeutic modalities for sports injuries,* American Orthopedic Society for Sports Medicine, St. Louis, 1989, Year Book.
7. DeRosa C, Porterfield JA: Lumbar spine and pelvis. In Richardson JK, Iglarsh ZA, editors: *Clinical orthopaedic physical therapy,* Philadelphia, 1994, WB Saunders.
8. Dietrich N, Kurowski P: The importance of mechanical factors in the etiology of spondylolysis: a model analysis of loads and stresses in the human lumbar spine, *Spine* 10(6):532-541, 1985.
9. Duda M: Elite lifters at risk of spondylolysis, *Phys and Sports Med* 15(10):57-58, 1987.
10. Edgelow PI: Dysfunction, evaluation, and treatment of the lumbar spine. In Donatelli R, Wooden MJ, editors: *Orthopaedic physical therapy,* New York, 1989, Churchill Livingstone.
11. Eismont FJ, Kitchel SH: Thoracolumbar spine. In DeLee JC, Drez D, editors: *Orthopaedic sports medicine: principals and practice,* vol 2, Philadelphia, 1994, WB Saunders.
12. Fulton M: *Lower-back pain: a new solution for an old problem,* Rolling Meadows, Ill., 1992, MedX Inc.
13. Goldstein TS: Treatment of common problems of the spine. In Lewis CB, editor: *Geriatric orthopaedics, rehabilitative management of common problems, Aspen series in physical therapy,* Gaithersburg, Md., 1991, Aspen Publishers.
14. Gould JA: The spine. In Gould JA, editor: *Orthopaedic and sports physical therapy,* ed 2, St. Louis, 1990, Mosby.
15. Hebert LA: *The neck-arm-hand book,* 1989, Greenville, Mass., IMPACC.
16. Hebert LA: *Your back for life,* IMPACC, 1993, Greenville, Me.
17. Holley TR: Biology of aging: the musculoskeletal system, Geriatric Physical Therapy course notes, February, Reno, Nev., 1995.
18. Iglarsh ZA, Snyder-Mackler L: Temporomandibular joint and the cervical spine. In Richardson JK, Iglarsh ZA, editors: *Clinical orthopaedic physical therapy,* Philadelphia, 1994, WB Saunders.
19. Jackson DW: Low back pain in young athletes: evaluation of stress reaction and discogenic problems, *Am J Sports Med* 7(6):364-366, 1979.
20. Kaiser RK, Rose SJ, Apts DW: An electromyographic analysis of two techniques for squat lifting, Washington University School of Medicine, Applied Kinesiology Laboratory, Program in Physical Therapy.
21. Kisner C, Colby LA: Scoliosis. In *Therapeutic exercise foundations and techniques* ed 2, Philadelphia, 1989, FA Davis.
22. Kisner C, Colby LA: The spine: treatment of acute problems. In *Therapeutic exercise foundations and techniques,* ed 2, Philadelphia, 1990, FA Davis.
23. Lewis CB, Bottomley JM: Orthopaedic treatment considerations. In *Geriatric physical therapy, a clinical approach,* New York, 1994, Appleton & Lange.
24. Macnab I: *Backache,* Baltimore, 1977, Williams & Wilkins.
25. McKenzie RA: The lumbar spine, mechanical diagnosis and therapy, Waikanae, New Zealand, 1981, *Spinal Publications.*
26. McRae R: *Practical fracture treatment,* ed 3, New York, 1994, Churchill-Livingstone.
27. Miller MD: Spine. In *Review of Orthopaedics,* Philadelphia, 1992, WB Saunders.
28. O'Sullivan JJ, Ellis JJ, Makofsky HW: The five "L's" of lifting, *Physical Therapy Forum* 10(14), April, Forum Publishing, 1991.

29. Panjabi M et al: A biochemical model, *Spine* 14(2), 1989.

30. Paris SV: The spine, etiology and treatment of dysfunction including joint manipulation, Atlanta Ga., 1979, Course notes.

31. Sawyer M, Zbieraneck CK: The treatment of soft tissue after spinal injury, *Clin in Sports Med* 5(2), April, 1986.

32. Shankman GA: Strengthening the lumbar spine in athletics, *NSCA J* 15(4):15-22, 1993.

33. Spengler DM, Szpalski M: Newer assessment approaches for the patient with low back pain, *Contem Ortho* 21(4), October, 1990.

34. Stratton SA, Bryan JM: Dysfunction, evaluation and treatment of the cervical spine and thoracic inlet. In Donatelli R, Wooden MJ, editors: *Orthopaedic physical therapy*, New York, 1989, Churchill-Livingstone.

35. Tan JC: Understanding lumbar strength testing In: *Advance for physical therapists*, October, 1992, Merion Publications.

36. U.S. Physical Therapy: Worksite partners, functional capacity evaluation system, industrial rehabilitation solutions, System Manual, U.S.P.T., Houston, 1994.

37. Watkins RG, Dillin WH: Lumbar spine injury in the athlete, *Clin in Sports Med* 9(2), April, 1990.

38. Wiltse LL: Spondylolisthesis in children, *Clin Orthop* 21:156-163, 1957.

39. Wiltse LL, Widell EH, Jackson DW: Fatigue fracture: the basic lesion in isthmic spondylolisthesis, *J Bone Joint Surg* 57A(1):17-22, 1975.

40. Wroble RR, Albright JP: Neck and low back injuries in wrestling. In *Clinics in sports medicine, injuries to the spine,* vol 5, no 2, Philadelphia, 1986, WB Saunders.

41. Yahara ML: Shoulder. In Richardson JK, Iglarsh ZA, editors: *Clinical orthopaedic physical therapy,* Philadelphia, 1994, WB Saunders.

Orthopedic Management of the Shoulder

LEARNING OBJECTIVES

1. Identify and describe methods, management, and rehabilitation for subacromial rotator cuff impingement.
2. Identify and describe methods of management and rehabilitation for tears of the rotator cuff.
3. Describe methods of management and rehabilitation for glenohumeral instability.
4. Discuss methods of management and rehabilitation for adhesive capsulitis.
5. Identify and describe common injuries of the acromioclavicular (A-C) joint.
6. Describe common methods of management and rehabilitation for injuries of the A-C joint.
7. Identify and describe common fractures of the scapula, clavicle, and proximal humerus.
8. Outline and describe methods of management and rehabilitation of fractures about the shoulder.
9. Describe methods of management and rehabilitation following shoulder arthroplasty.
10. Describe common mobilization techniques for the shoulder.

KEY TERMS

Subacromial rotator cuff
  impingement
Scapular stabilization
  exercises
Codman's pendulum
  exercises
Dislocation
Subluxation
Bankart lesion
Hill-Sachs lesion
TUBS
AMBRI
Capsulitis
Acromioclavicular (A-C)
  joint
Open reduction and
  internal fixation
  (ORIF)

CHAPTER OUTLINE

This chapter introduces common injuries, treatment, and rehabilitation procedures related to the glenohumeral joint, acromioclavicular joint, scapula, and proximal humerus. To fully understand the rationale for specific rehabilitation programs after injury or disease of the shoulder complex and surrounding tissues, the assistant is strongly encouraged to review pertinent anatomy and kinesiology of the glenohumeral, acromioclavicular, and scapulothoracic joints. Furthermore, the assistant should review the mechanisms of tissue healing because these principles will clarify tissue healing concepts and reinforce the need for early protected motion after injury, immobilization, and recovery of strength and function following injury to the shoulder complex. This section focuses on the recognition of certain orthopedic injuries and rehabilitation procedures used to reduce pain and swelling, improve motion, restore strength and power, and return the patient to normal function.

SUBACROMIAL ROTATOR CUFF IMPINGEMENT

A common cause of shoulder pain and dysfunction in laborers, athletes, and persons who do repetitive overhead lifting is **subacromial rotator cuff impingement**. In this disorder, the tendons of the rotator cuff are crowded, buttressed, or compressed under the coracoacromial arch, resulting in mechanical wear, stress, and friction (Fig. 16-1).[7,9] Clinically, distinction must be made between primary and secondary impingement because there are important differences in treatment related to the cause of the impingement:[7,9]

1. Primary shoulder impingement refers to mechanical compression of the rotator cuff tendons, primarily the supraspinatus tendon,[21] as they pass under the coracoacromial ligament between the acromion and the coracoid process.[7,13,21]
2. Secondary shoulder impingement is related to glenohumeral instability that creates a reduced subacromial space because the humeral head elevates and minimizes the area under the coracoacromial ligament.[7,9,13]

Age-related degenerative changes can also result in a decreased subacromial margin between the rotator cuff and the coracoacromial arch. Bony osteophyte formation can occupy space under the anteroinferior surface of the acromion, which therefore reduces the available space.[21] The supraspinatus tendon is the most common structure involved with rotator cuff impingement; the vascularity of the supraspinatus tendon is causative.[7,9,21] An area just proximal to the insertion on the greater tuberosity is hypovascular and is commonly referred to as a "watershed zone,"[21] "critical zone,"[7] or "critical portion."[25]

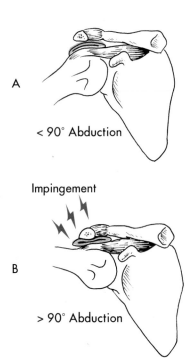

FIG. 16-1 Subacromial rotator cuff impingement. **A,** Less than 90 degrees of abduction, no impingement occurs. **B,** Greater than 90 degrees of abduction results in subacromial soft tissue impingement under the coracoacromial arch.

This area of relative transient hypovascularity occurs with repeated arm motions from abduction to adduction, which compromises the blood supply to the area.[7,25] The combination of reduced blood supply to the supraspinatus tendon and mechanical wear, stress, and friction as a result of repeated overhead motions can lead to primary impingement, supraspinatus tendinitis, and ultimately tears within the rotator cuff.[7,9,21]

The various stages of rotator cuff impingement are related to age and degenerative changes in the cuff itself. Neer[17] has identified three specific stages of impingement (tendinitis):[7,9,17,21,25]

Stage I: Occurs in younger patients (usually under 25 years of age), but can occur at any age. Clinical features are edema and hemorrhage. Pain is worse with shoulder abduction greater than 90 degrees.[2-5] Essentially a reversible lesion that responds to conservative physical therapy interventions.[4]

Stage II: The fibrosis and tendinitis stage, which usually affects patients between the ages of 25 and 40 years.[3,4] Classified as irreversible because of long-term repeated stress wherein the supraspinatus tendon, biceps tendon, and subacromial bursa become fibrotic.[21] Pain is the predominant feature and occurs with daily activities; it frequently causes the patient difficulty at night.[21,25]

Stage III: Affects patients over the age of 40 years. Is characterized by tendon degeneration, rotator cuff tears, and rotator cuff ruptures.[13,21] Usually associated with a long history of repeated shoulder pain and dysfunction as well as significant muscle weakness and atrophy.[21]

Various clinical tests can be used to identify the presence of pain related to specific maneuvers of the shoulder. During the initial evaluation performed by the physical therapist, tests are used to elicit impingement signs. Pain signifies impingement with an arc of shoulder abduction between 60 and 120 degrees, pain with forward shoulder flexion, and pain with forced internal rotation with the affected arm abducted to 90 degrees.[7] In most cases, flexion and/or abduction more than 80 or 90 degrees elicits pain. Therefore exercise and all activities that require the shoulder to flex and/or abduct past 80 or 90 degrees must be strictly avoided until all symptoms of pain have been eliminated.

Rehabilitation of Primary and Secondary Rotator Cuff Impingement

Kamkar, Irrgang, and Whitney[9] have identified scapular weakness as leading to "function scapular instability," which affects scapular position during activities that cause a "relative decrease in the subacromial space."[9] This secondary impingement requires the scapulothoracic muscles to be strengthened and stabilized before specific rotator cuff weakness can be addressed. To effectively stabilize the humeral head so that it does not migrate superiorly, causing "winging" or "tipping,"[9] the scapular muscles (serratus anterior, upper, middle, and lower trapezius, levator scapulae, and rhomboid muscles)[9] must be strengthened. Thein[22] describes the clinical features of humeral head migration (secondary impingement) as possibly confusing the typical impingement picture. She reports: "If the supraspinatus is overworked trying to stabilize the humeral head, then it is unable to effectively function to depress the humeral head. The resultant upward movement decreases the subacromial space and irritates the subacromial soft tissues thus perpetuating the impingement process."[22]

The initial evaluation performed by the physical therapist is crucial in determining which exercises are to be performed to help stabilize the scapula and which exercises should be avoided initially to reduce rotator cuff irritation with glenohumeral instability or superior migration of the humeral head.

Scapular stabilization exercises are only one component of a successful rehabilitation program. In general, a comprehensive rehabilitation program to address rotator cuff impingement, rotator cuff tendinitis (supraspinatus tendinitis), and degenerative tears of the rotator cuff tendons will include modification of activities, local and systemic methods to control pain and swelling (nonsteroidal antiinflammatory drugs [NSAIDs], corticosteroid injections, ice, ultrasound, iontophoresis, phonophoresis), stretching and strengthening exercises, and a return to normal function after reevaluation by the physical therapist and with continued maintenance of protective positions and general conditioning.[7,25]

The nonoperative treatment of impingement and symptomatic rotator cuff tears focuses on a three-phase criterion-based rehabilitation program advocated by Voight.[25] Phase I, the acute stage, concentrates on relief of symptoms and initiating exercises to improve or maintain motion. Because impingement symptoms are usually made worse with overhead activities, the patient must modify activities of daily living (ADLs) and all other motions that may place the shoulder at or above 80 to 90 degrees of abduction and/or forward flexion. Home activities that require modification include cleaning hard-to-reach places and painting overhead. Worksite tasks that must be adapted include heavy overhead lifting, manual labor, reaching, and climbing. Sporting activities such as tennis, golf, swimming, and baseball must also be modified to avoid impingement. The key to remember in each case is *modification,* not elimination, of compromising activities. For example, for a recreational tennis player, overhead serving should be avoided but all other ground strokes can be maintained. For household activities and worksite modifications, rearrangement and advanced planning of overhead tasks may be all that is needed to minimize the aggravating position of forward flexion or abduction past 80 or 90 degrees. The physical therapist assistant must constantly reinforce the concept of protective positioning and should encourage compliance throughout the course of rehabilitation.

In addition to activity modification, management of pain and swelling can be achieved with various physician-prescribed oral NSAIDs and physical therapy agents. Usually ice packs, ultrasound, and some type of pharmacophoresis (iontophoresis and phonophoresis)[25] help control symptoms.

Throughout phase I, stretching exercises are performed to increase blood flow and contractility[7] and to improve motion. The physical therapist assistant must pay particular attention to performing all stretching activities because many generalized shoulder stretches involve full forward shoulder flexion and abduction maneuvers. All phase I stretching should encourage nonballistic, slow, controlled, pain-free motion at less than 80 to 90 degrees of flexion and abduction. However, once symptoms are managed, the patient can perform all stretches involving flexion and abduction if these stretches do not produce symptoms. Depending on the initial evaluation data gathered by the physical therapist, the patient may be instructed in two specific stretches that authorities[7,25] suggest are effective in addressing posterior capsular tightness. Shoulder adduction across the chest (cross-body stretching) and internal shoulder rotation are used cautiously to improve posterior capsular tightness and overcome the limitations on motion of internal rotation of the shoulder.

Initial strengthening activities can begin during phase I but are generally reserved for phase II, the recovery stage. Once the patient demonstrates improved motion without pain and can do ADLs without pain, phase II can begin. It emphasizes regaining the strength of the rotator cuff and scapular stabilizers, improving motion, and maintaining activity modifications. Specific rotator cuff strengthening exercises focus on the supraspinatus muscle. Studies[4,23] demonstrate that the supraspinatus, infraspinatus, subscapularis, deltoid, latissimus dorsi, and pectoral muscles are effectively strengthened by arm elevation in the sagittal plane (Fig. 16-2), shoulder elevation with internal rotation in the plane of the scapula (Fig. 16-3), prone horizontal shoulder abduction with external rotation (Fig. 16-4), and seated press-ups (Fig. 16-5).[4,22,23]

Scapular stabilization exercises are also encouraged as part of a comprehensive glenohumeral and scapulothoracic strengthening program. Electromyographic

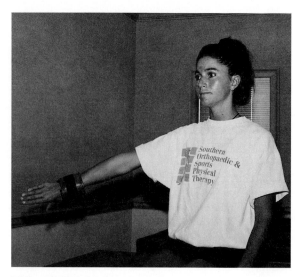

FIG. 16-3 Scaption. Shoulder elevation with internal rotation in the plane of the scapula.

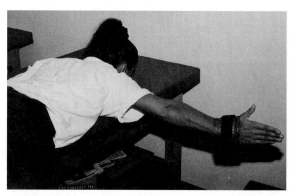

FIG. 16-4 Prone horizontal shoulder abduction with external rotation.

studies[16] have identified four basic scapular stabilization exercises that strengthen the upper, middle, and lower trapezius; the levator scapula; the rhomboid major; the pectoralis minor; and the middle and lower serratus anterior muscles.[16] The exercises are rowing, scapular plane elevation (scaption), press-ups, and push-ups followed by scapular protraction.[16] As strength improves and when motion increases, a gradual return to normal function signifies the beginning of phase III.

The process of functional recovery is slow and must be done cautiously. Overhead activities are introduced incrementally as the patient is able to demonstrate pain-free motion and the ability to perform strengthening activities.

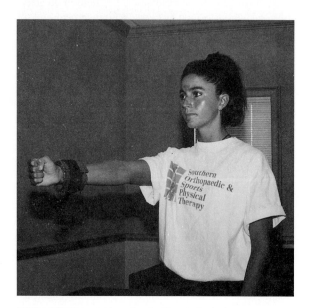

FIG. 16-2 Arm elevation in the sagittal plane.

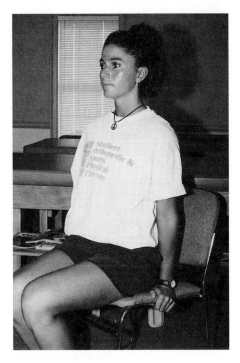

FIG. 16-5 Seated press-up.

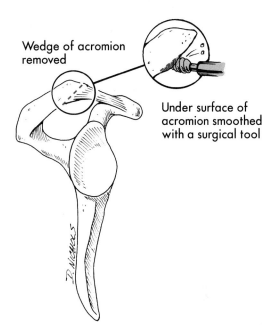

Wedge of acromion removed

Under surface of acromion smoothed with a surgical tool

FIG. 16-6 Subacromial decompression for impingement.

Surgical Management of Shoulder Impingement and Rotator Cuff Tears

When physical therapy interventions fail to provide long-lasting relief and in cases of rotator cuff tears (Neer's stage III impingement, tendon degeneration, and cuff tears), various surgical procedures can be used to correct the underlying pathologic condition. With subacromial impingement not involving a specific rotator cuff tear, subacromial decompression can be used to "eliminate or diminish the abnormality causing the impingement between the humeral head and the undersurface of the acromion, allowing freer movement of the tendons without irritation."[25] Miller[14] has outlined surgical options that comprise subacromial decompression. These options include coracoacromial ligament resection (Fig. 16-6), anterior acromioplasty, excision of the outer end of the clavicle, osteotomies of the glenoid and/or acromion, acromionectomy, and combinations of these procedures.[14,25] If there is an associated rotator cuff tear (small tear less than 1 cm, medium tear less than 3 cm, large tear greater than 5 cm),[14] a subacromial decompression procedure is used in conjunction with direct repair of the rotator cuff defect.[14] The subacromial decompression procedure can be performed as an open arthrotomy or as an arthroscopic procedure.[7]

Rehabilitation after subacromial decompression and/or rotator cuff repair closely parallels nonoperative rehabilitation of rotator cuff impingement. However, time must be allowed for healing of the soft tissues and bone after surgery.

Some clearly identified differences exist between rehabilitation procedures used for decompression and small cuff tears (less than 1 cm) and repairs of medium (less than 3 cm) and large (greater than 5 cm) cuff tears with subacromial decompression.[7,14,25] With a small cuff tear repaired in conjunction with a decompression procedure, active motion and pain-free exercise can begin as soon as the patient can tolerate these activities.[7,14,25] However, if the rotator cuff tear is between 1 and 5 cm, tissue protection must be longer to allow for extensive soft tissue healing. If full active range of motion (ROM) is allowed too early, healing of the rotator cuff may be compromised because of the stresses placed on the repaired tissues. Wilk and Mangine[28] state that "rehabilitation must match the surgical procedure"; therefore the physical therapist will choose procedures to parallel the size of the cuff defect, "the adequacy of the repair,"[25] the type of surgical procedure used (open procedure—anterior deltoid fiber resection; mini-open procedure—lateral deltoid fiber splitting and arthroscopic decompression),[28] as well as the healing constraints required for a secure repair. Thus larger cuff tears require longer periods of time for recovery to achieve improved healing.

Generally, recovery after subacromial decompression with or without rotator cuff repair follows a prescribed three-phase rehabilitation program.* Phase I, the early recovery period (acute stage) or maximum-protection phase, lasts approximately 6 weeks[28] and focuses on control of pain and swelling with NSAIDs, oral analgesics, ice packs, ultrasound, phonophoresis, iontophoresis, TENs, and various degrees and durations of immobilization, depending on the extent of tissue injury. Depending on the precise nature of the injury and which surgical procedure is used (if any), the concept of early protected motion applies. **Codman's pendulum exercises** can be used within the first few weeks to restore mobility and influence the mechanoreceptor system.

With small rotator cuff repairs (less than 1 cm),[28] isometric submaximal muscle sets of the shoulder abductors, external rotators, internal rotators, elbow flexors, and shoulder flexors can begin as early as pain allows. Active assisted ROM activities using a wall-pulley system begins during the first 3 weeks of recovery[28] and must be performed pain-free. As pain and swelling are controlled, ROM and strength gradually increase.

With increased strength and motion, phase II, the intermediate or fibroblastic phase, can begin.[25] It generally lasts from weeks 7 through 12 after surgery. During this moderate-protection phase, progressive motion can be used, although with caution for repetitive shoulder abduction and forward flexion above 90 degrees. Strength is increased using elastic tubing. In addition, dumbbell isotonic concentric and eccentric exercises, humeral head stabilization exercises (scapular stabilization exercises),[16] and the maintenance of pain and swelling control procedures are components of phase II management. Reinforcement of shoulder protection is then addressed, specifically avoiding repetitive motions that may slow the healing process. During phase II, local muscle resistance exercises are carried out in a pain-free, noncompromising position (above 90 degrees of shoulder abduction and/or flexion).

Phase III, the minimal-protection or maturation and tissue remodeling phase,[25] can begin once the patient can demonstrate increased motion without symptoms and with improved strength. This phase lasts approximately from week 13 to week 21[28] and is characterized by a gradual return to normal activities.

During each phase of recovery (maximal, moderate, and minimal protection), core rotator cuff strengthening exercises of forward flexion, scaption, prone horizontal abduction with external rotation, and press-ups,[23] as well as scapular (humeral head) stabilization[9] exercises of rowing, scaption, press-ups, and scapular protraction (push-ups with a plus),[9,16,25] form the foundation of improving strength that eventually leads to full functional recovery.

The recovery phases and periods of passive motion are rather extensive for rehabilitation after surgical repair of massive rotator cuff tears. Generally, no active shoulder motion or active concentric or eccentric strengthening is allowed for 3 to 4 months after surgery.[13,25] Extensive soft tissue healing must proceed unabated to foster the recovery of functional motion and strength.

Initially, after surgery, the patient is placed in a brace, splint (airplane splint), sling, or abduction pillow to allow the repaired tissues of the rotator cuff and deltoid to be shortened. Early active muscle strengthening and active motion are avoided to allow for appropriate healing. Generally, passive ROM with full motion restriction is allowed during the first several weeks of recovery. Codman's pendulum exercises as well as very gentle active assistive ROM activities can begin after the first 3 months following surgery.[13,25]

Submaximal isometrics and scapular stabilization exercises must be added cautiously 8 to 16 weeks after surgery.[13,25] Specific rotator cuff strengthening exercises[23] performed isotonically with dumbbells, Theraband, and so on are reserved until 3 to 4 months after surgery to accommodate the healing constraints of the tendons and muscles of the rotator cuff and deltoid. Full functional recovery of motion and strength may take up to 10 months after the repair of massive rotator cuff tears.[25]

GLENOHUMERAL JOINT INSTABILITY AND DISLOCATION

Dislocations and **subluxations** (partial dislocation) of the glenohumeral joint (the articulation between the humeral head and the glenoid fossa of the scapula) frequently occur after indirect trauma with the arm abducted, extended, and externally rotated[21] (anterior dislocation) and with the arm abducted, flexed, and internally rotated (posterior dislocation) (Fig. 16-7).[21] The shoulder is the most commonly dislocated joint in the body,[13] and dislocation occurs in men more often than women. Anterior dislocations occur more frequently than posterior dislocations.[13,21] Authorities classify shoulder instability based on frequency, cause,

---

*References 7, 12, 14, 22, 25, 28.

A

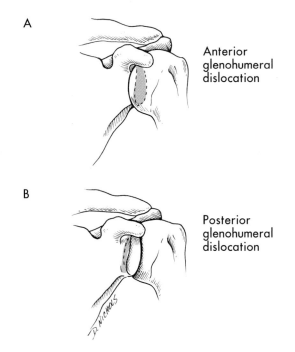

Anterior
glenohumeral
dislocation

B

Posterior
glenohumeral
dislocation

FIG. 16-7 Anterior and posterior glenohumeral dislocations. **A,** Anterior glenohumeral dislocation. **B,** Posterior glenohumeral dislocation.

direction, and degree of instability.[13,19] Also, rotator cuff tears of various dimensions (small less than 1 cm, medium less than 3 cm, and large greater than 5 cm) occur with relative frequency.[21] Strege[21] reports that

rotator cuff tears occur 30% of the time with acute anterior dislocations in patients over age 40 and 80% of the time in patients over age 60.

Two associated injuries may occur as a result of acute glenohumeral dislocation and instability. Because the shoulder is the most mobile joint in the body, bony restrictions do not provide substantial restraint.[19] Rather, the fibrocartilaginous glenoid labrum deepens the articulation between the humeral head and the bony glenoid fossa (Fig. 16-8). If forces are great enough to dislocate the humerus from its confines within the glenoid, injury to the labrum can occur. This injury is referred to as a **Bankart lesion**[7,13,19,21,22] and is defined as "an avulsion of the capsule and glenoid labrum off of the anterior rim of the glenoid resulting from traumatic anterior dislocation of the shoulder" (Fig. 16-9).[21]

The head of the humerus is subject to injury as a result of anterior shoulder instability. A **Hill-Sachs lesion** is a compression or "impaction fracture"[19] of the posterolateral aspect of the humeral head as a result of anterior shoulder instability (Fig. 16-10).* This lesion results from instability and is not the essential cause of glenohumeral instability.[19]

As previously stated, anterior dislocations are more prevalent than posterior dislocations. However, shoulder instability can be defined as multidirectional, wherein the humeral head may sublux or dislocate anteriorly, interiorly, and posteriorly.[14,19,21]

---

*References 7, 13, 14, 19, 21, 22.

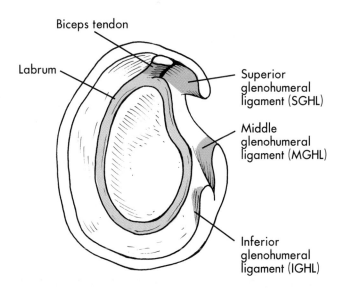

Biceps tendon

Labrum

Superior
glenohumeral
ligament (SGHL)

Middle
glenohumeral
ligament (MGHL)

Inferior
glenohumeral
ligament (IGHL)

FIG. 16-8 Anatomy of glenoid labrum.

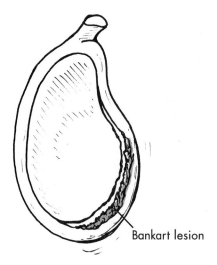

FIG. 16-9 Bankart lesion.

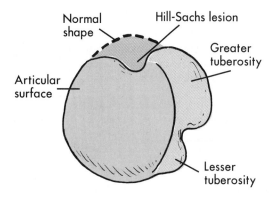

FIG. 16-10 Hill-Sachs lesion.

Nonoperative Management

The initial management of acute shoulder dislocations (anterior and posterior) calls for a period of immobilization lasting for up to 6 weeks.[19,27] All positions that may reproduce the mechanism of dislocation are avoided.

Management of pain and swelling is addressed with physician-prescribed NSAIDs, analgesics, ice packs, electrical stimulation, or other physical agents. While the patient is immobilized, the hand, wrist, and elbow of the affected shoulder must receive active motion and rudimentary strengthening exercises that do not compromise the shoulder. Also, a general conditioning program of strength, flexibility, and endurance activities can begin during immobilization. With an anterior shoulder subluxation (spontaneous reduction of the humeral head) or dislocation, the patient must avoid shoulder abduction and external rotation to allow proper capsular scarring and soft tissue healing to occur. Interestingly, patients older than age 40 who are not at significant risk of recurrent dislocation because of a relatively sedentary lifestyle may only need immobilization for a couple of weeks before rehabilitation can begin and motion can be regained.[19] Generally, after immobilization, ROM exercises are employed as the patient tolerates.

Codman's pendulum exercises, active assistive stretching for flexion, and cable pulleys help the patient regain lost motion after relatively lengthy immobilization while protecting the shoulder from excessive abduction and external rotation.

Initial strengthening begins while the patient is immobilized and pain is controlled. Submaximal isometric exercises can be safely started while the patient's shoulder and arm are adducted and internally rotated in the shoulder sling and immobilizer. Isometric shoulder adduction and abduction, internal and external rotation, and flexion and extension can be performed at a pain-free level while immobilized. Once the patient can demonstrate an increase from submaximal isometric contractions to near-maximal contractions, progressive internal and external rotation can begin using latex rubber tubing with the affected shoulder in zero degrees of abduction.[27]

When the symptoms of pain are reduced and the intensity and quality of muscle contractions are improved, the patient may increase ROM activities to forward flexion, extension, scapular mobility, and internal and external rotation and abduction. As the patient progresses through the moderate-protection phase, combined shoulder abduction and external rotation are avoided. In fact, some authorities recommend avoiding extremes of shoulder abduction and external rotation for 3 months after removal of the sling.[19] The hallmark of the moderate-protection and minimal-protection phases of recovery after anterior shoulder dislocation or subluxation is progressive strengthening of the rotator cuff, anterior shoulder muscles, and scapular stabilizers, paying particular attention to eccentric strengthening of the posterior rotator cuff (infraspinatus and teres minor).[22] Latex rubber tubing and cuff weights are effective because of the wide variety of motions that can be addressed and can carry over to home exercises.

Synchronous shoulder motion, or scapulohumeral rhythm, must be addressed before and throughout recovery from a shoulder dislocation. The 2:1 ratio of motion between the scapula and the glenohumeral joint (meaning that for every 2 degrees of glenohumeral flexion or abduction after the first 30 degrees of shoulder motion, the scapula must rotate upwardly 1 degree)[10] must be addressed early to prevent the facilitation of abnormal motions between the scapula and glenohumeral joint during strengthening activities. This can be adequately accomplished by focusing on normalized scapular motion and stabilization exercises during the early or maximum-protection phase as long as symptoms of pain and harmful glenohumeral joint positions are avoided.

Throughout each phase of recovery, various tissues that contain the humeral head in the glenoid fossa (glenoid labrum, capsule, and ligaments; superior, middle, and inferior glenohumeral ligaments; and musculotendinous rotator cuff) can be stressed or torn. By definition, glenohumeral instability identifies ligamentous and capsular restraints as being "attenuated,"[15] so the appropriate progressive application of strengthening activities for the rotator cuff and scapulothoracic muscles becomes central to the recovery of motion and function.

The criteria established by Wilk[27] to progress to the minimal-protection phase are described as follows:

- Full, nonpainful ROM
- No palpable tenderness
- Continued progression of shoulder strength

Thus the assistant must address functional motions and stimulate the afferent neural input system through closed kinetic chain activities. These enhance proprioception and promote dynamic joint stability.[25]

Initiating isotonic resistance exercises is quite challenging and stressful to the glenohumeral joint, and many appropriate exercises must therefore be modified to accommodate limitations of motion, pain, and the provocative positions of abduction and external rotation. For example, the overhead seated shoulder press can place the shoulder in a somewhat compromised position (Fig. 16-11), so the patient may need to turn and face the apparatus, thereby reducing shoulder abduction and creating a more adducted shoulder posture (Fig. 16-12). The seated or supine chest press is another example of isotonic exercise that promotes anterior shoulder strength. However, this particular exercise can place the shoulder in a horizontally abducted position that stresses the anterior shoulder capsule, causing the head of the humerus to rock forward within the glenoid (Fig. 16-13). This exercise can be modified by adjusting the starting ROM to a more adducted shoulder posture and changing the hand position to a more neutral location (Fig. 16-14).

Cable systems offer various exercises and positions that duplicate functional activities. Wall pulleys and cable systems are particularly useful in athletic patients,

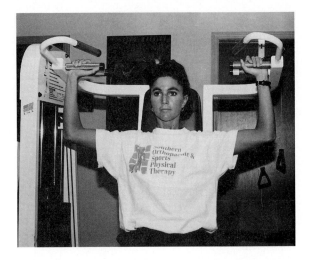

FIG. 16-11 Typical position for the performance of a seated overhead shoulder press. Notice the arms are held in an abducted and slightly externally rotated position.

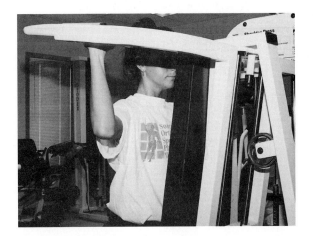

FIG. 16-12 By having the patient face the apparatus, the shoulder can be placed in a more protected position. Notice the upper arm is in a more adducted position, thereby reducing shoulder abduction and external rotation.

because sport-specific tasks can be reproduced with this equipment.

Local muscle endurance activities are done using an upper body ergometer, closed-kinetic chain "stepping" on a stair stepper, or "walking" on a treadmill (Fig. 16-15). Weight-bearing closed-chain exercises can be gradually introduced once the patient has regained sufficient strength and motion to tolerate these challenging activities. The

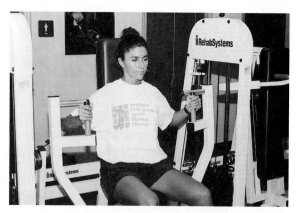

FIG. 16-14 Modification of the seated shoulder press can include adjusting the initial starting range of motion while also changing the hand position in order to avoid or limit horizontal abduction.

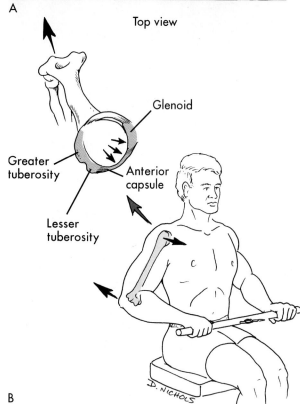

FIG. 16-13 A, Seated chest press. This initial position can place stress on the anterior shoulder capsule. **B,** In this figure, notice how the head of the humerus can rock forward within the glenoid causing stress to the anterior shoulder capsule.

physical therapist will identify the appropriate time table for each patient with regard to advanced closed-chain resistance exercises. Initially, simple wall push-ups can provide needed proprioceptive stimulation to the mechanoreceptor system. Gradually, more challenging weight-

bearing activities that demand progressive control of the glenohumeral joint in multiplane and diagonal motions are added (Fig. 16-16). A balance board can also help train the shoulder muscles to respond and "fire" quickly for sufficient stabilization (Fig. 16-17). In addition, a Plyo-ball can be used as part of a closed-chain proprioception exercise program during the minimal-protection phase. The Plyo-ball can be used in a seated, weight-bearing, or standing position (Fig. 16-18).

The process of recovery after shoulder dislocation matches the degree of injury (dislocation vs. subluxation), duration of immobilization (from 10 days to 6 weeks),[19] and any associated tissue damage (Bankart and/or Hill-Sachs lesion). Full functional recovery is not always possible. In some cases, after acute traumatic dislocation, minor stress causes the shoulder to dislocate again. With repeated episodes of shoulder dislocation or subluxation, recurrent anterior instability can result.[20] If patients fail to respond to an aggressive physical therapy program, the physician may choose one of several operative procedures to correct the instability.* Miller[13] reports that most surgical candidates have recurrent traumatic anterior dislocations. Two distinct factors have been identified as helping to guide treatment decisions regarding anterior shoulder dislocations.[13,19,22] Patients with a *T*raumatic *U*nidirectinal injury and a *B*ankart lesion frequently require *S*urgery (**TUBS**). Patients with *A*traumatic *M*ultidirectional *B*ilateral instability respond well to *R*ehabilitation, but

---

*References 7, 10, 13, 14, 19-22, 25.

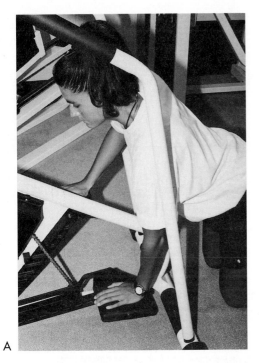
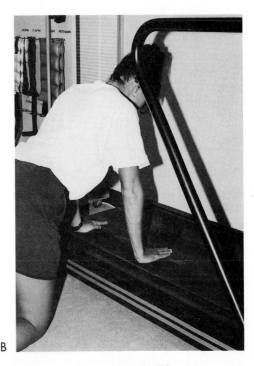

FIG. 16-15 A, Closed chain stair stepping activity. **B,** Side stepping on a treadmill for upper extremity reciprocal opened- and closed-chain "walking."

occasionally require an *Inferior* capsular shift surgical procedure (**AMBRI**).[13,22]

Operative Management and Rehabilitation

Because *posterior* shoulder dislocations account for only 2% to 4% of all shoulder dislocations,[19] this discussion focuses on repairs and rehabilitation procedures to enhance joint stability and promote function in patients with *anterior* glenohumeral instability. Surgical procedures for shoulder instability can be classified as open or arthroscopic techniques.[19] The three general categories of open stabilization techniques are as follows:[13,19]

- Surgical repairs of Bankart lesions
- Procedures used to limit external rotation of the shoulder
- Bone block procedures and coracoid process transfers

The Bankart procedure essentially reattaches the torn capsule to the glenoid.[13] Anterior shoulder staple capsulorrhaphy (staple or repair of a joint capsule) can be used to reattach and tighten the torn capsule. A potential complication of this particular procedure is migration of the staple used to secure the torn capsule.[13] In the Magnusen-Stack procedure, the surgeon moves the subscapularis from the lesser tuberosity to the greater tuberosity.[13,22] The primary disadvantage with this procedure is that the patient may be left with some residual decreased external rotation.[13,22]

An example of a coracoid transfer to increase anterior glenohumeral stability is the Bristow procedure.[13,22] This technique calls for the surgical repositioning of the coracoid process, the attached coracobrachialis, and the short head of the biceps to the glenohumeral neck[13,22] (Fig. 16-19). As with other transfer-type procedures that use bone and soft tissue stabilization hardware (screw, staples), a common complication is the potential for migration of the fixation devices and possible nonunion at the bone transfer site.[13] The capsular shift procedure transposes the capsule from an inferior position to a superior position and from superior to inferior position[13] (Fig. 16-20).

Anterior shoulder instability can also be corrected arthroscopically.[13,19,22] Interestingly, while arthroscopic techniques afford certain advantages over open surgical repairs (e.g., less postoperative pain and reduced soft tissue damage), there appears to be a higher risk for recurrent dislocations as compared to open surgical procedures.[19]

Rehabilitation after open or arthroscopic stabilization for anterior glenohumeral instability varies and must

text continued on pg. 256

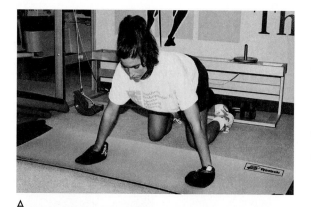

A

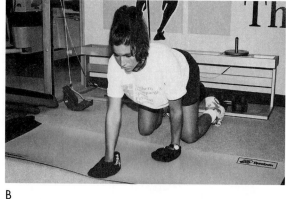

B

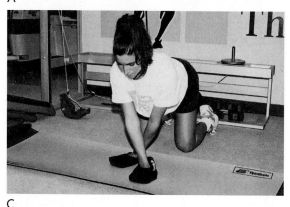

C

FIG. 16-16 Multiplane and diagonal closed-chain weight bearing activities. **A,** Shoulder abduction and adduction on a slide board in a kneeling position. Extreme caution must be taken to ensure that a limited range of abduction be allowed when initiating this activity. **B,** Shoulder flexion and extension in a kneeling position. When beginning all slide board activities the patient must be able to eccentrically and concentrically control the affected shoulder globally. **C,** Diagonal patterns on the slide board.

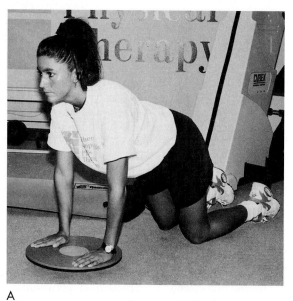

A

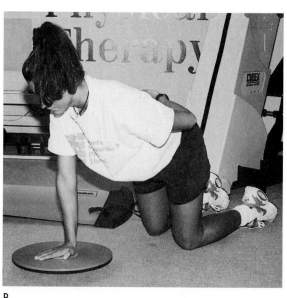

B

FIG. 16-17 Closed kinetic chain wobble board activity for stimulating shoulder stability. **A,** Initially both arms are used when introducing this exercise. **B,** When strength, control, and confidence improve, the patient can progress to one arm.

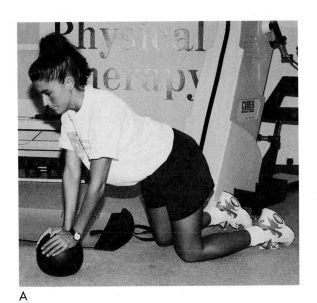

A

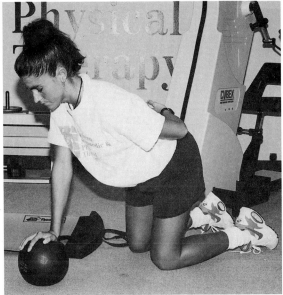

B

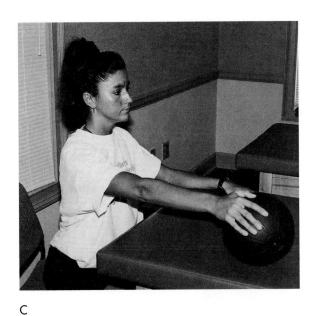

C

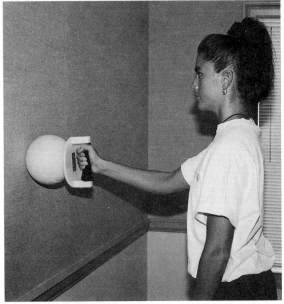

D

FIG. 16-18 Plyo-ball closed chain proprioception exercises. **A,** The patient is introduced to this activity by using both arms. **B,** As strength, balance, and confidence improve, the patient can progress to one arm. **C,** If the patient is unable to perform vertical loading on the Plyo-ball, then the patient may be started on this exercise in a seated position without vertical-compression loads. **D,** Standing wall pushes with the use of a Plyo-ball. Multiplanar stability is essential in order to perform any of these activities.

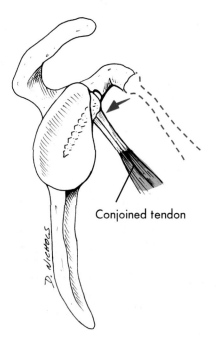

FIG. 16-19 Bristow procedure. Coracoid transfer to increase anterior glenohumeral stability.

specifically match the procedure.[27,28] While postoperative rehabilitation closely parallels nonoperative rehabilitation, specific limitations result from the process of bone and soft tissue healing. Each patient and each surgical procedure must be addressed differently, and the following rehabilitation plan represents general principles only. It is not meant to demonstrate precise physical therapy interventions for all surgical cases.

Initial postoperative care begins with a period of immobilization in a sling or shoulder immobilizer to allow for appropriate soft tissue healing.* During this period, medications for pain and swelling may be prescribed by the physician. Frequently, ice packs are applied to the shoulder for 15 to 20 minutes, 3 to 5 times daily as part of the home program to control postoperative pain and swelling. Also, the patient can actively perform finger, hand, wrist, and elbow mobility exercises. In addition, submaximal isometric exercises can be initiated while the arm is still in the sling. These must be performed pain-free.

The degree and direction of shoulder motion allowed are specific to the surgical procedure, the wishes of the

---

*References 7, 14, 19, 20, 22, 25, 27.

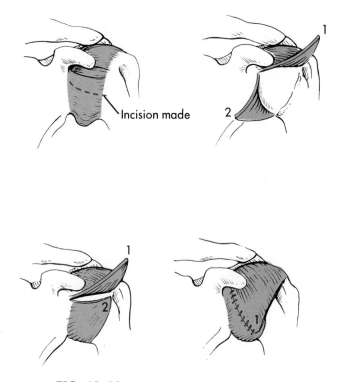

FIG. 16-20 Capsular shift surgical procedure.

physician, and the direction of the physical therapist. Generally, shoulder shrugs, scapular protraction and retraction, Codman's pendulum exercises, and various active assisted ROM exercises using a rope and pulley system, cane, or wand, as well as wall walking exercises, can be used to increase motion. The initiation of motion exercises is extremely important because faulty scapulothoracic and glenohumeral mobility can be affected early. Care must be taken to encourage scapular motion as well as glenohumeral mobility and to identify any limitations affecting normal scapulohumeral rhythm. With certain procedures (coracoid transfers, muscle transfers, and bone block procedures), avoiding shoulder abduction and external rotation (in various degrees) early is essential to allow bone and soft tissues to heal and not be overloaded. Therefore the assistant must be aware of the exact procedure used in order to understand the rationale behind limiting early active or passive shoulder abduction and external rotation.

As the patient is gradually weaned from the sling, progressive motion and strengthening exercises are allowed. Progressive shoulder strengthening must address both the glenohumeral and the scapulothoracic joints. To recover functional mobility of the shoulder, a program of "proximal stability for distal mobility"[24] is suggested. Because the scapula forms the base of support for glenohumeral motion, stabilization exercises[16] must be initiated. However, with some muscle transfer procedures, the initiation of strengthening for a specific muscle group (transferred muscle group) may be deferred for longer periods of time in order for secure healing to take place. As the patient demonstrates improved mobility without complaints of pain, the quality of muscle contraction (from submaximal to maximal) must be encouraged gradually. Progressive resistive exercises using surgical tubing or dumbbells within an active, pain-free ROM can begin, along with more challenging flexibility exercises, between 6 and 8 weeks after surgery.[20]

The eccentric contraction phase of each exercise must be encouraged. Hisamoto[8] reports: "Rehabilitation must incorporate eccentric loading to be successful with overhead activities." Applying this concept during the early recovery phase involves emphasizing the eccentric loading phase of all internal rotation, abduction, external rotation, adduction, and shoulder flexion exercises. Local muscle endurance must also be considered once the patient has achieved improved motion and strength. Usually an upper body ergometer or some other form of low-intensity, high-repetition shoulder-specific activity is appropriate. Functional activities, proprioception, and closed-kinetic chain exercises, although necessary for

functional recovery, may be delayed to allow for secure healing. However, weight-bearing, closed-chain resistance exercises, and proprioception activities are required during the moderate-protection to minimal-protection phases of recovery to stimulate the mechanoreceptor system and to encourage purposeful, functional motion that duplicates ADLs.

Generally, the total length of rehabilitation after surgical stabilization of the glenohumeral joint ranges from 3 to 6 months, depending on the exact procedure used.[2]

ADHESIVE CAPSULITIS

Adhesive **capsulitis,** which is also referred to as "frozen shoulder," is characterized by decreased shoulder ROM, pain, capsular inflammation, fibrous synovial adhesions, and reduction of the joint cavity (Fig. 16-21).[3,13,26,32] Adhesive capsulitis occurs more commonly in females and affects patients between 40 and 60 years of age.[3,13,32] The two distinct classifications of "frozen shoulder" are primary and secondary adhesive capsulitis.[26,32] Primary idiopathic frozen shoulder is the most common lesion and occurs spontaneously from unknown causes.[26,32] Secondary adhesive capsulitis generally occurs after trauma or immobilization.[26,32]

Among older patients, secondary adhesive capsulitis can develop because of limited immobilization for as

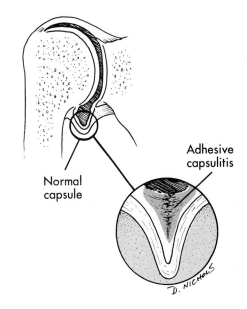

FIG. 16-21 Adhesive capsulitis or "frozen shoulder."

little as 1 or 2 days.[5] In the early stages of this disabling condition, pain occurs both at rest and during activity.[5,26] However, as the condition progresses, pain gradually subsides, then spontaneously disappears. Severely restricted motion and profound loss of function remain.[5,26,32] During the acute painful phase, treatment is focused on controlling inflammation and symptoms of pain. Physician-prescribed analgesics, NSAIDs, and intraarticular steroid injections can provide some pain relief.[26]

Physical therapy interventions during this acute painful stage include the judicious use of ice, heat, ultrasound, iontophoresis, phonophoresis, and TENS.[3] Also, central to this initial management phase is the stimulation of pain-free motion and relaxation of muscle guarding of the glenohumeral joint, cervical area, and scapulothoracic muscles.[3] Passive, active, and active assisted motion exercises must occur within a pain-free ROM to stimulate removal of metabolic waste, increase local blood flow, and assist in the reduction of edema in the local tissues.[3,26] Codman's pendulum exercises must be performed during this acute stage within a pain-free range. These exercises can be preceded by the use of thermal agents (ice, moist heat, ultrasound, phonophoresis, iontophoresis) to minimize spasm and pain. Both wand and rope and pulley systems can be used early if they are performed in a slow, controlled, pain-free ROM. For severely restricted glenohumeral motion, the physical therapist may prescribe the application of specific joint mobilization techniques to help modulate pain and reduce muscle guarding.[3,5,26,32] As addressed previously, grades I and II low-amplitude physiologic and accessory oscillations can help encourage relaxation while reducing pain.[3,5,26]

If the scapula is not stable and free from restriction while the patient attempts to regain shoulder motion and function, normal scapulohumeral rhythm cannot be obtained. Therefore early scapular stabilization exercises[16] can be employed as long as pain does not inhibit the correct performance of the exercise.[16] Normalized motion must precede specific strengthening activities to avoid developing faulty shoulder mechanics.

The complete restoration of glenohumeral joint mobility is the goal of treatment for the late stage of adhesive capsulitis.[3,26] The physical therapist must identify the appropriate application of increased joint mobilization techniques to address specific capsular restrictions and initiate more challenging progressive resistance exercises. When the patient demonstrates improved glenohumeral motion and appropriate scapulohumeral rhythm, strengthening exercises can begin for the deltoid, scapular muscles, rotator cuff, and upper-arm muscles.[5]

Although control of pain and inflammation is the primary feature of early physical therapy management, submaximal isometric exercise can be used to initiate strengthening if pain is not increased with exercise. Progressing from submaximal isometrics to maximal isometrics usually precedes the use of latex rubber tubing, cuff weights, or dumbbells for concentric and eccentric exercises. A comprehensive series of rotator cuff exercises[23] and scapular stabilization exercises[16] can be encouraged as early as pain and motion allow. To address normalized function, the patient does closed-chain resistance exercises and overhead loading along with proprioception exercises (balance board, slide board, Plyo-ball) in a sequential, orderly fashion once sufficient strength, improved motion, and scapulohumeral rhythm have been established. Local muscle endurance activities focus on purposeful, functional movements that duplicate ADLs.

Again, pain control, restoration of motion, and improved function must be continually reinforced to encourage compliance with a home exercise program and the avoidance of positions that may exacerbate pain and muscle guarding.

ACROMIOCLAVICULAR SPRAINS AND DISLOCATIONS

Ligamentous sprains of the **acromioclavicular (A-C) joint** usually result from a fall on the acromion (direct force)[1] or when force is transmitted from a fall on an outstretched arm proximally to the A-C joint (indirect force).[1,30] A-C joint sprains and dislocations are graded according to the degree of injury to specific ligamentous structures (A-C and coracoclavicular ligaments) as well as the position of the clavicle in complete rupture of both the A-C and coracoclavicular ligaments,[1,13,30,32] as follows:

First-degree, grade I A-C joint sprain: Characterized by partial tearing of the A-C ligaments, with resultant joint tenderness over the A-C joint, no joint instability or laxity of the ligament, and minimal loss of function (Fig. 16-22).[1,13,30,32]

Second-degree, grade II A-C sprain: Complete rupture of the A-C ligaments with partial tearing of the coracoacromial ligaments.[1,13,30,32] The patient has moderate pain, some dysfunction (reduction in shoulder abduction and adduction),[1] and a palpable gap between the acromion and the clavicle[1,13,30,32] (Fig. 16-23).

Third-degree, grade III A-C ligament injury: Dislocation between the acromion and the clavicle where both the A-C and coracoclavicular ligaments are ruptured and the distal clavicle becomes displaced superiorly (Fig.

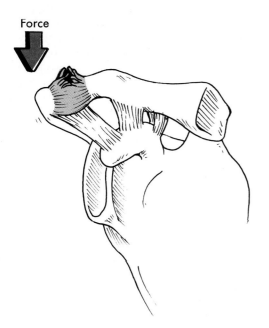

Force

FIG. 16-22 Grade I acromioclavicular (A-C) joint sprain. Partial tear of the acromioclavicular ligaments.

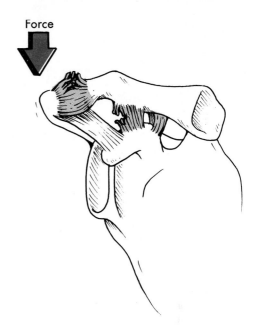

Force

FIG. 16-23 Grade II A-C sprain. Rupture of the acromioclavicular ligaments and partial tearing of the coracoacromial ligaments.

16-24). Patients demonstrate marked pain and severe limitation of shoulder motion.[1]

Three additional classifications have been proposed that describe the degree of vertical, posterior, and inferior separation of the clavicle in a grade III A-C dislocation.[1,13,30,32]

Rehabilitation and management of grade I A-C sprains focus on symptomatic relief. Typically, pain is controlled with the use of ice packs, NSAIDs, analgesics, and rest. Because the A-C ligaments have been partially torn, the A-C joint must be protected from further direct or indirect forces, which may stress the A-C ligaments. The patient may be allowed to resume activities within 2 weeks and usually does not require a rehabilitation program of significant duration.[1]

Grade II A-C sprains require more direct attention to approximate the torn A-C ligaments and allow for secure ligament healing. Usually this injury is managed nonoperatively using a shoulder harness or sling, which depresses the clavicle and supports the arm to provide close approximation of the torn ligaments. For A-C ligaments to heal, authorities advocate 3 to 6 weeks of "continuous uninterrupted pressure on the superior aspect of the clavicle"[30] after a grade II A-C sprain.

As noted previously, there is usually a palpable step-off between the acromion process and the distal clavicle with grade II A-C sprains. This deformity

represents a loss of joint continuity because of lost ligamentous support between the acromion and clavicle, and it remains permanently.[1]

The rehabilitation program for a grade II A-C sprain commences during immobilization. Symptomatic relief includes ice packs, NSAIDs, analgesics, ultrasound, phonophoresis, iontophoresis, and TENS to help minimize pain and inflammation. In the maximal-protection phase, immobilization is used, with patient education focusing on the avoidance of both direct and indirect forces that stress the A-C ligaments. During immobilization, submaximal isometrics can be performed for all muscles of the shoulder girdle. However, care must be taken to avoid contractions that stress the A-C joint in the sling or shoulder harness. After the immobilization device is removed, active shoulder motion can begin. Even after immobilization, the torn ligaments are not fully recovered and must still be protected from inappropriate stress.

The moderate-protection phase begins with active shoulder motions and active assisted rope and pulley activities. The patient is encouraged to perform active shoulder flexion, abduction to tolerance, and shrugs, which promote activation of the trapezius and levator scapula muscles. The patient must avoid downward displacement of the scapula or distraction of the humerus, both of which stress the A-C joint.

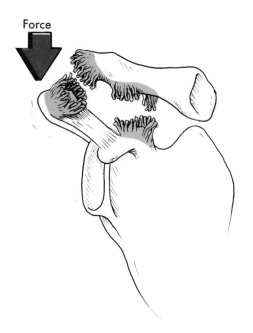

Force

FIG. 16-24 Grade III A-C sprain. Both the acromio-clavicular and coracoacromial ligaments are ruptured.

Progressive-resistive exercises are initiated during the moderate-protection phase and include scapular stabilization exercises, deltoid strengthening, and specific rotator cuff exercises. Latex rubber tubing, cuff weights, and dumbbells are effective and versatile for compliance and carryover to a prescribed home exercise program. As mentioned earlier, the performance of scapular and humerus elevation exercises helps approximate the torn ligaments and provides dynamic muscular support to the torn structures. However, with both active and resistance exercises the downward or "relaxation" phase of shoulder shrugs can create unwanted traction on the A-C joint. Therefore the patient must perform the contraction or elevation phase of the shoulder shrug to tolerance but limit the eccentric lowering phase to avoid distraction of the A-C joint. As with all other injuries, the whole person should be addressed during each phase of recovery. For example, during the maximum-protection phase of recovery, while the patient is immobilized, it is appropriate to encourage active and resistive exercises for the hand, wrist, and elbow of the affected arm if no excessive stress is directed to the A-C joint. In addition, a general conditioning program is warranted to improve or maintain aerobic fitness, strength, and flexibility.

The treatment of grade III A-C sprains (dislocation of the distal clavicle and acromion process) is quite controversial.[1,30] Although many surgeons advocate open surgical repair, others favor closed reduction, immobilization, and progressive rehabilitation. The nonoperative treatment of grade III A-C sprains is centered on reducing the dislocation and maintaining the reduction in immobilization for up to 6 weeks.[1,30] The goals of the initial course of treatment in physical therapy is to minimize pain and swelling, with the judicious use of ice, iontophoresis, phonophoresis, ultrasound, physician-prescribed NSAIDs, analgesics, and protection of the A-C joint from unwanted stress. To ensure proper healing of the ligaments, the rehabilitation team must continuously reinforce compliance using the immobilizer for the entire period prescribed by the treating physician.

While the patient is immobilized, submaximal isometric exercises can be initiated for the shoulder and scapula if no stress is applied to the healing ligaments. As with grade II A-C sprains, the hand, wrist, and elbow of the affected arm can be safely and effectively strengthened during immobilization. Generally, the nonoperative treatment of grade III sprains parallels the treatment plan for grade II sprains. The primary differences are the longer duration of immobilization, and the more cautious and delayed application of motion and resistance exercises so as not to adversely affect ligament healing. In some cases, nonoperative treatment is ineffective and surgical correction must be addressed.

Four general categories of grade III A-C repairs have been reported.[26] The surgeon may elect to insert pins directly through the A-C joint to stabilize and approximate the joint (Fig. 16-25). Another procedure calls for the surgeon to place sutures around the distal clavicle and the coracoid process to stabilize the joint (Fig. 16-26). The surgeon may also place a screw between the clavicle and coracoid process to provide more rigid stability to the A-C joint (Fig. 16-27). In addition, the distal clavicle may also be excised.[30]

In the early or maximum-protection phase, active motion and light resistance exercises for the hand, wrist, and elbow of the affected limb are encouraged. Isometric exercises focus on the shoulder and scapular muscles once the A-C joint is stabilized and protected from unwanted forces. Progressive active and active assisted shoulder motion is allowed as pain and soft tissue healing progresses. Bergfeld[1] advocates light resistive exercises after 3 weeks and more progressive weight lifting exercises 8 to 10 weeks postoperatively. Once the sling is removed, a progressive return to function closely follows the patient's level of motion and strength. As previously stated, heavy, intense resistance exercises must be delayed for 8 weeks until secure union has occurred, pain is abolished, and active shoulder motion returns.

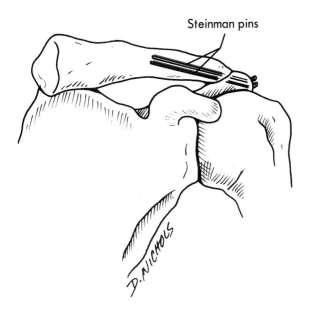

FIG. 16-25 Stabilization surgical procedure for the A-C joint. Steinman pins are inserted to stabilize and approximate the A-C joint.

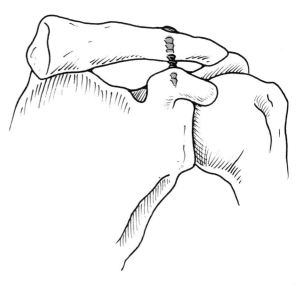

FIG. 16-27 A screw can be inserted between the clavicle and the coracoid process to stabilize the A-C joint.

SCAPULAR FRACTURES

Most scapular fractures result from direct, severe trauma.[11,29] Therefore there is a high incidence of significant associated injuries, including other fractures, glenohumeral dislocations, pneumothorax, and neurovascular injuires.[11,13,21,29] Interestingly, fractures of the scapular body (Fig. 16-28) are the most common (49% to 89%)[29] and demonstrate the highest incidence of associated injuries (35% to 98%).[21] However, the treatment of fractures to the scapular body is conservative if associated injuries have not occurred,[11,21,29] using ice and immobilization with a sling for 2 to 3 weeks.[21,29] During the immobilization period, hand, wrist, and elbow exercises can be initiated for the affected arm along with a general conditioning program. As the pain and swelling subside, early passive ROM exercises for the shoulder begin.

Isometric exercises performed submaximally can also be initiated early if the patient remains pain-free. As pain and swelling subside, strengthening exercises can be added within a pain-free ROM. Nonunion and malunion of this fracture are rare and are not usually associated with a loss of function or clinical symptoms.[21,29]

The second most common scapular fracture occurs to the glenoid neck (Fig. 16-29). If the fracture is extraarticular, Williams and Rockwood[29] suggest that healing can occur at 6 weeks and that management involves

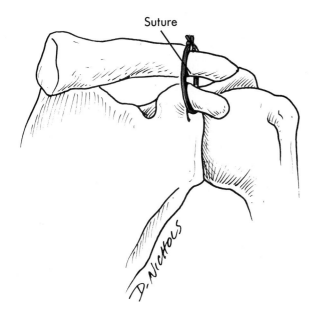

FIG. 16-26 Stabilization of the A-C joint by suturing the distal clavicle and the coracoid process.

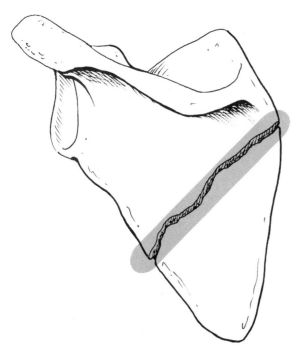

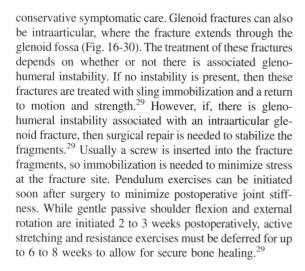

FIG. 16-28 Fracture of the scapular body.

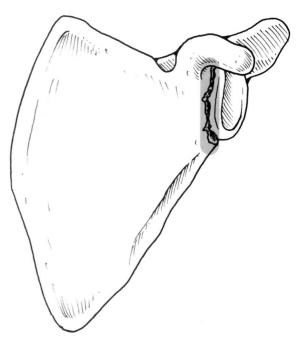

FIG. 16-29 Extraarticular fracture of the glenoid neck.

conservative symptomatic care. Glenoid fractures can also be intraarticular, where the fracture extends through the glenoid fossa (Fig. 16-30). The treatment of these fractures depends on whether or not there is associated glenohumeral instability. If no instability is present, then these fractures are treated with sling immobilization and a return to motion and strength.[29] However, if, there is glenohumeral instability associated with an intraarticular glenoid fracture, then surgical repair is needed to stabilize the fragments.[29] Usually a screw is inserted into the fracture fragments, so immobilization is needed to minimize stress at the fracture site. Pendulum exercises can be initiated soon after surgery to minimize postoperative joint stiffness. While gentle passive shoulder flexion and external rotation are initiated 2 to 3 weeks postoperatively, active stretching and resistance exercises must be deferred for up to 6 to 8 weeks to allow for secure bone healing.[29]

CLAVICLE FRACTURES

Fractures of the clavicle occur as a result of either direct or indirect trauma. These injuries are relatively common and primarily affect men under 25 years of age.[33]

Care is focused on achieving reduction of the fracture fragments, maintaining the reduction, and minimizing the immobilization of the glenohumeral joint of the affected arm.[33] Usually the patient is placed in a com-

mercially available figure-of-eight bandage (Fig. 16-31) to maintain proper alignment of the area. The duration of immobilization varies, but authorities suggest that healing takes 4 to 6 weeks or longer.[33]

During the initial period of immobilization, with the figure-of-eight bandage, the hand, wrist, and elbow of the affected arm are exercised with active motion and resistance exercises. Unwanted stress to the fracture site is avoided during this period. In addition, once pain has been controlled, the patient may perform gentle pendulum exercises and submaximal isometrics for the shoulder and scapula.

Active shoulder flexion must not be greater than 40 to 50 degrees until after 4 to 6 weeks[29] (although patients may be encouraged to perform gentle active shoulder motion no greater than 40 degrees when pain-free). As the healing process continues and when bone healing is confirmed radiographically (around 4 to 6 weeks), greater degrees of shoulder motion are allowed, with progressive resistive exercises added as tolerated.

If the fracture is located at the distal end of the clavicle, open reduction and internal fixation may be more appropriate, because these fractures tend to be unstable and do not maintain proper alignment with a figure-of-eight bandage.[21] The fracture fragments of a displaced distal clavicle fracture are usually secured with an intramedullary fixation pin.[21]

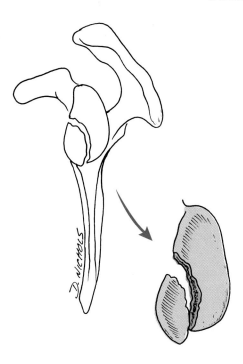

FIG. 16-30 Intraarticular fracture of the glenoid.

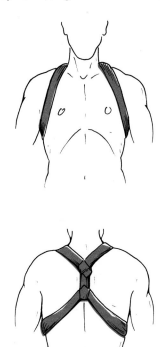

FIG. 16-31 Figure-of-eight bandage for alignment and stabilization of clavicle fractures.

PROXIMAL HUMERUS FRACTURES

Proximal humerus fractures are usually classified according to a four-part classification.[11,13,21] The four parts are the humeral head, the lesser tuberosity, the greater tuberosity, and the humeral shaft[13,21] (Fig. 16-32).

Physical therapy management of humerus fractures depends on the severity and complexity of the fracture as well as the means used to secure fixation of the fracture site. Generally, with nondisplaced one-part fractures (the most common type), the affected arm is placed in a sling for a period of time and the patient is given analgesics and encouraged to apply ice liberally to minimize pain and swelling. Within the first 2 or 3 weeks, gentle active motion is allowed, as well as active motion of the elbow, wrist, and hand of the affected arm.[11] In fact, the patient may be allowed to remove the sling for active motion exercises a few times each day.[11,13]

Submaximal shoulder isometrics are initiated as early as pain allows. Perhaps the most salient aspect of physical therapy care in proximal humerus fracture is the functional restoration of glenohumeral motion and strength after protracted periods of immobility to allow for appropriate bone healing. Early scapular motion exercises minimize the restriction of scapular mobility.

Submaximal scapular stabilization exercises[16] can also be encouraged early, as pain allows, to provide a stable base for glenohumeral motion exercises. Progressive motion and resistance exercises for the deltoid, rotator cuff, and upper arm muscles closely parallel bone healing and the patient's ability to demonstrate improved motion without pain.

Other, more complex fractures can require **open reduction and internal fixation (ORIF)** with screws and a plate (Fig. 16-33) as well as prolonged periods of immobilization. As with all fractures, during immobility the patient can participate in a total body conditioning program that does not compromise the healing of the fracture. In addition, the hand, wrist, and elbow of the affected limb must be exercised without stressing the fracture site.

The ultimate task after the healing of humerus fractures is regaining purposeful, functional strength and motion of the glenohumeral joint. Indeed, the time required to heal significant fractures may cause serious glenohumeral and scapular restrictions. The long-term healing restraints of bone form the primary guide for the physician and physical therapist in deciding when to employ progressive motion activities and when to initiate strengthening tasks without compromising the fracture site.

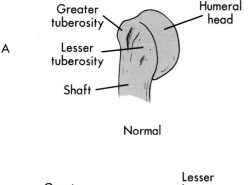

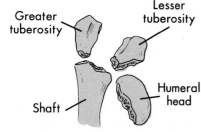

FIG. 16-32 A, Normal anatomy of proximal humerus. **B,** Four-part fracture of the proximal humerus.

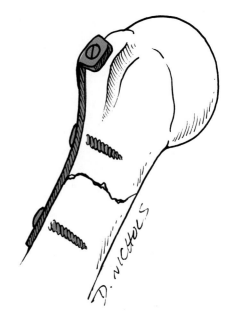

FIG. 16-33 ORIF procedure for transverse proximal humerus fracture. Fracture site fixation with side plate and screws.

With some significant fractures (displaced fractures of the anatomical neck), avascular necrosis (AVN) may be a risk.[11] For example, in an older population of patients with advancing osteoporosis who have a four-part proximal humerus fracture, internal fixation may be quite poor because of the osteopenic bone. In this case, a prosthetic humeral head may be more appropriate.[21]

As the fracture begins to stabilize, and under the direction and supervision of the physical therapist, some patients begin closed-kinetic chain exercises to stimulate the mechanoreceptor system (afferent neural input system) of the elbow, shoulder, and wrist and to effect proper bone healing (Wolff's law) by providing submaximal intermittent stress to the healing bone.

The physical therapist assistant participates in the rehabilitation process of proximal humerus fractures by following and supervising a comprehensive program of early protected limited ROM, submaximal isometrics for the scapular stabilizers,[16] rotator cuff, and upper arm muscles, and by providing continued protection for the injured site. As pain, motion, and bone healing progress, the physical therapist assistant must carefully observe the scapulothoracic and glenohumeral motion. If scapulohumeral rhythm is adversely affected, specific atten-

tion must be addressed to regain a stable scapula and proper glenohumeral motion. In many cases, if a restriction is noted, the physical therapist may use scapular and glenohumeral mobilization techniques to modulate pain and encourage improved motion. However, the fracture site must be secure and stable, with radiographic confirmation of this, and the physician must order this protocol before mobilization can commence.

Functional shoulder activities and resistance exercises are gradually added as bone healing advances and the patient demonstrates greater confidence, motion, and strength without pain. Proprioception and closed-kinetic chain activities may also be added during the minimal-protection phase of recovery in preparation for normalized purposeful motion and strength of the involved limb.

Total Shoulder Arthroplasty

With severe four-part fractures of the proximal humerus, avascular necrosis of the humeral head, osteoporosis, rheumatoid arthritis, and advanced osteoarthritis, the proximal humerus may be replaced with a prosthesis, or a total shoulder arthroplasty may be indicated[5,6,21] (Fig. 16-34). The condition of the rotator cuff is a significant feature in patients receiving either a hemiarthroplasty or total shoulder arthroplasty. Goldstein[5] reports that in patients suffering from rheumatoid arthritis, as many as 38% have a torn rotator cuff. If a rotator cuff tear is repaired in addition to the arthroplasty, postoperative

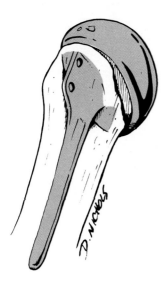

FIG. 16-34 Proximal humerus prosthesis.

immobilization may be as long as 6 to 8 weeks, with the affected arm held in an abduction splint to allow for healing of the repaired cuff.[5,6]

Thus a rotator cuff repair added to shoulder arthroplasty guides the course of rehabilitation and dictates the need for a protracted period of immobility in addition to a longer program of rehabilitation.[5] In addition, in terms of restoration of shoulder motion, if the rotator cuff is not repaired, postoperative abduction averages 143 degrees, whereas patients requiring rotator cuff repair may achieve an average of only 63 degrees of shoulder abduction.[6]

The course of rehabilitation after shoulder arthroplasty usually allows for early (day 1 or 2) gentle active assisted ROM and isometric exercises. Muscle contractions of the deltoid are contraindicated in cases of rotator cuff repair. In these cases, isometric exercise must be deferred until soft tissue healing has occurred to the repaired deltoid and cuff.[6] Usually during the first postoperative week, the patient is allowed active exercise of the wrist, hand, and elbow of the affected shoulder. The postoperative immobilizer is also frequently removed for hygiene and exercises.[5,6] By the end of the first week, the sling may be removed and Codman's pendulum exercises initiated while active assisted ROM exercises are continued.[5] At the end of the second postoperative week, the patient is introduced to scapular motion and stabilization exercises while the quantity and quality of isometric exercises and motion exercises are progressed.[5] The assistant must encourage compliance with a comprehensive home exercise program of motion and strength. The use of wand exercises

and rope and pulley systems at home is appropriate. By week 6 the use of light resistance exercise can begin.[5] Latex rubber tubing is an effective tool for the home exercise program.

If the patient has received a rotator cuff repair, the sequence of care and initiation of resistance exercise and active shoulder motion are delayed.[6] Functional use of the affected arm can be expected around 6 months postoperatively. However, Goldstein[5] suggests that for optimal results, the patient should participate in an active home exercise program for up to 2 years after surgery.[5]

MOBILIZATION OF THE SHOULDER

The precise application of specific peripheral joint mobilization techniques is extremely effective for pain reduction and restoration of normalized joint motion. In addition to various soft tissue injures and fractures, immobilization frequently causes limitations in scapulothoracic and glenohumeral mobility. To effect normalized scapulohumeral rhythm, any limitations in motion must be identified early in the rehabilitation period.

During the initial immobilization, the physical therapist documents all limitations of specific joint motion. Each limitation is addressed as part of the rehabilitation program. If, however, during the rehabilitation program, the physical therapist assistant recognizes delayed restoration of motion, reduced motion, or increased pain, he or she must immediately communicate this to the physical therapist.

The following scapular and glenohumeral mobilization techniques represent only a few of the many techniques available. The physical therapist will decide which specific technique is to be used, when to apply the technique, in which direction, and with what amplitude, grade, or oscillation.

Before using any mobilization technique, the position and comfort of the patient must be assessed. The use of oral physician-prescribed analgesics, thermal agents (heat, ultrasound, ice), and proper body and limb positioning enhances relaxation and compliance during treatment.

Mobilization of the Scapulothoracic Joint

While the patient is in a sidelying position on the unaffected side, the scapula can be effectively mobilized in a superior and inferior direction as well as distracted from the thorax.[31] To distract the scapula, stand facing the patient. Firmly grasp the medial or vertebral border of the affected scapula and purposefully distract the scapula away from the thorax[31] (Fig. 16-35). To glide the scapula superiorly and inferiorly, assume the same

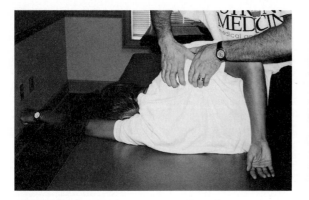

FIG. 16-35 Vertebral border scapular distraction.

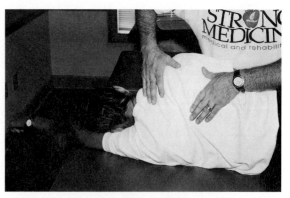

FIG. 16-36 Superior and inferior glide of the scapula.

position. Support the inferior border of the scapula with one hand while placing the opposite hand on the superior border of the scapula. Use the hand on the inferior border to direct a force to glide the scapula in a superior direction. Use the hand on the superior border to direct a force to glide the scapula in an inferior direction (Fig. 16-36).[31]

Mobilization of the Glenohumeral Joint

Anteroposterior glide of the glenohumeral joint can be accomplished with the patient supine. Sit toward the affected shoulder. In this position, Wooden[31] recommends putting towels under the elbow of the affected shoulder to place the humerus in a more horizontal position. Firmly grasp the humeral head with the thumb and fingers of one hand while actively stabilizing the scapula with the other hand. If the glenohumeral joint is stiff and motion is applied to the joint without stabilizing the scapula, the glenohumeral joint and scapula will move as a single unit. While stabilizing the scapula with one hand, use the other hand on the humeral head to provide an anteriorly and/or posteriorly directed force (Fig. 16-37).

Lateral distraction of the humeral head can also be achieved while the patient is supine. Sit toward the affected shoulder. The affected shoulder is abducted to 45 degrees and the elbow of the affected shoulder flexed to 90 degrees. Allow the flexed elbow to rest on and be supported by your shoulder. Use both open hands to firmly grasp the proximal humerus and direct a straight lateral force, effectively translating the humeral head from the glenoid (Fig. 16-38).

While the patient is supine and you are standing toward the affected shoulder, the motion of humeral head depression (inferior glide) can be accomplished. The arm of the affected shoulder is abducted as close to

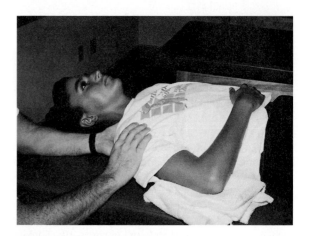

FIG. 16-37 Anterior and posterior glide of the glenohumeral joint.

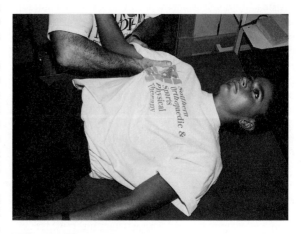

FIG. 16-38 Lateral distraction of the humeral head.

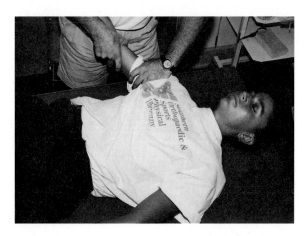

FIG. 16-39 Inferior glide of the glenohumeral joint.

90 degrees as possible. Firmly grasp the distal humerus with one hand and direct a straight axial force to distract the humeral head from the glenoid. Place the open palm of the other hand on the superior aspect of the humeral head and simultaneously direct an inferior force to the humerus (Fig. 16-39).

REFERENCES

1. Bergfeld JA: Acromioclavicular complex. In Nicholas JA, Hershman EB, editors: *The upper extremity in sports medicine,* St. Louis, 1990, Mosby.
2. Blackburn TA, Voight ML: Rehabilitation of the unstable shoulder. In *Advances in clinical education,* Mobile, Ala., 1994, course notes.
3. Boissonnault WG, Janos SC: Dysfunction, evaluation and treatment of the shoulder. In Donatelli R, Wooden MJ, editors: *Orthopaedic physical therapy,* New York, 1989, Churchill Livingstone.
4. Chandler TJ et al: Shoulder strength, power and endurance in college tennis players, *Am J Sports Med* 20 (4):455-458, 1992.
5. Goldstein TS: Treatment of common problems of the Shoulder Complex. In *Geriatric orthopaedics: rehabilitative management of common problems,* Gaithersburg, Md., 1991, Aspen Publications.
6. Halbach JW, Tank RT: The shoulder. In Gould JA, editor: *Orthopaedic and sports physical therapy,* ed 2, St. Louis, 1990, Mosby.
7. Hawkins RJ, Mohtadi N: Rotator cuff problems in athletes. In DeLee JC, Drez D editors: *Orthopaedic sports medicine: principals and practice,* vol I, Philadelphia, 1994, WB Saunders.
8. Hisamoto J: *Eccentric training: myth vs. reality in functional loading of the shoulder complex,* Atlanta, Ga., 1995, course notes.
9. Kamkar A, Irrgang J, Whitney SL: Nonoperative management of secondary shoulder impingement syndrome, *J Orthop Sports Phys Ther* 17:212-224, 1993.
10. Lippert L: Shoulder girdle. In *Clinical kinesiology for physical therapist assistant,* ed 2, Philadelphia, 1994, FA Davis.
11. McRae R: *Practical fracture treatment,* ed 3, New York, 1994, Churchill Livingstone.
12. Mendoza FX, Nicholas JA, Sands A: Principals of shoulder rehabilitation in the athlete. In Nicholas JA, Hershman EB, editor: *The upper extremity in sports medicine,* St. Louis, 1990, Mosby.
13. Miller MD: *Review of orthopaedics,* Philadelphia, 1992, WB Saunders.
14. Miller RH: Rotator cuff survery. In *Shoulder rehab,* Nashville, Tenn. 1990, course notes.
15. Morrison DS: The shoulder. In *Shoulder rehab 90,* Nashville, Tenn., 1990, course notes.
16. Moseley JB et al: EMG analysis of the scapular muscles during a shoulder rehabilitation program, *Am J Sports Med* 20:128-134, 1992.
17. Neer CS: Impingement lesions, *Clin Orthop* 173:70-77, 1983.
18. Neer CS, Rockwood CA: Fractures and dislocations of the shoulder. In Rockwood CA, Green DR, editors: *Fractures in adults,* ed 2, Philadelphia, 1984, JB Lippincott.
19. Pagnani MJ, Galinat BJ, Warren RF: Glenohumeral instability. In DeLee JC, Drez D, editors: *Orthopaedic sports medicine principals and practice,* vol I, Philadelphia, 1994, WB Saunders.
20. Skyhar MJ, Warren RF, Altchek DW: Instability of the shoulder, In Nicholas JA, Hershman EB, editors: *The upper extremity in sports medicine,* St. Louis, 1990, Mosby.
21. Strege D: Upper extremity. In Loth T, editor: *Orthopaedic boards review,* St. Louis, 1993, Mosby.
22. Thein LA: Rehabilitation of shoulder injuries. In Prentice WE, editor: *Rehabilitation techniques in sports medicine,* ed 2, St. Louis, 1994, Mosby.
23. Townsend H et al: Electromyographic analysis of the glenohumeral muscles during a baseball rehabilitation program, *Am J Sports Med* 19:264-272, 1991.
24. Voight ML: Overview of shoulder rehabilitation: a scientific biomechanical approach to the problem. In *Advances in clinical education, Mobile, Ala.* 1994, course notes.
25. Voight ML: Rotator cuff disorders. In *Advances in Clinical Education,* Mobile Ala., 1994, course notes.
26. Wadsworth CT: Frozen shoulder, *Phys Ther* 66(12):1878-1883, 1986.
27. Wilk KE: Conservative treatment for the unstable shoulder. In *Advances on the knee and shoulder,* 1993, Hilton Head, S.C., course notes.
28. Wilk KE, Mangine R: Post-operative rehabilitation of rotator cuff repairs. In *Advances on the knee and shoulder,* Hilton Head, S.C., 1993, course notes.

29. Williams GR, Rockwood CA: Fractures of the scapula. In DeLee JC, Drez D, editors: *Orthopaedic sports medicine: principals and practice,* vol I, Philadelphia, 1994, WB Saunders.

30. Williams GR, Rockwood CA: Injuries to the acromioclavicular joint. In DeLee JC, Drez D, editors: *Orthopaedic sports medicine: principals and practice,* vol I, St. Louis, 1994, WB Saunders.

31. Wooden MJ: Mobilization of the upper extremity. In Donatelli R, Wooden MJ, editors: *Orthopaedic physical therapy,* New York, 1989, Churchill Livingstone.

32. Yahara ML: Shoulder. In Richardson JK, Iglarsh ZA, editors: *Clinical orthopaedic physical therapy,* Philadelphia, 1994, WB Saunders.

33. Young DC, Rockwood CA: Fractures of the clavicle. In DeLee JC, Drez D, editors: *Orthopaedic sports medicine: principals and practice,* vol I, Philadelphia, 1994, WB Saunders.

Orthopedic Management of the Elbow

This chapter introduces the physical therapist assistant to common soft tissue injuries and fractures of the distal humerus and elbow. Specific attention is directed at identifying treatment programs used to control pain and swelling and improve motion, strength, and function of the elbow after injury and/or immobilization.

LATERAL EPICONDYLITIS

Commonly referred to as "**tennis elbow**,"[4] lateral epicondylitis[15] affects the common wrist extensor origin of the extensor carpi radialis longus, extensor carpi radialis brevis, extensor digitorum, and extensor digiti minimi.[4] The repetitive **overuse** of this area leads to tendinitis of the origin of the extensor carpi radialis brevis tendon[5,15] (Fig. 17-1).

Interestingly, lateral **epicondylitis** (tennis elbow) can affect anyone involved with repetitive activities of the wrist extensors.[14] Thus persons involved with the use of hand tools (hammer, screwdriver, pliers) and various activities involving wrist twisting, pulling, extending, and hand grasping can be affected by lateral epicondylitis.[14]

Generally, the patient suffering from lateral epicondylitis has pain with palpation of the lateral epicondyle, with active or resisted wrist extension, and occasionally with grasping of the affected hand.[4,12,14]

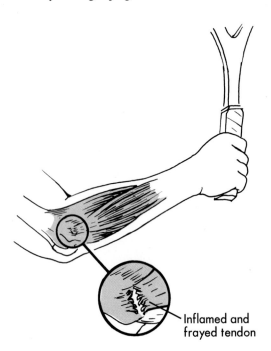

FIG. 17-1 Lateral epicondylitis, "tennis elbow," affects the common wrist-extensor origin.

Inflamed and frayed tendon

Because this is a chronic overuse tendinitis, the intense inflammatory response in the affected area of the lateral epicondyle is "an attempt to increase the rate of tissue production to compensate for the increased rate of tissue microdamage."[14]

Initial acute management focuses on resolving pain and swelling with the judicious use of ice massage directly over the affected area, phonophoresis or iontophoresis, physician-prescribed analgesics and nonsteroidal antiinflammatory drugs (NSAIDs), rest, and protection of the area from unwanted stress to allow for healing.[4,12,14]

"Relative rest" rather than strict immobilization is used. A wrist cock-up splint can be used in severe cases to minimize stress on the inflamed wrist extensor tendons. The patient is allowed to remove the splint as needed to participate in controlled motion exercises that do not produce pain. Long-term, rigid immobilization is *not* indicated, because treatment goals are to not only reduce pain and swelling but also to encourage proper collagen alignment and scar tissue maturation.[14] Without early protected motion, excessive tissue scarring and random collagen fiber alignment would severely limit normalized motion and function of the elbow and wrist.

During the initial healing stage, the assistant must encourage the patient to avoid any and all motions that may adversely affect healing. Short-term modifications in activities of daily living (ADLs), sports, and job-related activities must be addressed to provide a pain-free environment for healing. When this initial program fails to bring significant relief of symptoms, some physicians may elect to inject the area with a steroid to reduce the inflammation.[10,12]

In addition, active gentle static stretching is advised for the wrist extensors to produce normalized, pain-free wrist flexion and extension (Fig. 17-2). While specifically addressing treatment for the elbow, active motion and resistance exercises for the elbow and shoulder can be initiated if no wrist motion occurs to increase symptoms.

The physical therapist assistant can enhance the effectiveness of low-load, long-duration static stretching by applying moist heat packs (provided the acute inflammatory process has ended) and/or ultrasound to the lateral epicondyle to stimulate local circulation and relieve congestion caused by metabolic waste products and relax soft tissues in preparation for stretching.

As pain is reduced with active motion exercises, resistance exercise can begin. Generally, submaximal isometrics are used for wrist extension, flexion, forearm pronation and supination, and radial and ulnar deviation.

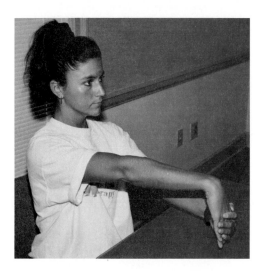

FIG. 17-2 Stretching of the wrist extensors.

The assistant must carefully instruct the patient to perform all exercises within a pain-free ROM. Throughout all phases of recovery, the patient must avoid stressful, pain-producing activities to prevent the continuation of the inflammatory condition. Progressive motion exercises and increased resistance exercise is the foundation for a return to functional activities. Once the patient can demonstrate increased quality of multiangle isometric contractions, concentric and eccentric muscle contractions are added. Care must be taken when initiating both concentric and eccentric resistance exercises because frequently these contractions produce symptoms. Very light resistance is advocated when having patients perform these exercises for the first time. A very important component for all resistance exercises used with lateral epicondylitis is the performance of slow, controlled eccentric contractions. As noted in Chapter 3, eccentric muscle contractions produce greater tension than either concentric or isometric exercise. In addition, energy use involving adenosine triphosphate (ATP) is less for eccentric exercise than for either concentric or isometric exercise. Eccentric muscle contractions are, in fact, advocated by Curwin and Stanish[4] for the treatment of "tennis elbow," and the rationale for the performance of eccentric exercise is described by Reid and Kushner[13] as follows: "Exercising the muscle eccentrically allows it to withstand greater resistance and prevent injury, which occurs by eccentrically loading an inflexible muscle."

Resistive exercises emphasizing the eccentric phase are described in Fig. 17-3. A hammer is an effective strengthening tool for the treatment of lateral epicondylitis. However, when instructing the patient to perform pronation and supination of the forearm for the first time, have the patient hold the hammer close to its head (Fig. 17-4). As the patient gains strength and can control the resistance of the hammer eccentrically, gradually have the patient hold the hammer at the mid-shaft. As strength improves further, allow the patient to hold the hammer at the end of the shaft, which requires greater eccentric muscle control, strength, and torque. In the same manner, strength can be gained for radial and ulnar deviation using the hammer. With a gradual return to functional activities, some physicians and therapists advocate the use of a counterforce brace to help dissipate the "**overload** forces" on the common origin of the wrist extensors[4,10,14] (Fig. 17-5).

Surgery is rarely required for this condition because physical therapy management is frequently very effective. In rare instances, when conservative means fail to reduce pain and improve function, the surgeon may elect to surgically excise the "angiofibroblastic tissue at the origin of the extensor carpi radialis brevis muscle."[15]

MEDIAL EPICONDYLITIS

This overuse condition affects the origin of the pronator teres, flexor carpi radialis, flexor digitorum sublimis, and flexor carpi ulnaris at the medial epicondyle of the elbow.[12] Although it occurs less often than lateral epicondylitis (lateral epicondylitis-to-medial epicondylitis ratio is 7:1),[14] it is no less incapacitating to the patient. Again, the dominant feature is pain with palpation over the medial epicondyle, active motion, and particularly with resisted wrist flexion and full passive wrist extension (Fig. 17-6).[12,13]

The acute management phase of this inflammatory overuse condition, also referred to as "golfer's elbow," concentrates on the management of pain and swelling. Usually the physician prescribes NSAIDs, ice (must protect the ulnar nerve), phonophoresis or iontophoresis, rest (not immobilization), protection, and gentle active motion exercises. The criteria-based treatment plan parallels that for lateral epicondylitis, while obviously focusing on the wrist flexors. Static low-load, long-duration stretching can proceed as pain allows. The physical therapist assistant must encourage the patient to avoid repetitive flexing of the wrist and pronating of the forearm if these motions produce pain. Modifications in lifting, twisting, pulling, or turning of the wrist and forearm must accompany each phase of recovery to avoid stress on the medial structures. Moist heat and ultrasound can be applied to the medial epicondyle

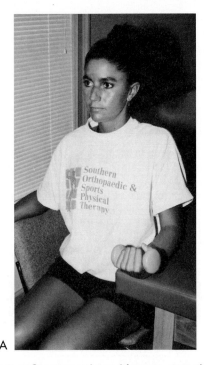
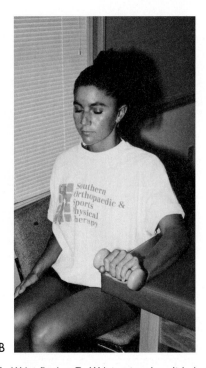

FIG. 17-3 Common wrist and forearm strengthening exercises. **A,** Wrist flexion **B,** Wrist extension. It is important to encourage slow, controlled, nonballistic concentric and eccentric contractions.

before stretching, once motion has improved without pain. Then resistance training can begin, first with submaximal isometrics, progressing to higher quality isometric multiangle contractions, and ultimately to concentric and eccentric isotonic and isokinetic resistance exercises. The patient is instructed in the active use of the shoulder of the affected limb and strongly encouraged to follow a conditioning program to maintain or enhance cardiovascular fitness, strength, and flexibility throughout the rehabilitation process.

Although the resolution of pain and swelling is paramount for active use of the wrist and forearm, regaining lost motion caused by pain and muscular dysfunction is critical for function and a return to normal daily activities. The normal ROM of the elbow is 0 degrees to approximately 145 degrees of flexion.[15] However, most daily activities can be carried out within a functional ROM of 30 to 130 degrees of flexion.[15] In addition, normal pronation of 75 degrees and supination of 85 degrees exceeds the functional arc of motion of 50 degrees needed to carry out most ADLs. Therefore the physical therapist assistant must encourage pain-free early protected motion to facilitate the collagen fiber alignment needed for both functional scar maturation and purposeful motion to perform daily activities.

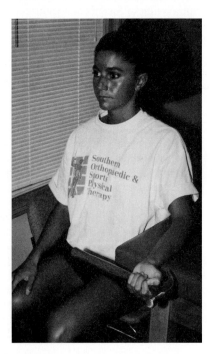

FIG. 17-4 Pronation exercise with a hammer. Notice that the grip is held close to the head of the hammer when first introducing this exercise.

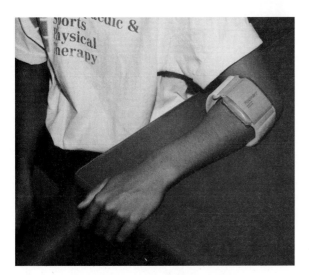

FIG. 17-5 Counterforce brace may help spread or dissipate overload force on the common wrist extensor origin.

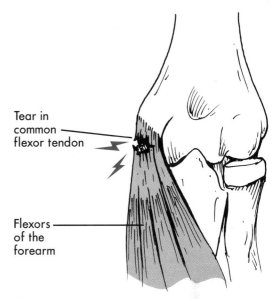

Tear in common flexor tendon

Flexors of the forearm

FIG. 17-6 Medial epicondylitis, "golfer's elbow." Repetitive overuse injury.

MEDIAL VALGUS STRESS OVERLOAD

Medial **valgus stress overload** occurs commonly among patients who participate in repetitive throwing and racquet sports such as javelin throwing, baseball, racquetball, and tennis.[5,11,12] Clinical differences exist between medial valgus stress overload and medial epicondylitis. While medial epicondylitis represents a chronic overuse syndrome affecting the soft tissue musculotendinous origin of the wrist flexors and pronators, medial valgus stress overload occurs to the capsuloligamentous structures (medial [ulnar] collateral ligament) as a result of repetitive valgus stress to the elbow[5,11,12] (Fig. 17-7).

Patients usually complain of pain over the medial aspect of the elbow and over the posterior aspect of the **olecranon.**[12,11] During the physical therapist's initial evaluation the assistant may observe the performance of ligament stability tests to confirm the presence of ulnar collateral ligament laxity. The affected arm is held in 10 to 30 degrees of flexion while the humerus is held in full external rotation. A medial or valgus stress is then applied to the elbow to assess the stability of the medial (ulnar) collateral ligament[11,12] (Fig. 17-8).

Management of valgus stress injuries must take into account the healing constraints of ligaments. The patient may receive physician-prescribed NSAIDs, analgesics, ice massage, phonophoresis, or iontophoresis to reduce pain and swelling. Rest and protection of the injured medial ligamentous structures, while avoiding valgus stress, are the hallmarks of management. Because most

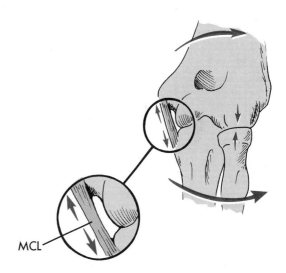

MCL

FIG. 17-7 Medial valgus stress overload. Repetitive valgus stress to the elbow may stress the capsuloligamentous structures of the elbow.

of these injuries occur to active sports enthusiasts, the patient must omit activities that produce medial valgus stress. To ensure compliance, it may be necessary to suggest short-term rest from the activity, during which the patient should participate in running, cycling, and strength training and should perform flexibility exercises as long as no valgus load is applied to the elbow joint. In addition, the wrist, hand, and shoulder of the

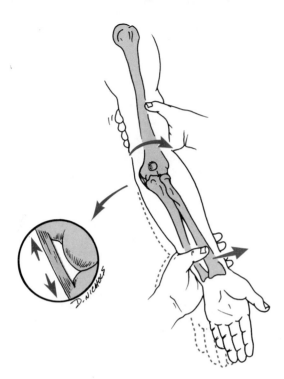

FIG. 17-8 Clinical valgus stress exam to test the stability of the medial (ulnar) collateral ligament.

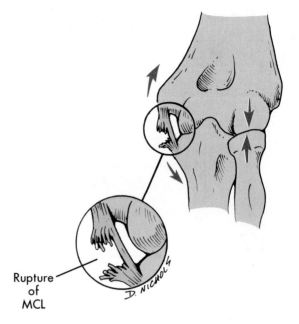

Rupture of MCL

FIG. 17-9 Sudden valgus force applied to a skeletally mature adult may result in rupture of the medial collateral ligament.

affected limb must be exercised during each phase of recovery.

Gentle low-load static stretching begins as soon as pain allows. All valgus stress must be eliminated for spontaneous ligamentous healing to occur. Therefore the stretching regimen focuses on all wrist motions, forearm pronation and supination, and elbow flexion and extension as long as no symptoms of pain occur with these activities.

The strengthening component of recovery must be modified to prevent any valgus stress. Full ROM (flexion-extension) concentric and eccentric resistance exercise is allowed with light weights as motion and pain dictate. Wrist and hand exercises are encouraged early and pose no threat to the healing ligament. In addition, forearm pronation and supination using a hammer, as previously outlined, is employed as the patient is able to demonstrate improved motion without pain.

With time, the physical therapist reassesses the stability of the medial collateral ligaments. If these structures demonstrate improved stability without pain, a very gradual return to throwing can begin.

If conservative treatment fails to restore function and eliminate pain, surgery is considered. Degenerative changes, which are usually present in the adult, *must* be

addressed surgically.[11,13] In general, an osteotomy is performed to remove osteophytes (bone spurs) and fibrotic, degenerated tissue.[11,13]

In skeletally mature adults, if valgus stress is applied suddenly with sufficient force, acute rupture (grade III—ligament rupture) of the medial (ulnar) collateral ligament can occur (Fig. 17-9).

First, these patients are managed conservatively with ice, NSAIDs, analgesics, and, most importantly, rest and protection. The progression from the acute, maximal-protection phase to return-to-normal function parallels treatment outlined for valgus stress injuries. However, because the ligament has been ruptured, a longer period of recovery is needed and rest and joint protection from valgus stress will last longer. Normal elbow function, which means flexion, extension, pronation, and supination, should be encouraged as early as pain and motion allow.

If early active protected joint motion and progressive resistance exercise have been used, authorities suggest that the injured patient can resume throwing activities approximately 3 months after injury.[11] However, if the patient does not demonstrate improved valgus stability and continues to have dysfunction, surgery may be required to stabilize the joint.

Generally, if the ulnar collateral ligament is ruptured midsubstance, then either a direct repair is carried out or a reconstructive procedure is used wherein a free tendon graft of the palmaris longus is routed through drill holes to reconstruct the medial stabilizers of the elbow.[11,12]

Postoperative rehabilitation begins immediately, with the patient's affected limb immobilized in a brace to protect against valgus stress. Instructions are given to perform hand, wrist, and shoulder exercises to maintain motion. Usually, by the third week postoperatively, ROM should approach 20 to 110 degrees.[5] The continuous use of ice and therapeutic agents (ultrasound, TENS, galvanic stimulation)[13] are prescribed as needed. Progressive resistance concentric and eccentric contractions are used for the wrist of the involved limb, whereas submaximal isometrics can begin for elbow flexion and extension.

Shoulder strengthening and flexibility exercises can also begin during the third week of recovery.[5] However, care must be taken to avoid external shoulder rotation exercises because this motion produces valgus stress on the elbow.[5]

Usually, by 4 to 6 weeks after surgery, ROM should be 0 to 130 degrees.[5] In addition, concentric and eccentric resistance exercises for elbow flexion and extension are added progressively as tolerated. Gentle forearm pronation and supination exercises can also be made more challenging. From 2 to 4 months after surgery, functional training can begin with an emphasis on shoulder, elbow, and wrist strengthening, motion exercises, and gentle throwing for the athlete. Ultimately, it takes 12 months after elbow reconstruction and rehabilitation for valgus instability before a functional return to competitive sports is allowed.[11]

FRACTURES OF THE DISTAL HUMERUS (SUPRACONDYLAR FRACTURES)

By definition a **supracondylar fracture** is a transverse fracture of the distal third of the humerus.[7] These frequent injuries usually occur in children.[7,11,14] Supracondylar fractures are generally of two types.[3,7,15] Type I is the most common and refers to an injury that occurs as a result of a fall on an extended, outstretched arm in which the distal humerus fragment is displaced posteriorly and is maintained in that position because of the strong pull of the triceps[3,15] (Fig. 17-10). Type II is considered a flexion injury and occurs after direct trauma to the posterior aspect of the elbow in which the distal humeral fragment lies anterior to the humerus (Fig. 17-11).[3,15]

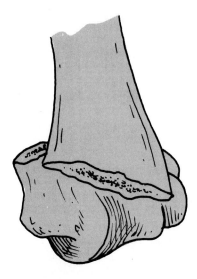

FIG. 17-10 Supracondylar fracture type I or extension-type fracture in which the distal humeral fragment is displaced posteriorly.

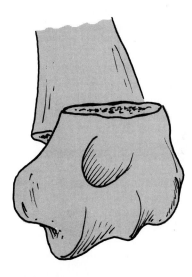

FIG. 17-11 Supracondylar fracture type II, or flexion-type in which the distal humeral fragment is displaced anteriorly.

The most common treatment of these fractures is by closed reduction and immobilization for 4 to 6 weeks. The affected arm is held in a flexed position to allow the triceps to help maintain the fracture in a stable position.[7,15]

As with all other fractures, the initial phase of recovery focuses on motion and strengthening exercises for the contralateral limb, general body conditioning, and active motion of the hand, wrist, and shoulder of the injured limb, as along as no undue stress is directed at the fracture site.

Physical therapy treatment after immobilization focuses on gentle active motion exercises, which can be preceded by the use of moist heat or a warm whirlpool to encourage relaxation, removal of wastes, and improved local circulation. In most cases, progressive active motion of the elbow and resistance exercises proceed as radiographic evidence confirms solid union, a minimum of 6 weeks has elapsed since surgery (consistent with the healing constraints of bone tissue), and the patient demonstrates improved motion without pain.

Complications arising from supracondylar fractures[8] include nonunion, malunion, and joint contracture. Perhaps the most disastrous complication results from vascular compromise.[3,7,8,15] As the fracture fragments are displaced, hemorrhage beneath the deep fascia produces an ischemic injury that creates an arterial and venous obstruction (usually affecting the brachial artery), leading to **Volkmann's ischemic contracture** (Fig. 17-12).[3,8,14] Most importantly, the clinical signs and symptoms of ischemic obstruction may not be noticed until the end of immobilization.[3] The symptoms of Volkmann's ischemic contracture can occur throughout each phase of recovery after a supracondylar fracture.

Stralka and Brasel[14] outline six symptoms authorities define as indicating vascular obstruction:
- Severe pain in the forearm muscles
- Limited and extremely painful finger movement
- Purple discoloration of the hand with prominent veins
- Initial paresthesia followed by loss of sensation
- Loss of radial pulse and later loss of capillary return
- Pallor, anesthesia, and paralysis

Restoration of elbow function (flexion, extension, pronation, and supination of the forearm) after supracondylar fractures initially focuses on motion exercises that do not stress the fracture site. Therefore passive stretching is contraindicated during the early healing phase.[7] Gentle active exercises for the upper arm, wrist, and shoulder should, of course, be performed to the patient's tolerance. Resistance exercises using submaximal isometrics and progressing to concentric and eccentric muscle contractions are allowed, pending confirmation of secure union of the fracture fragments.

INTERCONDYLAR "T" OR "Y" FRACTURES

In addition to nondisplaced or displaced transverse supracondylar fractures, potentially more significant fracture patterns can occur with falls or direct trauma to the elbow. **Intercondylar fractures** describe injuries that extend between the condyles of the humerus and involve the articular surfaces of the elbow joint.[3,7,8,15] According to Strege[15] and Miller[8], there are four classifications of intercondylar fractures that display a T or Y configuration:

Type I: A nondisplaced fracture that extends between the two condyles (Fig. 17-13) [3,7,11,15]

Type II: A displaced fracture without rotation of the fracture fragments (Fig. 17-14)[3,7,11,15]

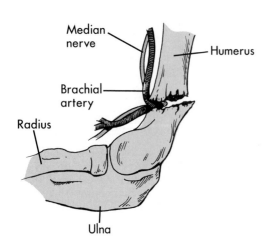

FIG. 17-12 Volkmann's ischemic contracture.

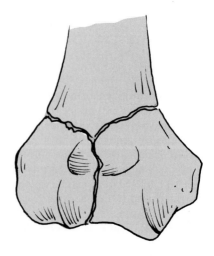

FIG. 17-13 Intercondylar fracture, type I—nondisplaced.

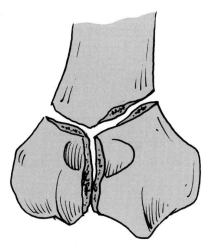

FIG. 17-14 Intercondylar fracture, type II—displaced without rotation.

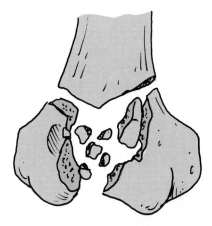

FIG. 17-16 Severely comminuted type IV intercondylar fracture with significant displacement.

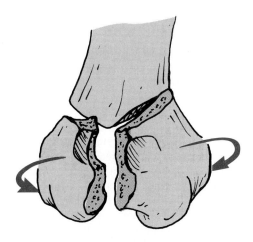

FIG. 17-15 Intercondylar fracture, type III—displaced with rotation of fragments.

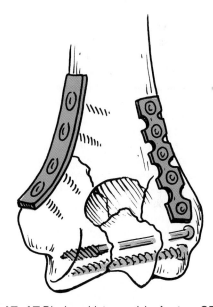

FIG. 17-17 Displaced intercondylar fracture ORIF.

Type III: A displaced fracture with a rotational deformity (Fig. 17-15) [3,7,11,15]

Type IV: A severely comminuted fracture with significant separation between the two condyles (Fig. 17-16) [3,7,11,15]

The type of fracture dictates a course of treatment that parallels the significance of the injury. With a type I nondisplaced fracture, treatment can be immobilization for approximately 3 weeks, followed by progressive, gentle active motion. Resistance exercises are deferred until secure bone union has been confirmed radiographically. With types II and III displaced fractures, the treatment is open reduction and internal fixation (ORIF)

with the use of Kirschner wires, side plates, and lag screws to secure and stabilize the displaced fracture fragments (Fig. 17-17).[7,8,15] Type IV comminuted intercondylar fractures are treated differently for adults and elderly patients with poor bone quality (osteoporosis).[8,15] In adult patients the treatment is usually with an ORIF procedure to stabilize the fragments. However, in the elderly patient, because of generally poor bone quality (osteopenic bone), a treatment procedure referred to as the "**bag of bones technique**" is used.[7,8,15]

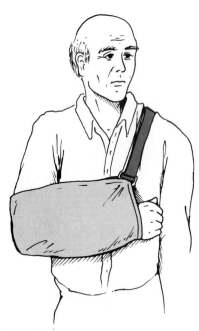

FIG. 17-18 In cases where elderly patients with osteoporosis suffer a severely comminuted intercondylar fracture, a treatment referred to as the "bag of bones" technique is used.

This technique calls for the use of a "collar and cuff"[15] sling with the affected elbow flexed as far as the limits of swelling and circulatory compromise allow.[15] With the elbow flexed and able to hang freely within the sling, gravity is used to help obtain possible reduction of the fracture fragments (Fig. 17-18).[8,15]

With intercondylar fractures of the elbow, during immobilization, the patient is instructed in a general conditioning program while close attention is paid to avoiding all stress to the affected arm. In addition, the wrist, hand, and shoulder of the affected limb may be exercised with active motion if prescribed by the physician and physical therapist. With intercondylar fractures, the anatomic relationship of the elbow (being extremely compact, with significant bony stability) dictates that the restoration of purposeful, functional motion becomes paramount during recovery. Soft tissue scarring and bone callus formation can lead to early joint stiffness, arthrosis, and contractures.

During the early postimmobilization period, no passive manipulation or passive stretching can be performed.[15] Strege[15] reports an appreciable risk of joint ankylosis when passive stretching and manipulation are performed during early postinjury elbow rehabilitation.

Once wound closure has occurred after an ORIF procedure, the use of a whirlpool bath may aid local circulation, removal of waste, reduction in soft tissue congestion, and enhancement of soft tissue relaxation in preparation for protected active motion. Elbow flexion and extension as well as forearm pronation and supination are encouraged as prescribed by the physician and directed by the physical therapist. Stable union of the fracture signifies more active involvement with progressive motion exercises and the initiation of resistance exercise training to regain strength. If the patient demonstrates loss of motion, the physician and physical therapist may decide to perform specific joint mobilization techniques once bone union is secure. This does not conflict with the previously mentioned contraindication for passive manipulation and stretching immediately after immobilization. Some patients may ultimately have residual loss of motion. However, functional activities can be performed with flexion and extension of 30 to 130 degrees and pronation and supination of 50 degrees.[15]

RADIAL HEAD FRACTURES

Another common fracture that occurs as a result of a fall on an outstretched arm is a radial head fracture. These fractures represent approximately one-third of all elbow fractures and nearly 20% of all elbow trauma.[6]

The definition of the "**carrying angle**" of the elbow and the difference noted between males and females are important in understanding radial head fractures. The carrying angle is formed between the intersection of the long axis of the humerus and the axis of the ulna with the elbow joint in full extension.[15] A normal carrying angle for males is 10 degrees of valgus; in females, it is 13 degrees of valgus[15] (Fig. 17-19). The clinical relevance is that a fractured radial head can lead to an increased valgus deformity as well as the varus elbow malalignment called a "gunstock deformity."[6]

Radial head fractures are generally classified into four types, as follows:

Type I: A nondisplaced fracture
Type II: A marginal fracture with displacement
Type III: A comminuted fracture of the entire radial head
Type IV: Any radial head fracture with elbow dislocation[15] (Fig. 17-20)

Treatment options parallel the significance of the injury and dictate the course of rehabilitation. Type I nondisplaced radial head fractures usually require a period of immobilization ranging from 5 to 7 days[15] up to 3 to 4 weeks.[7] Usually, early active motion is allowed as soon

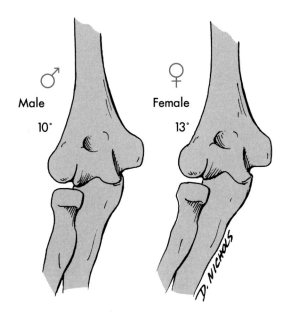

FIG. 17-19 Elbow carrying angles.

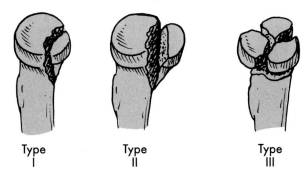

FIG. 17-20 Radial head fractures: type I—nondisplaced, type II—displaced, type III—comminuted.

as pain subsides. Because these fractures are generally stable (nondisplaced), healing occurs with very good results.[7] Terminal elbow extension may be recovered many months after type I radial head fractures.[7]

With a type II displaced fracture, the radial head can either be excised or stabilized with an ORIF procedure. With a type III comminuted radial head fracture, the fractured area is excised.[6-8,15]

Rehabilitation after an ORIF or radial head excision usually calls for immobilization in a hinged splint to protect the healing bone (ORIF procedure) and soft tissues (excision). As noted previously, excision of the radial head can lead to increased varus or valgus

deformity. In either case, migration of the radial shaft may occur after excision and place stress on the distal ligamentous radio-ulnar articulation.[6-8] Therefore if discomfort is expressed by the patient at the distal radio-ulnar joint following excision of the radial head, it usually results from added stress on this area created by the disrupted proximal radial segment.[6-8] When the patient is immobilized, the hand, wrist, and shoulder of the affected limb are exercised as tolerated. The patient is also encouraged to participate in a general conditioning program of aerobic exercise, strength training, and flexibility exercises. Pain and swelling are usually managed satisfactorily by placing ice packs directly over the painful area. Early active ROM exercises are advocated 3 to 5 days postoperatively by some[15] or deferred for up to 3 weeks by others.[6] Restoration of motion is the cornerstone for recovery after radial head fractures. As noted earlier, joint restrictions secondary to arthrofibrosis and contractures can occur, with pronation and supination most commonly affected after radial head fractures.

The physical therapist may elect to perform specific joint mobilization techniques to enhance pronation and supination if secure fixation has occurred after an ORIF procedure. Once wound closure has occurred, a whirlpool bath can be an effective adjunct preceding motion exercises. After excision of the radial head, resistance exercises of elbow flexion and extension and forearm pronation and supination can begin as soon as pain and motion allow. These exercises may need to be deferred for longer periods if an ORIF procedure was used so that stable bone union and soft tissue healing can occur.

OLECRANON FRACTURES

Olecranon fractures commonly result after a fall on the point of the elbow (olecranon process) or indirectly from forceful contraction of the triceps.[7] They are generally classified as either nondisplaced or displaced fractures. Displaced fractures of the olecranon have four subclassifications:[8]
- Avulsion fracture—displaced
- Oblique or transverse fracture
- Comminuted fracture
- Fracture-dislocation

The treatment for nondisplaced olecranon fractures requires immobilization for 6 to 8 weeks,[3,7] although as little as 3 weeks or less is used in some cases (particularly elderly patients).[8,15] The position in which nondisplaced olecranon fractures are immobilized is somewhat controversial, in that some authorities advocate placing the affected arm in extension or slight flexion,[1,3,6,7] whereas others recommend placing the affected arm in 45 to 90 degrees of flexion.[8,15] The rationale for placing the elbow in 45 degrees of flexion is the likelihood of the loss of flexion after immobilization.[15] In addition, Strege[15] suggests that immobilization should not exceed 45 degrees because of the risk of displacing fracture fragments.[15]

Usually, nondisplaced olecranon fractures are allowed gentle active ROM exercises after 3 weeks of immobilization. Flexion of the affected arm should not exceed 90 degrees for the first 6 to 8 weeks after injury so that fracture fragments can heal.[6,15]

Displaced or comminuted fractures of the olecranon can be treated with an ORIF procedure to secure the fragments. With severely comminuted fractures, excision of as much as 80% of the olecranon can occur without loss of joint stability.[8,15]

Physical therapy can begin during the initial stages of immobilization. Active motion of the ipsilateral hand, wrist, forearm (pronation and supination), and shoulder can commence once acute pain has subsided. A general physical conditioning program is allowed as soon as tolerated by the patient. Active elbow flexion must not exceed 90 degrees for the first 2 months after injury. Active resistance exercises for elbow extension must be minimized because the forceful contraction of the triceps can displace the fracture fragments before secure bone healing at 8 weeks. Resistance exercises for elbow flexion can begin earlier if motion is limited and the muscle contractions are submaximal. Submaximal isometric triceps extensions can proceed once bony union has been verified. Progressive concentric and eccentric loading is added as motion increases and secure fixation of the fragments has occurred.

Progressive flexion and extension movements must proceed cautiously and slowly to prevent displacement of the fragments. In addition, the patient must be carefully instructed to initially perform resistance exercises well within the limits of pain and motion restrictions to allow for proper bone healing. The strong contractions of the biceps during flexion and the triceps during extension activities are effective to gradually overcome most motion limitations observed early after injury or surgery. Full recovery after olecranon fractures may take 6 months to 1 year.[6]

Fracture-dislocations

A fall on an extended outreaching arm causes isolated elbow dislocations and combined fracture-dislocations (Fig. 17-21).[5,7,9,13,14] Conwell[3] reports that "with the exception of the shoulder, the elbow is the most frequently dislocated joint in the body." This injury occurs

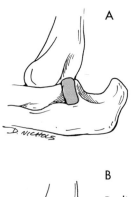

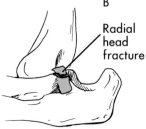

Radial head fracture

FIG. 17-21 A, Posterior elbow dislocation without radial head fracture. **B,** Posterior elbow dislocation with radial head fracture.

most often in males, with the nondominant arm representing about 60% of these injuries.[9]

Posterior elbow dislocations are the most common, whereas anterior dislocations represent only 1% to 2% of all elbow dislocations.[9] Associated fractures of the radial head occur in approximately 10% of elbow dislocations.[9,14] In addition, associated neurovascular injuries can occur with either isolated elbow dislocations or with fracture-dislocations.[7,9,14,15] Injuries involve the median, radial, and ulnar nerves as well as the brachial artery with elbow dislocations.[9,15]

Isolated posterior elbow dislocations are managed with closed reduction and immobilization.[3,5,7-9,14] The elbow is placed in 90 degrees of flexion in a splint for 3 to 6 weeks.[3,7,15] During this period, hand and shoulder motion is allowed if no offensive stress is applied to the elbow. Early active ROM exercises can begin during the first week after reduction.[15] However, no passive ROM or stretching is allowed because of the risk of myositis ossificans,[7,14] which results from aggressive passive stretching and mobilization. Active motion is not believed to cause this condition.[14] Therefore gentle active flexion and extension exercises are added as pain, swelling, and soft tissue healing dictate. Because this injury represents a hyperextension trauma that significantly affects the joint capsule, muscle, tendon, and frequently ligamentous restraints, extensive soft tissue healing is required for a stable, functional joint. The joint capsule of the elbow may require 8 to 10 weeks to heal satisfactorily.[5] Restoration of elbow extension must therefore proceed cautiously because the mechanism of injury is usually elbow hyperextension. As soft tissue healing progresses, resistance exercises can begin. Eccentric and concentric resistance exercises for the biceps can be emphasized to reduce hyperextension forces.[5] Resistance-type exercises are deferred for at least 3 weeks to allow for acute symptoms to subside. However, aggressive elbow extension must be prevented until 8 to 10 weeks have elapsed.[5,9]

The most common complication after elbow dislocation is loss of extension.[9,14,15] Ten weeks after dislocation, a 30-degree flexion contracture is common, and a 10-degree flexion contracture is typically observed 2 years after injury.[9] However unacceptable this loss of motion may be, it does not represent an "overwhelming functional deficit."[15]

The treatment of fracture-dislocations centers on the appropriate management of the fracture (most commonly the radial head) and reduction of the elbow. In most cases, radial head excision is performed to minimize the development of myositis ossificans.[14] Therefore with radial head excision, proximal migration of the radius can result in stress and pain to the distal radioulnar ligamentous articulation.[7,8,15]

Rehabilitation after fracture-dislocation of the elbow gains focus on early protected active motion. Passive stretching is again strictly avoided during the early recovery phases of healing. With radial head excision, a loss of 25 to 30 degrees of pronation and supination can be expected if postoperative immobilization lasts longer than 4 weeks.[14] As with isolated dislocation, loss of full elbow extension is not uncommon.

MOBILIZATION OF THE ELBOW

The rationale for specific joint mobilization is to avoid joint restrictions or hypomobility.[2] In many instances, arthrofibrosis occurs as a result of immobilization and internal fixation methods used to stabilize fracture fragments.

The physical therapist determines if mobilization is indicated after injury, surgery, or immobilization based on tissue healing constraints; the nature of the joint restriction (hypomobility of noncontractile tissue or articular surface dysfunction);[2] and whether passive motion is indicated for the treatment of joint limitations (see Chapters 11 and 12, Common Mobilization Techniques of the Ankle, Foot, and Toe). The physical therapist must clearly define the specific indications for mobilization with reference to the exact technique to be employed, the rate of movement, the amplitude of force,

and the direction of the force applied to the elbow. To obtain relaxation, the assistant must place the patient in a comfortable position, with specific attention paid to the support and stability of the shoulder, elbow, and arm of the patient. Before applying joint mobilization, thermal agents are employed to reduce tissue congestion, aid in the removal of wastes, and enhance relaxation of the patient and the affected joint.

Injuries to the elbow that require mobilization need to increase in flexion, extension, or both. Wooden[16] outlines three techniques used to enhance general motion, flexion, and extension of the elbow.

To enhance general mobility of the elbow, the patient is supine with the affected elbow flexed to 90 degrees. Hold the shoulder of the affected limb at the patient's side or in an abducted position. Place both hands at the proximal aspect of the forearm, and direct a straight lateral distraction force that directs the forearm away from the humerus (Fig. 17-22).

To promote elbow extension, humeral-ulnar abduction is employed.[16] The patient is supine with the affected arm abducted and the elbow slightly flexed. Sit to the patient's affected side with one hand stabilizing the distal lateral humerus and the other hand firmly grasping the ulnar aspect of the distal forearm. In this position, direct a valgus or abduction force to the elbow (Fig. 17-23).[16]

To increase elbow flexion, an adduction technique is applied.[16] The patient remains supine with the affected arm abducted. Sit to the patient's affected side and stabilize the distal humerus on the medial aspect with one hand, while placing the opposite hand on the distal radial aspect of the forearm. In this position, direct a varus or adduction force to the elbow (Fig. 17-24).

Although these few techniques are representative of the more common motions requiring mobilization, other

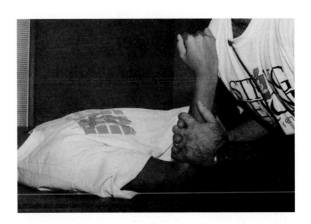

FIG. 17-22 Elbow distraction.

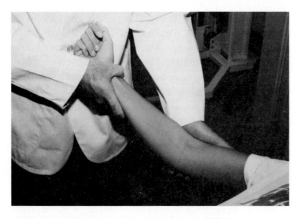

FIG. 17-23 Valgus or humeral-ulna abduction.

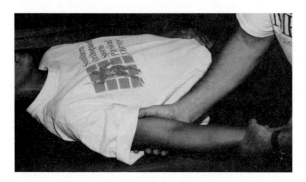

FIG. 17-24 Varus or humeral-ulna adduction.

positions and techniques can be used to enhance elbow motion.

REFERENCES

1. Bennett JB, Tullos HS: Acute injuries to the elbow. In Nicholas JA, Hershman EB, editors: *The upper extremity in sports medicine,* St. Louis, 1990, Mosby.
2. Bowling RW, Rockar PA: The elbow complex. In Gould JA, editor: *Orthopaedic and sports physical therapy,* ed 2, St. Louis, 1990, Mosby.
3. Conwell HE: Injuries to the elbow, Clinical symposia, Ciba-Geigy, 1969.
4. Curwin S, Stanish WD: *Tendinitis: it's etiology and treatment,* Lexington, Mass., 1984, DC Heath.
5. Dickoff-Hoffman S, Foster D: Rehabilitation of elbow injuries. In Prentice WE, editor: *Rehabilitation techniques in sports medicine,* ed 2, St. Louis, 1994, Mosby.
6. LaCroix E: Treatment of common problems of the elbow, forearm, and wrist joints. In Goldstein TS, editor: *Geriatric orthopaedics: rehabilitative management of common problems,* Gaithersburg, Md., 1991, Aspen Publications.
7. McRae R: Injuries about the elbow. In *Practical fracture treatment,* ed 3, New York, 1994, Churchill-Livingstone.
8. Miller MD: *Review of orthopaedics,* Philadelphia, 1992, WB Saunders.
9. Morrey BF: Elbow dislocation in the athlete. In DeLee JC, Drez D, editors: *Orthopaedic sports medicine: principles and practices,* vol 1, Philadelphia, 1994, WB Saunders.
10. Morrey BF, Regan WD: Tendinopathies about the elbow. In DeLee JC, Drez D, editors: *Orthopaedic sports medicine: principals and practices,* vol 1, Philadelphia, 1994, WB Saunders.
11. Morrey BF, Regan WD: Throwing injuries. In DeLee JC, Drez D, editors: *Orthopaedic sports medicine: principles and practice,* vol 1, Philadelphia, 1994, WB Saunders.
12. Parks JC: Overuse injuries of the elbow. In Nicholas JA, Hershman EB, editors: *The upper extremity in sports medicine,* St. Louis, 1990, Mosby.
13. Reid DC, Kushner S: The elbow region. In Donatelli R, Wooden MJ, editors: *Orthopaedic physical therapy,* New York, 1989, Churchill-Livingstone.
14. Stralka SW, Brasel JG: Elbow. In Richardson JK, Iglarsh ZA, editors: *Clinical orthopaedic physical therapy,* Philadelphia, 1994, WB Saunders.
15. Strege D: Upper extremity. In Loth TS, editor: *Orthopaedic Boards Review,* St. Louis, 1993, Mosby.
16. Wooden MJ: Mobilization of the upper extremity. In Donatelli R, Wooden MJ, editors: *Orthopaedic physical therapy,* New York, 1989, Churchill-Livingstone.

Orthopedic Management of the Wrist and Hand

KEY TERMS

Carpal tunnel syndrome
Compression neuropathy
Nerve entrapment
De Quervain's
   tenosynovitis
Cumulative trauma
   disorder
Colles' fracture
Smith's fracture
Dinner fork deformity
Scaphoid fracture
Anatomic snuffbox
Avascular necrosis
   (AVN)
Nonunion
Skier's thumb
Boxer's fracture
Fighter's fracture
Bennett's fracture
Dupuytren's contracture
Mallet finger
Boutonniere deformity
Flexor tendon
Reflex sympathetic
   dystrophy (RSD)

LEARNING OBJECTIVES

1. Identify and describe common compression neuropathies of the wrist.
2. Discuss methods of management and rehabilitation of compression neuropathies of the wrist.
3. Identify and describe common ligament injuries of the wrist.
4. Describe and discuss methods of management and rehabilitation of ligament injuries of the wrist.
5. Describe methods of management and rehabilitation for distal radial and ulnar fractures.
6. Identify methods of management and rehabilitation for scaphoid fractures.
7. Identify and describe common metacarpal fractures and methods of management and rehabilitation.
8. Describe methods of management and rehabilitation of Dupuytren's contracture.
9. Identify and describe common extensor and flexor tendon injuries.
10. Discuss methods of management and rehabilitation of extensor tendon and flexor tendon injuries.
11. Identify methods of management and rehabilitation for reflex sympathetic dystrophy.
12. Describe common mobilization techniques for the wrist and hand.

CHAPTER OUTLINE

This chapter will introduce common soft tissue injuries and fractures affecting the wrist and hand. The focus is on general therapeutic interventions to control pain and swelling and specific techniques to enhance motion, strength, and functional restoration of the wrist and hand after injury, surgery, and immobilization. The study of hand and wrist anatomy, kinesiology, and pathomechanics of injury is a difficult task. The physical therapist assistant must understand the interrelationships between the foundations of basic science (anatomy, kinesiology, injury, immobilization, and tissue healing) of the wrist and hand to effectively carry out and supervise rehabilitation programs prescribed by the physical therapist. Therefore before reading this chapter, the assistant is strongly urged to thoroughly review pertinent anatomy and kinesiology of the wrist and hand to more fully appreciate the rationale for immobilization, surgery, and rehabilitation after injuries to these areas.

CARPAL TUNNEL SYNDROME

Carpal tunnel syndrome refers to an entrapment **compression neuropathy** of the median nerve within the wrist[4-6,9,15](Fig. 18-1). This syndrome represents the most common compression neuropathy of the wrist.[4-6,9,15] It is caused by repetitive motions of the wrist

(flexion, ulnar deviation, supination, gripping, pinching)[4] as well as specific job tasks, occupations, and various leisure and sporting activities that place great repetitive demand on the wrist.[4-6,9,15] With repetitive motions, the carpal tunnel (formed by the transverse carpal ligament and the carpal bones, through which neurovascular structures pass) may become swollen and irritated, thereby "entrapping" and "compressing" the median nerve, which is located between the transverse carpal ligament and the carpal bones. There are many clinical symptoms of carpal tunnel syndrome; some of the more common ones include numbness; tingling; pain; clumsiness in hand activity; weakness of grip, pinch, and thumb actions; swelling in the hand and forearm; atrophy of the thenar muscles; and symptoms that become worse at night.[4,5] The effect of this overuse injury (also referred to as cumulative trauma disorder or repetitive motion injury)[4] is rather startling, with estimates that overuse injuries, in general, occur in approximately 4% of the entire United States' work force.[4]

Physical therapy management of carpal tunnel syndrome focuses on eliminating the motions that produce symptoms, using physician-prescribed nonsteroidal antiinflammatory drugs (NSAIDs), and splinting the affected wrist in 0 to 20 degrees of extension.[5,9,15] Wrist cock-up splints are commonly advocated nocturnally and as needed during the day.[5,9,15] Obviously, occupational tasks must be modified and those activities of daily living (ADLs), jobs, and recreational activities that call for repetitive motions of the wrist identified. In many cases, the use of NSAIDs and splinting is enough to minimize the inflammatory condition and reduce symptoms of pain, swelling, and tingling. However, if symptoms do not respond to this initial course of action, the physician may elect to inject the area with a corticosteroid to reduce pain and swelling. Furthermore, if a history of constant sensory loss, atrophy, and weakness of the thenar muscles is present, surgery may be indicated.[7] In general, the transverse carpal ligament is cut using an open technique or with endoscopic instrumentation.[5,9]

Physical therapy management during nonoperative splinting, rest, and antiinflammatory medications usually calls for active motion and resistance exercises for the elbow and shoulder of the affected limb, as well as a general conditioning program. Usually a course of specific motion and resistance exercises for the affected wrist is deferred for 4 to 5 weeks to allow the acute inflammation to subside.[5] Finger, hand (gripping), and wrist range of motion (ROM) and gentle resistance exercise must proceed cautiously once the patient can tolerate active motion of the wrist and hand without

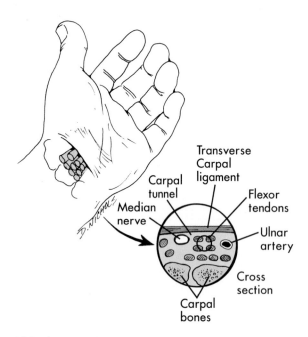

FIG. 18-1 Carpal tunnel syndrome. Compression neuropathy of the median nerve.

Transverse
Carpal
ligament

Carpal
tunnel

Median
nerve

Flexor
tendons

Ulnar
artery

Cross
section

Carpal
bones

pain. All aggravating motions that produce symptoms must be avoided.

If a surgical release is performed, the affected wrist is immobilized for as long as 10 to 14 days[9] or as little as 2 to 7 days.[5] During wrist immobilization, the patient is encouraged to actively use the elbow and shoulder of the affected limb and to participate in a general physical conditioning program. In addition, the patient should flex and extend the fingers and use the hand of the affected wrist.[9] As the surgical wound heals (sutures removed in 10 to 14 days),[9] active wrist motion exercises are initiated, along with motion and resistance exercises for the fingers and hand. Because a decompression surgical procedure was employed to reduce **nerve entrapment** and compression, the prevention of postoperative scarring to the wrist area is of paramount concern. Therefore the patient should be instructed in active motion exercises and massage of the tissues around and through the incision (scar management).[5,9] Once the sutures are removed, the wound is closed, and the patient is able to tolerate massage to the area, along with wrist motion and strengthening, a program of functional activities begins. In some instances, a full return to activities (particularly those duties that caused the problem in the first place) may need to be restricted or modified to accommodate the healing of the soft tissue.

DE QUERVAIN'S TENOSYNOVITIS

De Quervain's tenosynovitis is a repetitive motion injury or a **cumulative trauma disorder** that affects the tendons of the abductor pollicis longus and extensor pollicis brevis as they pass within the first dorsal compartment (Fig. 18-2).[5,6,9,15] Generally, motions that produce repetitive ulnar deviations can create tenosynovitis at the first dorsal compartment of the wrist. This condition is characterized by pain and swelling at the radial styloid, as well as reduced motion of the thumb.[5,9,15]

This overuse syndrome is managed conservatively at first with the use of NSAIDs and wrist and thumb immobilization. Any motions that produce pain must be eliminated for appropriate soft tissue inflammation to subside. The elbow and shoulder of the affected limb must be exercised with active ROM and resistance exercises from the time immobilization begins. In addition, ice and iontophoresis or phonophoresis may be effective adjuncts to reduce pain and swelling during the acute phase of recovery.[6] If after a few weeks of immobilization pain and swelling are much improved, active motion of the wrist and thumb can commence.

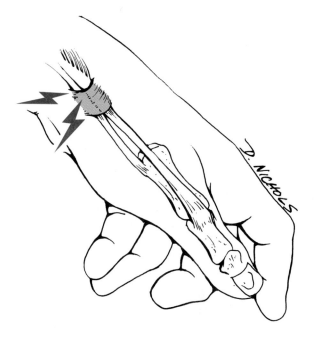

FIG. 18-2 De Quervain's tenosynovitis.

Resistance exercises must focus on slow, controlled concentric and eccentric muscle contractions that do not produce symptoms. Usually, all motions of the wrist and forearm are addressed, including flexion, extension, radial and ulnar deviation, pronation, and supination. Limited ulnar deviation motion may be needed when initiating ROM and resistance exercises. The volume and rate of activity involving radial and ulnar deviation may also require modification to accommodate soft tissue healing.

When conservative care fails to relieve symptoms, the physician may elect to inject the first dorsal compartment with a corticosteroid to reduce pain and inflammation.[5,9,15] Chronic cases of De Quervain's disease may also require surgical decompression of the affected area.[9] The postoperative care closely parallels care for carpal tunnel syndrome. The affected wrist is immobilized for approximately 1 week[5,9] with a compression bandage.

Some authorities recommend immediate ROM exercises,[9] whereas others suggest that active ROM exercises of the thumb and wrist begin after 3 to 5 days.[5] The important common denominator remains the management of normalized, pain-free motion (ulnar deviation) without undue scar formation, which would congest and occlude the surgically released and decompressed first dorsal compartment. Therefore motion exercises must be encouraged as directed by the physical therapist, with specific attention directed at scar management once the sutures are removed and wound closure occurs. Pain-free resistance exercises can commence once the patient demonstrates improved wrist and thumb motion without pain.

LIGAMENT INJURIES OF THE WRIST

Stability of the wrist depends primarily on intracapsular ligaments and not on intrinsic dynamic support from musculotendinous tissue.[15] Ligament sprains with varying degrees of carpal instability usually result from a fall with the wrist hyperextended (Fig. 18-3).[5,6,9,15]

With partial ligament sprains not involving carpal instability, the wrist should be immobilized to allow for proper alignment, stability, and healing of the partially torn ligament. Concurrent with immobilization, oral NSAIDs, and ice packs may be prescribed to control pain and swelling. Without question, a major factor in healing is the elimination of motions that stress the torn ligaments (most commonly the end ROM of wrist extension).

During immobilization, the elbow and shoulder of the affected limb are exercised with active motion and resistance exercises if no stress is applied to the healing ligaments of the wrist. To maintain or enhance fitness, a general conditioning program is encouraged throughout each phase of recovery. The hand and fingers of the ipsilateral limb should also be exercised during immobilization. Once the splint is removed, gentle active, pain-free motion can begin, with specific attention paid to avoiding full wrist extension. As motion improves and pain subsides, resistance exercises are employed to promote a gradual return to function. Both concentric and, especially, eccentric muscle contractions contribute to strengthening of the wrist flexors. To encourage eccentric control and dynamic support of wrist flexion and to enhance muscle control of wrist extension (usually the mechanism of wrist ligament injuries), a progressive resistance exercise program focusing on the eccentric phase of wrist flexion is gradually added.

The restoration of functional motion and strength after incomplete or partial ligament sprains (grades I and II) of the wrist generally follows the course of ligament healing constraints (see Chapter 3).

With more significant ligament injuries accompanied by carpal instability, the treatment is more complex. Options include rigid cast immobilization, closed reduction with percutaneous pinning, and open reduction and internal fixation (ORIF).[9,15] If cast immobilization is used to stabilize the joint, the patient is placed in a cast for approximately 6 to 12 weeks.[15] However, authorities question the ability of rigid immobilization to maintain the reduction satisfactorially to effect functional stability.[9,15] With closed reduction and pinning with wires, the wrist is immobilized for about 2 months, the pins are removed, and the arm is placed in a cast for an

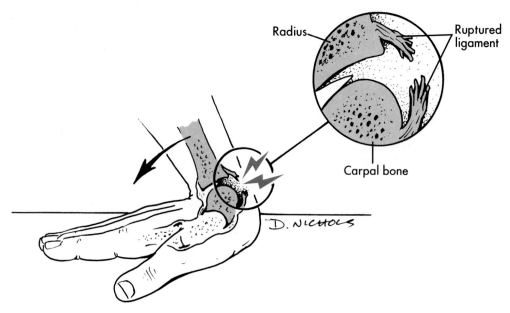

FIG. 18-3 Hyperextension ligament sprain of the wrist.

additional 4 weeks (Fig. 18-4).[15] With an ORIF procedure, the ligaments are directly repaired and the unstable carpal articulations are stabilized with wires or pins. The duration of immobilization is similar to that for closed reduction with percutaneous pinning.[15] Rehabilitation after cast immobilization or surgical repair begins during immobilization. The fingers and hand of the affected wrist, the elbow, and the shoulder should all be exercised with active pain-free motion (cautiously avoiding unwanted stress to the wrist) and resistance exercises. A general body conditioning program is universally encouraged.

Immediately after removal of the cast, splint, or immobilizer, active pain-free protected (limited ROM) activities are begun. If wound closure is complete, the use of a whirlpool before active mobility exercises can effectively reduce tissue congestion and aid in soft tissue extensibility. Initially, the injured or surgically repaired wrist should be protected from unwanted pressure, motions, and from extremes of active motion, consistent with long-term ligament healing constraints. Active assisted ROM exercises can be gradually added once active motion has increased and pain is controlled. Resistance exercises can be initiated once active motion has improved and pain is reduced. Submaximal isometric contractions can be used initially, then gradually progressing to maximal multi-angle isometric contractions and concentric and eccentric contractions. Protection of the wrist continues well into the final recovery

stages of rehabilitation. The use of functional, protective wrist splints is encouraged to protect the repaired and healing ligaments. A generalized wrist rehabilitation program after ligament injury or repair is shown in Box 18-1.

DISTAL RADIAL AND ULNAR FRACTURES

Radius

The most common distal radius fractures are extra-articular **Colles' fractures** and **Smith's fractures.**[5,10,11] A Colles' fracture is defined as a radius fracture within 2.5 cm of the wrist in which the distal radius is displaced in a dorsal direction (Fig. 18-5).[5,10,11] This fracture is recognized as the most common of all fractures, affecting mainly middle-aged and elderly women, with the mechanism of injury being a fall on an outstretched arm.[5,10] As with other types of fractures, the various treatment options generally parallel the degree of significance of the fracture type. Generally, Colles' fractures can be managed with closed reduction and rigid immobilization if the fracture is minimally displaced and stable.[10,12] If, however, the fracture is comminuted

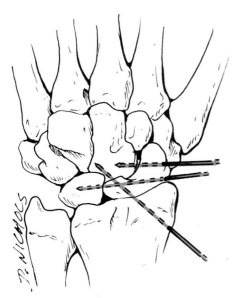

FIG. 18-4 Insertion of pins for stabilization following ligament sprain with carpal instability.

BOX 18-1 General Wrist Rehabilitation Program Following Ligament Injury

Maximum Protection Phase–Acute

a. Immobilization–protection–rest
b. NSAIDs–analgesics
c. Ice packs
d. Active, gentle finger, hand, elbow, shoulder motion and resistance exercise
e. General conditioning

Moderate Protection Phase–Subacute

a. Continue protection—slowly reduce immobilization
b. If no inflammation, then use whirlpool before active, gentle protected ROM
c. Active–assisted ROM
d. Resistance exercise for the hand, fingers
e. Sub-max isometric wrist exercises
f. Continue elbow, shoulder exercises and general conditioning program

Minimum Protection Phase–Maturation

a. Functional splint for protection
b. Active motion–whirlpool prior to exercise
c. Active assisted motion
d. Concentric–eccentric resistance
e. Hand, finger resistance exercise

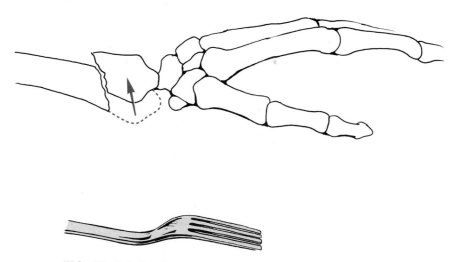

FIG. 18-5 Colle's fracture with resultant **dinner fork deformity.**

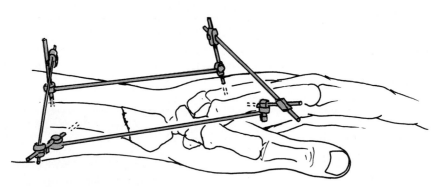

FIG. 18-6 External fixator for stabilization of severely displaced, unstable comminuted fractures.

and unstable, an ORIF procedure or an external fixator (for severely comminuted fractures) can be used to stabilize the fracture (Fig. 18-6).[5,10,12]

Rehabilitation after a Colles' fracture begins immediately, during immobilization. The hand, elbow, and shoulder of the ipsilateral wrist undergo active motion and resistance exercises as directed by the physical therapist. The contralateral limb is allowed to exercise freely, and a general conditioning program is employed, provided no undue stress is allowed to the affected wrist. Restoration of purposeful, functional motion is the foundation of the rehabilitation program during each phase of recovery. Therefore gentle active pain-free motion is encouraged after immobilization, with radiographic confirmation of secure bone healing, and under the direction of the physical therapist. However, extreme

caution is urged to ensure the patient performs the active motion exercises pain-free.

Once the sutures are removed (after an ORIF procedure) a whirlpool can be effective to reduce edema and encourage soft tissue extensibility before the performance of active motion exercises. Resistance exercise is deferred until secure bone union has occurred, which is reported to take 5 to 8 weeks.[5]

Colles' fractures can result in a loss of reduction of the fracture fragments, nonunion, malunion, tendon adhesions, median nerve compression, instability, Volkman's ischemic contracture, and reflex sympathetic dystrophy.[5,12] Therefore the assistant must be able to identify the need to advance patients' exercises gradually without increasing symptoms and to immediately communicate slow progress, reduced motion, and signs of neurovascular compromise to the physical therapist. Recovery may take up to a year.[5]

Smith's fracture is also referred to as a "reverse Colles' fracture."[10] The fracture usually occurs from a fall on the dorsum of the hand, with resultant distal radial fragment displaced in a palmar direction (Fig. 18-7). The course of treatment is either closed reduction with rigid cast immobilization or ORIF in cases of unstable, displaced, or comminuted fractures. The rehabilitation program after these injuries is similar to that of Colles' fracture.[5,10-12]

Ulna

Fractures of the distal ulna rarely occur as isolated injuries.[11] Usually distal ulnar fractures occur in combination with distal radius fractures.[11] In fact, Melone[11] reports that avulsion fracture of the ulnar styloid occurs in nearly 90% of unstable distal radius fractures.[11] In general, "successful treatment of the fractured radius results in accurate reduction and uncomplicated healing of the ulnar component with a favorable recovery of radioulnar and ulnocarpal joint function."[11] Therefore rehabilitation of distal ulnar fractures closely parallels treatment for fractures of the radius.

SCAPHOID FRACTURES

Before discussing treatment for fractures of the scaphoid, it is important to outline the vascular anatomy of the scaphoid because the location and degree of fragment displacement profoundly affects treatment and rehabilitation. Usually fractures of the scaphoid occur within the proximal pole, midportion, or distal pole of the bone.[5] The distal portion and midportion of the scaphoid are vascular, whereas the proximal pole, be-

cause of the distal to proximal direction of blood flow, if fractured is more likely to result in nonunion and avascular necrosis (Fig. 18-8).[5,7] Therefore the intrinsic ability of the scaphoid to heal is directly related to the location of the fracture and the resultant impact on the blood supply to the fractured area.

Scaphoid fractures are universally recognized as the most common fracture that occurs to the carpal bones, affecting nearly 60% of all carpal fractures.[5,9] Interestingly, the initial injury is frequently minor, with the mechanism of injury being wrist hyperextension with ulnar deviation.[9] Perhaps the most significant clinical feature of this fracture is pain localized to the "**anatomic snuffbox.**"[9] When the fracture is stable and nondisplaced, treatment is usually with closed reduction and rigid cast immobilization for approximately 6 weeks,[9] whereas proximal pole nondisplaced fractures may require immobilization for 12 to 24 weeks.[5]

Generally, displaced fractures require ORIF with wires and rigid immobilization.[5,9,11] Because of the increased risk of **avascular necrosis (AVN)** and **nonunion** occurring with proximal pole fractures, immobilization lasts quite long. Fracture site protection and immobilization form the cornerstone of recovery after fracture of the scaphoid. When nonunion and avascular necrosis ensue, bone grafts from the distal radius may be required as an osteogenic stimulus.[11] Noninvasive, pulsed electrical stimulation is used to expedite recovery after bone graft surgery.[11] When used in conjunction with bone grafting, electrical stimulation can reduce the time to union and eventual healing "regardless of fracture location or the presence of avascular necrosis."[11]

Rehabilitation must proceed cautiously during immobilization and on removal of the cast. Finger, elbow, and

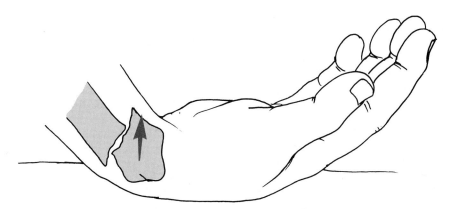

FIG. 18-7 Smith's fracture, also referred to as a reverse Colle's fracture. The mechanism of injury is usually a fall on the dorsum of the hand.

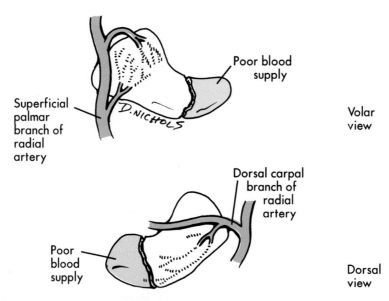

FIG. 18-8 Vascular anatomy of the scaphoid. The proximal pole of the scaphoid has a poor blood supply. If fractured in the proximal pole, there is the likelihood of avascular necrosis and resultant nonunion.

shoulder motion is encouraged during immobilization, as is a general conditioning program. Early, pain-free active thumb and wrist motion is allowed once immobilization has ended. However, caution is needed so that no undue stress or extremes of motion that produce pain occur during recovery. The full return to functional motion is affected by the protracted period of immobility and methods of bone fixation. After wound closure, the use of a whirlpool may aid in soft tissue extensibility. Passive stretching or mobilization exercises are contraindicated after immobilization. Passive exercise and joint mobilization techniques must be deferred until solid bone union has been confirmed radiographically. Resistance exercises for the wrist can begin gradually as pain allows, as motion increases, and when bone union occurs. As a general rule, every effort should be made to eliminate undue forces that may negatively affect bone healing.

SKIER'S THUMB

Skier's thumb is an acute sprain of the ulnar collateral ligament of the thumb. The mechanism of injury is usually sudden valgus stress and hyperextension of the thumb, which results in either a partial ligament tear (grade I or II) or a complete rupture (grade III) (Fig. 18-9).[3,5,6]

Partially torn ligaments can be treated nonsurgically with a thumb spica cast or rigid immobilization. Usually immobility lasts 3 to 6 weeks.[3] On removal of the splint, gentle active thumb motion, while avoiding extremes of abduction (valgus) and hyperextension, can proceed cautiously. Resistance exercises for the elbow and shoulder of the involved limb are prescribed throughout each phase of recovery. The initiation of progressive resistance exercises for the involved thumb must be deferred for approximately 2 months after injury for appropriate ligament healing to occur.[5] Generally, a series of submaximal isometrics is used to encourage adduction of the thumb. As motion and pain improve, more demanding exercises are added that include the use of putty for resistance. If the ulnar collateral ligament is ruptured, gross instability occurs that profoundly affects function. In this case, surgical stabilization may be indicated. Generally an ORIF procedure is used where wires and pins help approximate and stabilize the joint for ligament healing to proceed. A short arm, thumb spica cast is applied for approximately 4 to 6 weeks.[3,5] On removal of the cast, active, pain-free motion of the fingers, wrist, and thumb is advocated, being ever cautious to avoid thumb abduction (valgus stress) and hyperextension. With complete ligament sprains, the patient must avoid harmful stress to the healing ligaments. After cast removal, the injured thumb is placed in a protective splint that is removed only for active, protected motion exercises for about 10 weeks.[5] Once active motion is

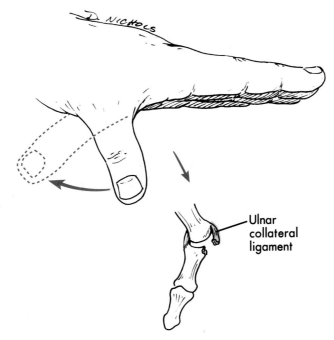

FIG. 18-9 Game keeper's thumb, also referred to as skier's thumb. Sudden valgus stress and hyperextension can result in partial or complete rupture of the ulnar collateral ligament of the thumb.

increased and pain does not affect activity, gentle resistance exercises are used to enhance purposeful, functional use of the thumb.

METACARPAL FRACTURES

Two of the more common metacarpal fractures are **boxer's fractures ("fighter's fracture")**[3] and **Bennett's fracture.** A boxer's fracture is a fracture to the neck of the second, third, fourth, or fifth metacarpal.[12] It is aptly named because of the incidence of this fracture among fighters (Fig. 18-10).[3,5] Treatment can be with closed reduction and rigid immobilization or with an ORIF procedure to rigidly fix and stabilize the fracture site. Generally the following indications are recognized to pursue ORIF procedures with metacarpal fractures:[17]

Unstable fractures
Inadequately reduced fractures
Open fractures
Associated soft tissue problems
Multiple fractures
Articular fractures
Bone loss

However, with a boxer's fracture, the physician may elect closed reduction and immobilization rather than an ORIF procedure, depending on the degree of angulation demonstrated at the fracture site.[3,5,12] If closed reduction is used, fracture consolidation is noted between 3 to 5 weeks after injury.[17] Throughout immobilization, the digits, elbow, and shoulder of the involved limb are exercised. On removal of the cast, active motion of the hand is encouraged if radiographic evidence confirms solid union and active motion poses no threat to displace the fracture segments. Progressive resistance exercises must be added gradually as pain, motion, and stable bone union dictate. Putty exercises, pinching, and sand can be used to encourage functional strength of the hand after fractures.

A Bennett's fracture is a "fracture-subluxation"[3] of the proximal first metacarpal.[3,5,12] As with a boxer's fracture, treatment can be with closed reduction and rigid cast immobilization or with an ORIF procedure, depending on the severity of the fracture. In either case, before active motion, there must be nondisplaced solid union at the fracture site. If closed reduction is used, immobilization lasts 6 to 8 weeks to promote stable union.[5] If an ORIF procedure is used, immobilization is

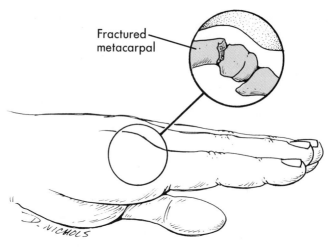

Fractured metacarpal

FIG. 18-10 Boxer's fracture, or fighter's fracture.

slightly shorter because of the rigid internal fixation. Rehabilitation closely parallels the treatment for a boxer's fracture and depends on the degree of bone healing, presence of pain, and amount of active motion demonstrated by the patient.

DUPUYTREN'S CONTRACTURE

Dupuytren's contracture is a disease process that affects the palmar fascia.[5] Miller[12] describes this disease as "proliferative fibrodysplasia of the palmar connective tissue; can lead to contractures from nodules and cords that progressively develop." A common characteristic of this disease is the development of immature type III collagen (normal fascia is composed of type I collagen); it is associated with myofibroblast proliferation (Fig. 18-11).[5,7,12] Usually this disease affects males 40 years or older; it is bilateral in 45% of cases; and it most frequently involves the ulnar digits.[12] Although tender nodules are occasionally present,[7] this disease is generally not painful.[5] Therefore treatment is centered on the correction of deformity and restoration of function rather than resolution of pain. Loth[7] notes that a 20- to 30-degree flexion contracture of the ulnar metacarpophalangeal (MCP) joint is an indication for surgery because this degree of flexion contracture is associated with an inability to lay the hand flat.[7] Even a small degree of contracture of the proximal interphalangeal (PIP) joint necessitates surgical correction.[7]

The treatment of contractures and functional limitation secondary to Dupuytren's disease is to surgically excise the palmar fascia or perform a fasciectomy (Fig. 18-12).[1,5] In many cases the surgical incision is left open

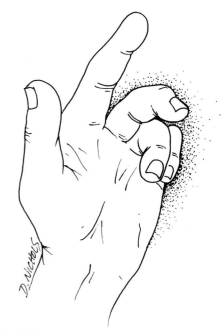

FIG. 18-11 Dupuytren's contracture most commonly affects the ulnar digits with flexion contracture of the ulnar metacarpal phalangeal joint (MCP).

rather than sutured together.[1,5] Historically, procedures that closed the tissue after excision of the palmar fascia resulted in scar tissue formation, tendon adhesions, tissue necrosis, and infection.[1,5] Leaving the surgical wound open means that skin care, wound cleansing, and infection control become central to the initial course of

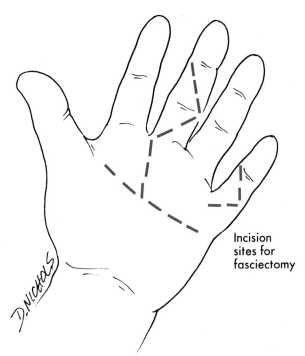

FIG. 18-12 Fasciectomy for Dupuytren's contracture. The dotted lines represent the surgical incision that is usually left open and not sutured together.

physical therapy management. The open incision may require 4 to 6 weeks to close completely.[1]

Maintenance of motion (extension) after palmar fascia release is essential for a good functional outcome. Fietti and Mackin[1] recommend the use of a whirlpool on the fifth day postoperatively to promote healing through removal of surface eschar and bacteria, enhance circulation, and provide for greater soft tissue extensibility.[1,5] During the whirlpool treatment the patient performs active hand and finger extension ROM exercises to maintain freedom of motion gained through surgical release. During each phase of recovery, the wrist, elbow, and shoulder of the affected hand must be actively exercised, and a general physical conditioning program is encouraged.

Along with the concept of maintaining or increasing function and motion of the hand and digits after surgical release, the fabrication, application, and close daily supervision and possible revision of a static resting splint is used to provide stretching of the palmar fascia and affected digits. Usually the occupational therapy rehabilitation team designs and fabricates the static and dynamic splints required to enhance function, but physical therapists with specific experience and training in

splint fabrication for hand and finger injuries can also initially design and apply static and dynamic splints.

In conjunction with daily whirlpool treatments, active ROM movements, and static splinting, the following general exercises can be used to enhance early motion and a return to function:[1]

> Thumb opposition to all fingers
> Flexion of each finger to distal palmar crease
> Full flexion of the PIP joints
> Making a fist
> Abduction and adduction of the fingers
> Finger extension
> Full wrist and thumb motion
> Crossing the fingers

The application of scar tissue massage is appropriate once the surgical wound is healed. Retrograde massage as well as specific cross fiber scar massage can be performed as soon as pain, swelling, and wound healing allow.[1,5] The patient is instructed to perform automassage techniques a few times daily to enhance tissue extensibility, prevent adhesions, and reduce edema.

The ultimate restoration of function after surgical care of Dupuytren's contracture is achieved by maintaining and enhancing hand and finger extension, controlling swelling and edema, reducing scar tissue proliferation, and promoting active motion while enhancing static soft tissue stretching using splints.

MALLET FINGER

Mallet finger is a tendon injury (rupture) or avulsion fracture (tendon-bone) of the extensor tendon that results in a distal interphalangeal (DIP) joint flexion contracture (Fig. 18-13). Usually this injury occurs as a result of direct trauma to the distal end of the phalanx, causing the terminal tendon or digit to rupture or fracture.[5] With either tendon rupture or avulsion fracture, the treatment is essentially the same. Continuous, uninterrupted splinting of the DIP joint for 6 to 10 weeks in 0 degrees of extension allows for appropriate tendon and/or bone healing.[3,5] Throughout immobilization, the patient actively exercises all noninvolved joints of the upper extremity. The affected joint begins active exercise at the sixth to eighth week. Passive flexion exercises of the DIP are contraindicated to protect the healing tendon and bone from extremes of motion and unwanted forces. Instead, the patient performs only gentle active DIP flexion to 20 degrees to avoid excessive stretch of the healing tendon.[5] Extension lag may develop. If the patient is unable to actively extend the DIP when the splint is removed, active flexion exercises are terminated and continuous splinting in 0 degrees of extension to 10

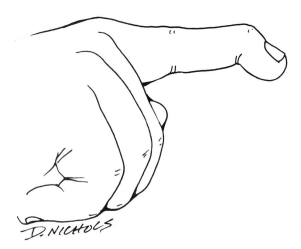

FIG. 18-13 Mallet finger. Avulsion fracture or tendon rupture results in distal interphalangeal (DIP) joint flexion contracture.

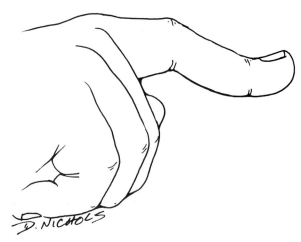

FIG. 18-14 Boutonniére deformity, PIP flexion with DIP extension.

degrees of hyperextension resumed for an additional 2 to 4 weeks before active exercises are re-initiated.[3,5] Extension lag may recur.[3] If no extension lag is noted during early (6 to 8 weeks) active flexion of the DIP, during the following weeks, active flexion is gradually allowed with progressions in 5- to 10-degree increments. The physical therapist assistant must continue to observe for any extension lag of the DIP.

As motion gradually improves, the strength of the involved digit must be increased. Tendon and/or bone healing must not be overstressed before secure union occurs, so active resistance exercises are deferred for up to 12 weeks after injury and are begun only in the absence of extension lag.[5]

BOUTONNIERE DEFORMITY

Direct trauma to the terminal phalanx can also resut in a rupture or stretch of the central extensor tendon at the PIP joint, which creates PIP flexion with DIP extension and the recognizable **boutonniere deformity** (Fig. 18-14).[3,16] When the tendon is ruptured and no associated avulsion fracture is present, the treatment is to immobilize the PIP joint in full extension for a minimum of 6 to 8 weeks.[3,16] The DIP joint is not immobilized; the patient performs both active and passive DIP flexion with the PIP in extension.[3] As with DIP extensor tendon injuries (mallet finger) the course of recovery follows the course of tendon and/or bone healing.

FLEXOR TENDON INJURIES

Although extensor tendon injuries occur approximately five times more often than flexor tendon injuries,[5] **flexor tendon** injuries, repair, and rehabilitation are universally considered more complicated and challenging.[3,5,16] To apply appropriate motion and stress after flexor tendon injuries and subsequent surgical repair, the assistant must be aware of the dynamic nature of tendon healing while focusing on the desired outcome of functional motion and strength via normal tendon glide and excursion as a result of inhibition by adhesions.[2,5,13]

Adhesions generally form early in the recovery stage of tendon healing and affect both motion and function. Without appropriate stress and directed motion, scar tissue forms in a random pattern and does not attain normal intact tendon strength.[2] Therefore to preferentially develop mature collagen fibers, which align in the direction of applied forces, mechanical stimuli are required during remodeling, similar to Wolff's law for bone healing.[2] Specifically, intermittent purposeful stress and motion enhance tendon healing and collagen fiber alignment. Because the ultimate goal of recovery after flexor tendon injury and repair is to achieve motion and strength of the involved tendon, early, controlled passive motion and stress are used to influence the organization, maturation, and remodeling of collagen fibers.[2,5,13]

The most salient features of rehabilitation after flexor tendon repair involve the interrelationship between immobilization and the application of early, protected, limited passive motion.[2,5,13] After flexor tendon repair, "carefully applied early protected motion can produce a consistent range of gliding in the early postoperative period that is not associated with significant repair site deformation."[2]

Although a detailed description of the various tendon repair procedures is beyond the scope and intent of this discussion, general rehabilitation procedures parallel tendon healing and motion influences appropriate cellular response in the injured tendon tissue.[2] Two to 3 days after repair, gentle motion is allowed.[5] Progressive motion is encouraged within the limits of postoperative protective plaster splinting and rubber band traction (Fig. 18-15). The purpose of this postoperative immobilization arrangement is to maintain the interphalangeal (IP) joint in 30 to 50 degrees of passive flexion while encouraging active IP extension within the limits of the plaster splint.[5] This is consistent with the "concept that a limited, immediate mobilization program improves the quality of the biologic repair response after flexor tendon repair within the digital sheath by effectively eliminating the associated adhesion formation."[2]

Jacobs[5] advocates that more "aggressive" flexion and extension exercises can begin around 6 weeks and that manual resistance exercise can be initiated at 8 weeks. As motion and strength improve, more challenging resistance exercises using incremental degrees of putty tension, rubber balls, and spring and cable hand exercises are employed. At approximately 12 weeks, functional ADLs and specific job tasks requiring repetitive hand motions are begun, with all motion restrictions eliminated.[5]

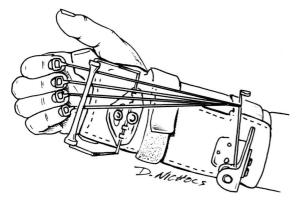

FIG. 18-15 Postoperative protective splint with rubber band traction following flexor tendon repair.

REFLEX SYMPATHETIC DYSTROPHY

Reflex sympathetic dystrophy (RSD) is a vasomotor dysfunction[5,8] or reflex vasomotor response to a chronic sensory stimulus.[14] Perhaps one of the most complex and challenging conditions to treat, RSD is characterized by pain (predominant feature), hyperesthesia, edema, discoloration, and loss of motion and function.[8] This pain syndrome develops gradually after various fractures, soft tissue injuries, and surgery.[8,14] Interestingly, there is no direct relationship between the injury and the degree of pain experienced by persons suffering from RSD.[5,8,14] Generally, persons who are susceptible to RSD demonstrate a low pain threshhold and dependent personality.[14] The mechanism of RSD is not completely clear, but it has been proposed that the vasoconstriction occurring after an injury becomes severe and prolonged, developing into a painful stimulus that perpetuates abnormal vasomotor reflexes.[14]

Jacobs[5] identifies three stages of RSD. Stage I represents the acute episode, which may last as long as 3 months. During the acute stage, pain and edema are the dominant clinical symptoms. Discoloration and excessive sweating (hyperhydrosis) are obvious, as are temperature changes.[5] Stage II lasts from the third month to approximately 1 year after injury.[5] Classically, pain and edema increase during this period, and skin coloration changes from red to a "pale cyanosis."[5] In addition, the skin becomes dry (changing from hyperhidrosis) and tissue atrophy becomes more apparent. Radiographic examination frequently reveals the development of osteoporosis.[5,8,14] Stage III involves increasing trophic changes, severe motion restrictions, atrophy, and the production of inelastic fibrous tissue.[5,14]

Treatment focuses on controlling pain and swelling and completely eliminating all pain-producing activities. Treatment must be initiated as soon as a diagnosis is confirmed. Initially, medical management focuses on using sympathetic nerve blocks that do not affect numbness, weakness, or paralysis, but rather significantly reduce hypersensitivity and pain.[8] Moist heat, gentle massage, TENS, and electrical stimulation are effective tools to use for pain and swelling control. Most importantly, protection of the involved extremity from activities that produce pain is critical to successful treatment. Aggressive exercise or passive motions that produce pain are strictly avoided during each phase of recovery. Splints can be used to modify motions and allow for intermittent gentle active pain-free motion. The management of swelling can be enhanced if the patient elevates the involved extremity, uses compression wraps or garments, and applies therapeutic gentle retrograde massage and electrical stimulation.[5,8,14] Unfortunately, for persons suffering from RSD, many therapeutic exercises perpetuate the pain. Therefore use of active exercises is determined by the patient's tolerance of pain with passive motion and control of edema, as well as the ability to demonstrate continued pain relief with splints to eliminate unwanted motions. At no point in the course of recovery from RSD is aggressive, active motion prescribed in the presence of pain.

MOBILIZATION OF THE WRIST AND HAND

The use of peripheral joint mobilization techniques can be quite effective to modulate pain and increase motion of the wrist and hand. The specific applications of these techniques are determined by the physical therapist, and the appropriate direction and amplitude of force are dictated by the specific injury and degree of soft tissue and bone healing (see Chapters 11 and 12).

Moist heat, paraffin baths, whirlpools, electrical stimulation, and gentle active exercise can be used immediately before mobilization to encourage soft tissue relaxation and evacuation of waste from the injured area. In addition, physician-prescribed analgesics, muscle relaxants, and NSAIDs may be effective before beginning mobilization techniques.

The position of the patient is a critical feature of effective mobilization. The injured extremity must be positioned to provide comfort, relaxation, and support while affording the clinician access to the extremity.

As with other joints, many different techniques are used. This discussion introduces only a few of the more common and easily performed techniques. The intricate and complex nature of the wrist and hand demands mastery of anatomy, kinesiology, pathomechanics of injury, and biomechanics to effectively perform the more difficult techniques described in orthopedic texts.[18]

Mobilization of the Wrist

Anterior, posterior, medial, and lateral glides of the wrist are performed with the patient either sitting with the affected arm supported or supine. Use one hand to stabilize the distal radius and ulna on the dorsal aspect while firmly grasping the proximal row of carpal bones with the other hand.[18] Using the hand supporting the carpal bones, direct an anterior and posterior force or a medial and lateral force to "glide" the carpal bones from the stabilized distal radius and ulna (Fig. 18-16).[18]

Distraction of the carpals is done with the patient either sitting or supine. The hand position is exactly the

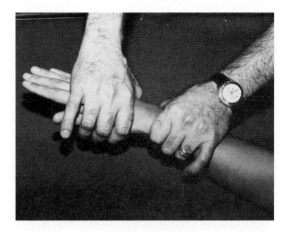

FIG. 18-16 Anterior-posterior medial and lateral glides of the wrist.

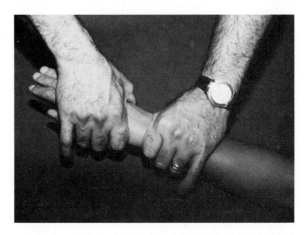

FIG. 18-17 Long axis or longitudinal distraction of the wrist.

same as described above, but the direction of force is distal or longitudinal to the radius and ulna. This direction of force distracts or displaces the carpal bones from the stabilized radius and ulna (Fig. 18-17).[18]

Mobilization of the Hand

Anterior, posterior, medial, and lateral glides of the MCP joint can be performed with the patient supine or sitting. Use one hand to stabilize the shaft of the affected metacarpal while firmly grasping the proximal phalanx with the other hand. With the metacarpal firmly stabilized, use the hand contacting the phalanx to direct an anterior, posterior, or medial and lateral force that glides the MCP joint (Fig. 18-18).[18]

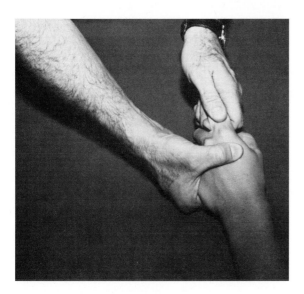

FIG. 18-18 Anterior-posterior, medial and lateral glides of the metacarpal phalangeal (MCP) joint.

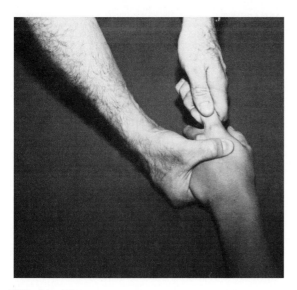

FIG. 18-19 Long axis or longitudinal distraction of the metacarpal phalangeal (MCP) joint.

Distraction of the MCP joint occurs with the patient in the same position as described above. With the hand placement the same, the direction of force is applied to distract the phalanx from the stabilized metacarpal (Fig. 18-19).[18]

REFERENCES

1. Fietti VG, Mackin EJ: Dupuytren's disease. In Hunter JM, Schneider LH, Mackin EJ, Bell JA, editors: *Rehabilitation of the hand,* St. Louis, 1978, Mosby.
2. Gelberman R et al: Tendon. In Woo S L-Y, Buckwalter JA, editors: *Injury and repair of the musculoskeletal soft tissues,* Rosemont, Ill., 1988, American Academy of Orthopaedic Surgeons.
3. Green DP, Strickland JW: The hand. In DeLee JC, Drez D, editors: *Orthopaedic sports medicine: principles and practice,* vol I, Philadelphia, 1994, WB Saunders.
4. Hebert LA: *The neck-arm-hand book,* Greenville, Me., 1989, IMPACC.
5. Jacobs JL: Hand and wrist. In Richardson JK, Iglarsh ZA, editors: *Clinical orthopaedic physical therapy,* Philadelphia, 1994, WB Saunders.
6. Lephart S: Injuries to the hand and wrist. In Prentice WE, editor: *Rehabilitation techniques in sports medicine,* ed 2, St. Louis, 1994, Mosby.
7. Loth TS: Hand and wrist. In Loth TS, editor: *Orthopaedic boards review,* St. Louis, 1993, Mosby.
8. Mayer AV, McCue FC: Rehabilitation and protection of the wrist and hand. In Posner MA, editor: *The upper extremity in sports medicine,* hand section, St. Louis, 1990, Mosby.
9. McCue FC, Bruce JF: The wrist. In DeLee JC, Drez D, editors: *Orthopaedic sports medicine: principles and practice,* vol I, Philadelphia, 1994, WB Saunders.
10. McRae R: The wrist and hand. In *Practical fracture treatment,* ed 3, New York, 1994, Churchill Livingstone.
11. Melone CP: Fractures of the wrist. In Nicholas JA, Hershman EB, editors: *The upper extremity in sports medicine,* St. Louis, 1990, Mosby.
12. Miller MD: *Review of orthopaedics,* Philadelphia, 1992, WB Saunders.
13. Nissenbaum M: Early care of flexor tendon injuries: application of principles of tendon healing and early motion. In Hunter JM, Schneider LH, Mackin EJ, Bell JA, editors: *Rehabilitation of the hand,* St. Louis, 1978, Mosby.
14. Omer GE: Management of pain syndromes in the upper extremity. In Hunter JM, Schneider LH, Mackin EJ, Bell JA, editor: *Rehabilitation of the hand,* St. Louis, 1978, Mosby.
15. Wilgis EFS, Yates AY: Wrist pain. In Nicholas JA, Hershman EB, editors: *The upper extremity in sports medicine,* St. Louis, 1990, Mosby.
16. Wilson RL, Carter MS: Joint injuries in the hand: preservation of proximal interphalangeal joint function. In Hunter JM, Schneider LH, Mackin EJ, Bell JA, editors: *Rehabilitation of the hand,* St. Louis, 1978, Mosby.
17. Wilson RL, Carter MS: Management of hand fractures. In Hunter JM, Schneider LH, Mackin EJ, Bell JA, editors: *Rehabilitation of the hand,* St. Louis, 1978, Mosby.
18. Wooden MJ: Mobilization of the upper extremity. In Donatelli R, Wooden MJ, editors: *Orthopaedic physical therapy,* New York, 1989, Churchill Livingstone.

Glossary

A-C joint Acromioclavicular joint.

Abductor "lurch" Gluteus medius gait due to weak or non-functioning hip abductor muscles. The patient lurches toward the weak side to place the center of gravity over the hip.

Accessory movements Joint movements that are necessary for a full range-of-motion, but that are not under direct voluntary control of the individual.

Accountability Being accountable or responsible for the moral and legal requirements of proper patient care.

Actin A protein found in muscle fibers that acts with myosin to bring about contraction and relaxation. Also called actinin.

Adhesions Tissue structures normally separated that adhere together because of injury.

Aerobic capacity Degree of aerobic fitness. Also referred to as cardiovascular endurance, cardiovascular fitness, or cardiorespiratory fitness.

Afferent neural input Nerves and sensory organs that carry or transmit information from the periphery to the Central Nervous System (*see also* mechanoreceptor system).

Age-adjusted maximum heart rate (AAMHR) Expressed as 220–Age=MHR.

Allograft Transplant tissue used from cadavers. Commonly, the ACL can be reconstructed with an allograft.

AMBRI Atraumatic multidirectional bilateral instability that responds to rehabilitation, but occasionally requires an inferior capsular shift surgical procedure.

Amplitude Width or breadth of range or extent, such as amplitude of accommodation or amplitude of convergence.

Annulus Any ring-shaped structure, such as the outer edge of an intervertebral disc.

Antalgic gait Due to pain in the stance phase (while walking through on the foot), the time spent on the affected side is shortened compared with that on the normal side.

Anterior cruciate ligament (ACL) Deep ligament within the knee that crosses the posterior cruciate ligament.

AO classification of fracture fixation devices: Also referred to as ASIF (the Association for the study of International Fixation). A group of general and orthopedic surgeons was founded in 1956 by Dr. Maurice E. Müller to develop a series of screws, plates, and other internal fixation clevices. In addition, the AO group (Arbeitgemeinschaft für Osteosynthesefragen) established a system of fracture classification and management.

Arthroplasty Surgery to reconstruct joints.

Arthroscopy Examination of a joint interior using an arthroscope.

Articular cartilage Thin layer of hyaline cartilage on joint surfaces.

Atrophy Reduction in size of an anatomic structure, frequently related to disuse or decreased blood supply.

Autograft A tissue or organ removed from one site and placed in another within the same individual.

Avascular necrosis (AVN) Tissue death from a lack of blood supply.

Back school Education model to inform individuals about spine anatomy, injury, self-care, fitness, ADLS, and ergonomic modifications.

"Bag of bones technique" Sling and swath procedure used to help stabilize severe comminuted intercondylar fractures of the elbow in elderly people with poor bone quality.

Ballistic stretching Method of dynamic stretching involving rapid bouncing.

Bankart lesion Seen surgically as a detachment of the glenoid labrum and sometimes a bone fragment from the glenoid.

Base of support The distance between a person's feet while standing and during ambulation.

Bennett's fracture Fracture-subluxation of proximal first metacarpal.

Biomechanical ankle platform system (BAPS) A commercial or hand-made disc used to challenge a patient's balance.

Bone callus Subsequent scarring of bone following a fracture.

Bone to bone end-feel A sudden, hard, nonyielding sensation that is felt at the end range-of-motion. An example is terminal elbow extension.

Borg scale A scale of measurement of relative perceived exertion.

Boutonniere deformity A fixed deformity of the finger consisting of flexion of the proximal interphalangeal joint and extension of the distal interphalangeal joint. A result of rheumatoid destruction of the extensor tendon mechanism at the proximal interphalangeal joint and also secondary to trauma without arthritis.

Boxer's fracture Volarly displaced impacted fracture of the neck of the fifth and/or fourth metacarpal, caused by striking a close-fisted hand on a hard object.

Bursitis Inflammation of a bursa.

Cadence Number of steps or strides taken per unit of time.

Calcaneal gait Weakness of gastroc-soleus muscle groups that results in reduced foot propulsion during the toe-off period of the stance phase of gait.

Cancellous bone Spongy, porous, lattice-like tissue within midshaft of long bone.

Capsular and noncapsular pattern Every synovial joint under muscular control possesses a characteristic pattern of limitation. An example of a capsular pattern is described by Barak, Rosen, and Sofer. The capsular pattern of the shoulder "involves external rotation as the most limited movement, abduction as less limited, internal rotation still less limited, and flexion as the least limited movement." If a lesion exists that does not correspond to a characteristic, predetermined capsular pattern, it is called a noncapsular pattern. (From Barak T, Rosen ER, Sofer R: Basic concepts of orthopaedic manual therapy. In Gould JA, editor: *Orthopaedic and sports physical therapy*, ed 2, St. Louis, 1990, Mosby.)

Capsular end-feel An abnormal feel encountered during the performance of mobilization techniques. An elastic resistance is encountered prior to the normal range-of-motion. Usually, this end-feel is related to a specific capsular restriction.

Capsulitis Inflammation of the capsule.

Cardiovascular endurance The capacity of the aerobic energy system to perform work. Also referred to as cardiovascular fitness, aerobic capacity, and cardiorespiratory fitness.

Carpal tunnel syndrome A compression entrapment neuropathy of the median nerve within the wrist, most commonly caused by repetitive motions of the wrist.

Carrying angle Viewing the upper extremity in the anterior-posterior (AP) frontal plane, the angle observed at the axis of the elbow between the upper arm and lower arm.

Center of gravity Point in a body where the body mass is centered.

Cervical spondylosis Chronic degenerative disc disease of the cervical spine. Occurs most often in the fourth and fifth decades of life and characteristically affects men more often than women. Commonly affects the C_5–C_6 and C_6–C_7 segments.

Chondrocytes Cartilage cells.

Circuit training A method of physical exercise in which activities are arranged in sets so that the participant moves quickly from one activity to another with minimum rest between sets.

Claw toe Dorsiflexion of the metatarsophalangeal joints associated with hammer toe deformities and often with a clavus foot.

Closed kinetic chain exercise (CKC) Any exercise where the distal or terminal exercising segment is weight bearing or "fixed." Functional exercises that use concentric and eccentric muscle contractions in a synchronous fashion to produce functional movement in which motion at one joint will produce motion at all of the other joints in the kinetic chain in a predictable manner.

Close-packed The most congruent position of a joint. The joint surfaces are aligned and the capsule and ligaments are taut.

Codman's pendulum exercises Exercises for a stiff shoulder in which the patient is bent over at the waist (90 degrees) and the hand hangs like a pendulum toward the floor. A weight may be placed in the hand and the arm is then moved through various arcs to increase the range-of-motion in that shoulder.

Collagen Fibrous protein of connective tissue, ligament, cartilage, bone and skin.

Colles' fracture Fracture of the distal end of the radius with the lower fragment displaced posteriorly.

Communication Any process in which a message containing information is transferred, especially from one person to another, via any of a number of media.

Compact bone The thick outer portion of bone that surrounds the medullary (marrow) cavity. Also called cortical bone.

Compression neuropathy Loss of motor or sensory nerve function (acute or chronic) due to extrinsic compression. Entrapment can occur within tight fibroosseous tunnels or as a result of tumor, hemorrhage, or metabolic changes, causing swelling of soft tissues around the nerve.

Compression fracture Crumbling or smashing of cancellous bone by forces acting parallel to the long axis of the bone. (Applied particularly to vertebral body fractures.)

Concentric contraction Tension produces a shortening contraction of muscle that results in the approximation of the origin and insertion of the contracting muscle.

Constrained A type of total joint implant (TKR) that sacrifices the cruciates (ACL, PCL, or both). Also referred to as a conforming implant.

Continuous passive motion (CPM) A technique for maintaining or increasing the amount of movement in a joint with the use of a mechanical device that applies force to bring about motion in a joint without normal muscle function.

Contracture Shortening of muscle tissue, joint capsule, ligament, tendon, and other soft tissues due to paralysis, spasm, or fibrosis of tissue around the joint.

Controlled-protected motion Therapeutic technique that calls for gentle, specific motion that does not place unwanted force or stress on injured or healing tissue. The joint or joints affected can be protected with a cast-brace or range limiting hinge brace.

Contusion Bruise of any tissue but without disruption.

Convex-concave rule "When the concave surface is stationary and the convex surface is moving, the gliding movement in the joint occurs in a direction opposite to the bone movement." If the convex surface is mobile, the gliding motion occurs in the same direction as the bone movement. (From Barak T, Rosen ER, Sofer R: Basic concepts of orthopaedic manual therapy. In Gould JA, editor: *Orthopaedic and sports physical therapy*, ed 2, St. Louis, 1990, Mosby.)

Cortical bone The thick outer portion of bone that surrounds the medullary (marrow) cavity. Also called compact bone.

Cumulative trauma disorder A soft tissue injury that is characteristically caused by overuse or repetitive motion.

De Quervain's tenosynovitis Repetitive motion injury that affects the tendons of the abductor pollicis longus and extensor pollicis brevis as they pass within the first dorsal compartment of the wrist.

Deceleration A decrease in the speed or velocity of an object or reaction.

Delayed union   The speed of callus formation (fracture healing) is slower than anticipated, but this does not imply expectancy of either total healing or a nonunion.

Delayed onset muscle soreness (DOMS)   Muscle weakness, restricted range-of-motion, and diffuse tenderness that occurs 24 to 48 hours after intense or prolonged muscle activity.

Dinner fork deformity   Resultant characteristic angular deformity of the radius following a Colle's fracture.

Direct muscle injury   Lacerations, surgical incisions, contusions, or blunt trauma.

Disc   An avascular and aneural (except that the outer fibers are innervated) structure comprised of the annulus (fibroelastic cartilage) and the nucleus (mucopolysaccharide gel) that provides stability and movement between the vertebral bodies within each segment.

Dislocation   Complete displacement of a bone from its normal position at the joint surface, disrupting the articulation of two or three bones at that junction and altering the alignment.

DJD   Degenerative joint disease. Also called osteoarthritis.

Double support   The point within the gait cycle in which both feet are in contact with the ground and weight transfer occurs from one foot to the other.

Dupuytren's contracture   Disease affecting the palmar fascia of the hand, causing the ring and little finger to contract toward the palm.

Eccentric contraction   A muscle contraction in which tension is produced but lengthening of the muscle occurs. The origin and insertion of the contracting (lengthening) muscle will move further apart during the contraction. Also referred to as a negative contraction or negative work.

Elastic deformation   The viscoelastic property of soft tissues to "deform" under slow rates of stress then return to normal resting length and tension.

Empty end-feel   An abnormal end-feel encountered during the performance of mobilization techniques. Motion that is very limited by significant pain without muscle spasm. This end-feel is not characterized by any mechanical block or restriction.

Endomysium   A fibrous sheath of connective tissue that enfolds striated muscle fiber within a fasciculus.

Epicondylitis   Inflammation of the common wrist extensor origin or inflammation of the common flexor tendon and pronator teres at the medial epicondyle of the elbow.

Epimysium   A fibrous sheath that enfolds a muscle and extends between the bundles of muscle fibers, such as the perimysium. It is sturdy in some areas but more delicate in others, such as those areas where the muscle moves freely under a strong sheet of fascia. The epimysium may also fuse with fascia that attaches a muscle to a bone.

Ergonomics   A scientific discipline devoted to the study and analysis of human work, especially as it is affected by individual anatomy, psychology, and other human factors.

Extruded disc   An injury to the intervertebral disc in which the nucleus extends through the annulus but the nuclear material remains confined by the posterior longitudinal ligament.

Fasciculus   Small bundle or cluster (referring to muscle, tendon, or nerve fibers).

Fast twitch (type II-white glycolytic) muscle fiber   Muscle fiber type with high levels of myosin- ATPase. These muscle fibers are recruited for activities that require speed, strength, and power.

Fibroelastic cartilage   A type of cartilage that is composed of water, four types of collagen (of which type I represents approximately 90%) and proteogylcans and elastin. The menisci of the knee is an example of fibroelastic cartilage.

Fighter's fracture   A fracture to the neck of the second, third, fourth, or fifth metacarpal. Also referred to as a boxer's fracture.

Foot-flat   The point in the gait cycle when the entire foot is in contact with the floor. Shock absorption is a primary action during the foot-flat period.

Four-point gait pattern   Using crutches as an example, the patient will advance the crutch opposite the involved limb first, followed by the involved limb, then advance the crutch toward the uninvolved limb, then finally advance the uninvolved limb.

Free nerve endings   A receptor nerve ending that is not enclosed in a capsule. A typically free nerve ending consists of a bare axon that may be myelinated or unmyelinated. They are often found in fibrous capsules, ligaments, or synovial spaces and may be sensitive to mechanical or biochemical stimuli.

Full weight bearing (FWB)   Weight bearing status that allows no restrictions.

Functional capacity evaluations   Specific functional testing procedure designed to identify and quantify physical limitations, restrictions, and risk factors associated with specific job tasks.

Gait   Walking pattern.

Gamekeeper's thumb   A traumatic rupture of the ulnar collateral ligament of the metacarpophalangeal joint of the thumb, usually a hyper abduction injury. Also called skier's thumb.

Glide   An accessory joint motion.

Golgi tendon organs (GTO)   Inhibitory sensory receptors located within the myotendonous junction.

Hallux valgus   The big toe bends toward the other toes.

Hammer toe   Descriptive of a variety of deformities of the second to fifth toes; increased flexion of the distal toe, causing prominence of the bones of the dorsal aspect of the proximal interphalangeal joint.

Hard or springy tissue stretch   A normal end-feel encountered during the performance of mobilization techniques. The most common normal end-feel at the end range-of-motion of joints. Examples are terminal knee extension and wrist flexion where elastic resistance and a springy stretch are felt at the end range-of-motion.

Heel-off   When the heel of the weight bearing limb initially raises from the floor. At this point, weight is unloaded from the weight bearing limb and is shifted or transferred to the opposite limb.

Heel-Strike   The instant foot contact is made with the ground. Ideally, the heel should initiate contact.

Hemi-arthroplasty   Partial reconstructive surgery of a joint. The hip is an example of when the femoral head is replaced and not the acetabulum. A total hip replacement is when both the femoral head and the acetabulum are replaced.

Hill-Sachs lesion   Seen radiographically as an indentation of the posteromedial humeral head, which occurs at the time of the dislocation. Also called hatchet head deformity.

HNP   Herniated nucleus pulposus. A broad term referring to more specific nomenclature concerning various stages of disc injury. Three general categories of HNP include: disc protrusion, extruded disc, and sequestrated disc.

Hyaline cartilage   Flexible, glassy, translucent cartilage.

Hypertrophy   Increase in diameter of structure.

Immobilization   Method of stabilizing a structure, limb, or joint by internal fixation, casting, bracing, splinting, traction, or any means to limit motion and to protect healing tissues.

Impingement   Pressure transmitted from one tissue to the next, such as subacromial rotator cuff impingement.

Indirect muscle injury   An injury where the muscle or musculotendinous junction becomes injured by sudden stretch or concentric or eccentric muscle contraction.

Inflammation   Localized increase in blood supply, resulting in small vessel dilation and/or migration of white blood cells into the tissue. Inflammation is the normal response of living tissue to an injury with tissue alteration. The inflammatory process mobilizes the body's defense mechanism to initiate the healing process and react against any microbes that may be introduced at the site of the injury with resultant heat, pain, swelling, and loss of function.

Intercondylar fractures   Fractures that extend between the condyles of the humerus and involve the articular surfaces of the elbow joint.

Isometric contraction   A type of muscle contraction where tension is developed but no joint motion takes place.

"Joint play"   The application of accessory joint motion (glide, roll, slide, spin) "as a response to an outside force but not as a result of voluntary movement." (From Barak T, Rosen ER, Sofer R: Basic concepts of orthopaedic manual therapy. In Gould JA, editor: *Orthopaedic and sports physical therapy,* ed 2, St. Louis, 1990, Mosby.)

Joint congruency   Articular position regarding concave and convex joint surfaces. A joint is in congruence when both articulating surfaces are in contact throughout the total surface area of the joint.

Karvonen method   An equation used to establish a training heart rate. The training intensity range for the Karvonen method is 50% to 85% of the VO_2 MAX. The Karvonen method uses the difference between the maximal heart rate (HR MAX) and the resting heart rate (HR rest), which is known as the maximum heart rate reserve (HR MAX reserve).

Kinesthesia   The recollection of movement, weight, resistance, and position of the body or parts of the body.

Kyphosis   Round shoulder deformity; humpback; dorsal kyphotic curvature; may refer to any forward-bending area or deformity in the spine.

Lauge-Hansen classification   Based on five possible positions of the foot at the time of injury: supination-adduction, supination-eversion, pronation-eversion, pronation-abduction, and pronation-dorsiflexion.

Legg-Calvé-Perthes disease   Aseptic epiphyseal ischemic necrosis of the capital femoral epiphysis in children.

Ligament   Bands of strong fibrous connective tissue that bind together the articular ends of bones and cartilage at the joints, to facilitate or limit motion.

Loose end-feel   An abnormal end-feel felt during the performance of joint mobilization techniques. Primarily, this end-feel is characterized by joint hyper mobility. Typically, no resistance is felt at the end range-of-motion, signifying extraordinary joint looseness.

Loose-packed   Also referred to as the joint resting position. In a loose-packed position, the joint capsule and supporting ligaments are not stressed. For example, when the knee joint is flexed 30 degrees, the intracapsular space is increased and supporting ligaments become more relaxed. The joint loose-packed position is ideal for applying joint mobilization techniques.

Low-load prolonged stretch   Therapeutic technique used to enhance tissue extensibility by preheating the affected area, applying an external load (0.5% of body weight) to the area to stretch soft tissue contractures, and maintaining a passive, pain-free stretch for 20 to 60 minutes.

Mallet toe   Flexion of the distal joint of the second to fifth toes, such that the toenails are pointing into the ground when walking.

Mallet finger   Acute rupture of the terminal end of the distal extensor tendon. This may be intratendinous or bony. This arises as a result of a direct axial blow to the digit. This digit is left with an inability to extend the distal interphalangeal joint (extensor lag). There is usually full passive movement of the digit.

Malunion   Bone heals in abnormal position and/or alignment.

Mechanical instabilities   Chronic laxity of the ankle ligaments. A functional instability defines a subjective "giving way" of the ankle, but does not demonstrate instability or laxity of the supporting ligaments.

Mechanoreceptor system   Joint receptors that provide information concerning joint displacement, velocity and amplitude of joint movement, pressure, stretch, and pain. The mechanoreceptor system includes Ruffini mechanoreceptors, Pacinian mechanoreceptors, type III mechanoreceptors, and free nerve endings. This afferent neural input system is important in regulating adaptive changes in joint movement and body position.

Medial collateral ligament   Strong fibrous ligament on the medial side of the knee connecting the femur with the tibia.

Meniscal repair   Surgical technique that attempts to suture and approximate torn portions of the meniscus. If a tear is present in a vascularized portion of the meniscus, the repair technique is favored over subtotal meniscectomy in order to maintain as much viable meniscus tissue as possible.

Meniscectomy   Excision of the medial or lateral meniscus. There are other menisci in the body but meniscectomies are usually done on the knee. A partial meniscectomy is the removal of the torn portion only or a definite attempt to leave meniscal margins of an even width.

Meniscus   A crescent-shaped fibrocartilaginous disc between two joint surfaces. There are three groups of menisci in the body.

Midstance   The period during stance where the body is directly over the weight-bearing leg. This action serves to "roll-over" the foot into single-limb support during stance.

Midswing   The action where the nonweight bearing limb is advanced to where the limb passes directly beneath the body.

Miserable malalignment syndrome   An anatomic malalignment of the lower extremity, which is characterized by femoral anteversion (internal femoral rotation), "squinting" patella (patallae face toward each other), proximal external tibial rotation, and foot pronation. This malalignment syndrome is commonly seen with extensor mechanism disorders of the knee.

Mobilization An attempt to restore joint motion or mobility and/or decrease pain associated with joint structures via manual selective grades of passive accessory joint movement.

Muscle spindle A specialized proprioceptive sensory organ composed of a bundle of fine striated intrafusal muscle fibers innervated by gamma nerve fibers. Their nuclei are gathered together near the center of each fiber to form a nuclear sac, which is surrounded in turn by sensory, annulospiral nerve endings, all enclosed in a fibrous sheath.

Muscle spasm Sudden contraction of muscle, usually in reflexive response to stimulus from an external source.

Myofibrils Individual muscle fibers are composed of myofibrils, which lie parallel to each other and to the muscle fiber itself.

Myosin A cardiac and skeletal muscle protein that makes up close to one half of the proteins that occur in muscle tissue. The interaction of myosin and actin is essential for muscle contraction.

Nerve entrapment Compression of nerve tissue related to bony overgrowth, inflammation, disc bulge, muscular hypertrophy, and repetitive motion.

Neuroma Benign tumor of the nerve.

Nonconstrained A type of implant used for joint reconstruction (TKR). This type of implant retains the cruciate ligaments (cruciate sparing implant).

Nonunion Failure of progression of healing with expectation of no further healing.

Nonweight-bearing (NWB) Weight bearing status that does not allow contact or loading of the involved limb.

Nucleus pulposus A mucopolysaccharide gel contained within the concentrically arranged rings of fibroelastic cartilage called the annulus fibrosus of the intervertebral disc.

Olecranon Curved process of the ulna at the elbow.

Open reduction and internal fixation (ORIF) A surgical technique where a fracture is visualized by surgical exposure (open), manually realigned into anatomic apposition (reduction), then stabilized with an internal fixation device.

Osteoarthritis Degenerative joinn disease affecting articular cartilages and the synovial membranes.

Osteoblasts Bone-forming cells.

Osteoclasts Remodeling cells of bone.

Osteocytes Bone cells.

Osteomalacia Softening of bones.

Osteoporosis Abnormal loss of bone density.

Osteotomy Excision of all or part of a bone.

Overload A system of progressive, incremental demand in order to stimulate growth and strength.

Pacinian mechanoreceptors Encapsulated afferent nerve tissue that responds to changes in joint position and pressure. Type II mechanoreceptors.

Partial weight-bearing (PWB) Weight bearing status assigned to a patient that is frequently graded in a percentage of the patient's body weight.

Pathologic fractures A group or classification of fractures caused by tumors (malignant or primary bone disease), osteoporosis (most common), microtrauma from repetitive overload (stress fractures), or metastatic bone disease (second most common).

Pelvic "list" Rotation of the pelvis within the frontal plane of the body during gait.

Perimysium Noncontractile connective tissue that surrounds the fasciculus.

Physiologic movement Movement that occurs as a result of either active or passive joint range-of-motion. This type of joint motion can be visualized and measured by goniometric assessment.

Piccolo traction Manually applied traction used to minimize joint compressive forces during mobilization. Piccolo traction is used to describe a stage I traction technique. The force used to deliver a grade I traction is not enough to actually separate the joint surfaces, but rather to only neutralize joint pressure.

Piezoelectric effect A negative electric charge toward the concave, or compression side of a force applied to a bone. An electropositive charge is seen on the tension or convex side of the bone. The negative charge side responds by stimulating osteoblasts, whereas the positive charge side (tension side) responds by increasing osteoclast activity.

Pilon fractures Distal tibia compression fracture where a vertical or axial load compresses the tibia into the talus.

Plantar fasciitis A chronic inflammatory reaction of the plantar aponeuroses (fascia) at the insertion into the calcaneus. Also referred to as heel spur syndrome due to the occasional development of a calcaneal exostosis (spur).

Plyometrics A system of physical exercise that is based on the neurophysiological responses from the golgi tendon organs (GTO) and muscle spindles that involve ballistic, high velocity movement to develop power and speed of movement.

Posterior cruciate ligament A deep ligament within the knee that crosses the anterior cruciate ligament.

Progressive resistance exercise (PRE) A system or program of resistance exercise that systematically and incrementally prescribes progressive amounts of externally applied stress or resistance to stimulate adaptive physiological responses to enhance strength. Examples are the DeLorne PRE program, the Oxford technique, and the daily adjustable progressive resistance exercise (DAPRE) technique.

Proprioception Sensibility to position, whether conscious or unconscious.

Proprioceptive neuromuscular facilitation (PNF) Stretching and facilitation technique that uses the neurophysiological organs (GTO) and muscle spindles to enhance muscle contraction and joint motion and to inhibit resistance to increase muscle flexibility.

Protected motion Therapeutic principle and technique where specific motion limitations are allowed but unwanted motions are avoided or eliminated in order to protect healing tissues.

Protrusion Displaced nuclear material causes a discrete bulge in the annulus, but no material escapes through the annular fibers (protrusion of disc).

Proximal femoral intertrochanteric osteotomy A specific surgical procedure used to reduce pain and improve function of the hip related to advanced osteoarthritis by surgically changing the femoral neck-shaft angle in order to expose healthy articular cartilage thereby improving joint surface congruity.

Q-angle Made by intersection of lines drawn from anterosuperior iliac spine (ASIS) to midpatella and from midpatella to anterior tibial tuberosity.

Radicular signs Neurological signs of radiating pain and parathesias (numbness and tingling).

Range-of-motion (ROM) Extent of movement within a given joint.

Red-on-red A zone classification concerning location of a tear within the meniscus. Red-on-red refers to the tear being vascular on both sides of the tear. Zone I.

Red-on-white A zone classification concerning location of a tear within the meniscus. Red-on-white refers to the tear being vascular on one side (red) and avascular (white) on the other side. Zone II.

Reflex sympathetic dystrophy (RSD) Usually post-traumatic (major or minor) pain dysfunction syndrome. Thought to be due to abnormal modulation of afferent pain signals with possible short circuiting of somatic and autonomic nervous fibers. Attendant autonomic nervous system hyperactivity will produce abnormal peripheral small vessel response to cold and heat stimulus. Symptoms include hyperpathia (increased pain at rest), allodynia (painful response to a nonpainful stimulus), erythema (brawny edema), joint stiffness, and loss of skin elasticity. Osteoporosis and complete loss of dexterity result.

Remodeling The process of tissue restructuring in response to stress.

Roll An accessory joint motion.

Ruffini mechanoreceptors Type I mechanoreceptors that respond slowly to static joint position.

SAID principle Specific adaptations to imposed demands. A fundamental exercise principle that states that tissues respond and adapt specifically to the type of stress or demand placed on the tissue. For example, high intensity exercise of short duration will yield specific physiologic adaptations specific to this type of stress.

Salter-Harris fracture Epiphyseal fracture in children involving epiphyseal growth plate, the seriousness of which could arrest growth or cause deformity.

Scaphoid fracture A fracture of the scaphoid bone of the carpals. Recognized as the most common fracture to the carpal bones. Fractures of the scaphoid are related to a high incidence of avascular necrosis and nonunion due to the vascular anatomy of the proximal pole of the scaphoid.

Scar tissue The healing or union of torn or injured tissue with connective tissue.

Scoliosis Abnormal lateral curvature of the spine.

Sequestrated disc Injury to the intervertebral disc in which the nucleus is free within the canal.

Single-support The time during the stance phase when only one foot is in contact with the ground.

Skier's thumb A traumatic rupture of the ulnar collateral ligament of the metacarpophalangeal joint of the thumb, usually a hyper abduction injury. Also called gamekeeper's thumb.

Slide An accessory joint motion.

Slow twitch (type I-red oxidative) muscle fiber Muscle fiber type that possesses more mitochondria, triglycerides, and enzymes. These fatigue-resistant fibers are recruited for muscular endurance activities.

Smith's fracture Reverse Colles' fracture. Distal fragment displaced volarly.

Snuffbox The anatomical snuffbox is an area on the dorsum of the thumb formed by extension of the thumb.

Soft-tissue approximation A normal joint end-range feel. This type of joint end-range feel is characterized by a yielding compression of muscular tissue compression during joint flexion.

Specificity Specific and predictable physiologic adaptations a muscle goes through in response to a specific training stimulus.

Spin An accessory joint motion.

Spinal stenosis Narrowing of the spinal canal, constricting and compressing nerve roots that give rise to symptoms of neurogenic or spinal claudication. This condition is most commonly acquired from degenerative arthritic changes that encroach on the diameter of the canal producing symptoms of nerve root compression.

Spondylolisthesis Not a true dislocation because it rarely occurs as a result of trauma or muscle imbalance, but is a forward displacement of one vertebral body over another; usually occurs as a result of a defect in the pars interarticularis.

Spondylolysis Disruption of the pars interarticularis (a portion of bone between each of the joints of the back), allowing one vertebral body to slide forward on the next. May be referred to as pars interarticularis defect, acute (traumatic) dissociation of pars interarticularis, or posterior elements (lamina) with or without spondylolisthesis

Spongy bone Spongy bone is less dense and is more elastic than compact or cortical bone. Approximately 20% of the adult skeleton is spongy or cancellous bone.

Sprain Stretching or tearing of ligaments (fibrous bands that bind bones together at a joint) varying in degrees from being partially torn (stretched) to being completely torn (ruptured). After a sprain, the fibrous capsule that encloses the joint may become inflated, swollen, discolored, and extremely painful. Involuntary muscle spasm, and sometimes a fracture, may occur.

Springy block An abnormal end-feel in which full motion is limited by a soft or springy sensation occasionally accompanied by pain.

Step length Linear distance between two consecutive contralateral contacts of the lower extremities.

Steppage gait Muscular weakness of the ankle dorsi flexors that is characterized by extreme hip flexion and knee flexion during swing through in order to prevent dragging the toes on the ground.

Strain Stretching or tearing of a muscle or its tendon (fibrous cord that attaches the muscle to the bone it moves) that may result in bleeding into the damaged muscle area, which causes pain, swelling, stiffness, and muscle spasm, followed by a bruise.

Strength The maximal load that a structure can withstand before functional failure occurs (load strength) or the maximal energy that a structure can withstand before functional failure occurs (energy strength).

Stress The force per unit area of a structure and a measurement of the intensity of the force. Units of measure are newtons per square meter or pound force per square foot. The amount of tension or load placed on tissues.

Subtotal meniscectomy Surgical removal of part of a torn meniscus.

Subacromial rotator cuff impingement The tendons of the rotator cuff are crowded, buttressed, or compressed under the coracoacromial arch resulting in mechanical wear, stress, and friction.

Subchondral bone Bone directly under any cartilaginous surface.

Subluxation   Incomplete or partial dislocation in that one bone forming a joint is displaced only partially from its normal position, also a chronic tendency of a bone to become partially dislocated.

Subluxing peroneal tendon   Either an acute or chronic subluxation of the peroneal tendons due to a loose retinaculum or from a shallow peroneal groove, which results in instability.

Supracondylar fractures   A transverse fracture of the distal third of the humerus.

Swing phase   The time in which one limb is entirely nonweight bearing throughout the gait cycle. The swing phase occupies approximately 40% of the gait cycle.

Tendinitis   Inflammation of a tendon.

Tennis elbow   Inflammation of the wrist and finger extensor muscles at the lateral epicondyle.

Tenocytes   Tendon cells.

Tenosynovitis   Inflammation of the tendon sheath. Causes are multifactorial. Rheumatoid and nonspecific overuse are implicated.

Three-point gait pattern   The advancing of both crutches and the involved limb. The noninvolved limb is advanced and then the sequence repeated.

Thoracic outlet (inlet) syndrome   Mechanical problem related to the exit of arteries and nerves at the base of the neck leading down the arm, and can also involve the vein bringing blood back from the arm (inlet).

THR   Total hip replacement

Tibial plateau fractures   Various fracture patterns related to the proximal tibia. Generally classified as nondisplaced or displaced.

Toe-off   The instant where the knee of the weight-bearing limb flexes and preparation occurs for the swing phase. Also referred to as preswing.

Toe-touch weight-bearing (TTWB)   Minimal contact of the involved limb with the ground during gait. Also referred to as touch-down weight-bearing.

Total hip precautions   Postoperative precautions following total hip replacement that involve patient education on avoiding hip flexion greater than 90 degrees, avoiding hip and leg adduction past midline, and avoiding internal hip rotation.

Traction   Pull on a limb or a part thereof. Skin traction (indirect traction) is applied by using a bandage to pull on the skin and fascia where light traction is required; skeletal traction (direct traction), however, uses pins or wires inserted through bone and is attached to weights, pulleys, and ropes.

Trendelenburg gait   Weakness of the gluteus medius is characterized by the pelvis dropping toward the unaffected limb during the single limb support period of the stance phase.

TUBS   Traumatic unidirectional injury with a bankart lesion; frequently requires surgery.

Two-point gait pattern   The patient characteristically uses each crutch with opposing leg.

Valgus overload   Medial valgus stress overload occurs to the capsulo ligamentous structures as a result of repetitive valgus stress to the elbow.

Vascular access channel   A surgical incision created to provide blood flow (vascular access) to a part of the meniscus that is avascular.

Velocity   Displacement divided by the time taken for that displacement (cm/sec).

VO₂ MAX   Maximum oxygen uptake.

Volkmann's ischemic contracture   Contracture of the fingers, and sometimes the wrists, with loss of muscle power caused by vascular blockage.

Weight bearing as tolerated (WBAT)   This weight bearing status is assigned to patients for whom pain tolerance is the predominant limiting factor.

White-on-white   A zone classification of an injury to the meniscus. White-on-white refers to the injury being avascular on both sides. Zone III.

Wolff's law   The scientific law that states bone will form and remodel in the direction of forces acting on it.

Work   The product of force multiplied by the displacement through which the force moves.

Zone I   Red-on-red zone of the meniscus where both parts of the torn meniscus are vascular.

Zone II   Red-on-white zone where one part of the torn meniscus is vascular and the other part is avascular.

Zone III   White-on-white avascular zone of the meniscus.

Index